The Neurobiologic Mechanisms in Manipulative Therapy

Edited by

Irvin M. Korr
Michigan State University

With the assistance of
Ethel H. Huntwork

PLENUM PRESS · NEW YORK AND LONDON

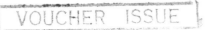
Library of Congress Cataloging in Publication Data

Research Workshop on Neurobiologic Mechanisms in Manipulative Therapy, Michigan State University, 1977.
 The neurobiologic mechanisms in manipulative therapy.

 Includes index.
 1. Manipulation (Therapeutics)—Congresses. 2. Neurobiology—Congresses. I. Korr, Irvin M. II. Huntwork, Ethel H. III. Michigan. State University, East Lansing. College of Osteopathic Medicine. IV. Title. [DNLM: 1. Neurophysiology—Congresses. 2. Manipulation, Orthopedic—Congresses. 3. Physical therapy—Congresses. WB535 N494 1977]
 RD736.M25R47 1977   615'.82   78-4667
 ISBN 0-306-31150-X

Proceedings of a workshop, held at the Kellogg Center
for Continuing Education, Michigan State University,
East Lansing, Michigan, October 23—26, 1977

Planning Committee: Thomas Adams, Martin Balaban, James
Cunningham, Philip E. Greenman, Irvin M. Korr (Chairman),
all of Michigan State University; Horace W. Magoun, UCLA;
and Sidney Ochs, University of Indiana

Sponsored by The Michigan State University College of
Osteopathic Medicine

The Workshop was funded by Grant R13 NS13320 from the National
Institute of Neurological and Communicative Disorders and Stroke,
National Institutes of Health

Acknowledgments

The editor wishes to thank all persons who contributed to the success of the Workshop, most particularly:

> The other members of the Planning Committee;
> Ann E. Tsiminakis, Conference Coordinator – Kellogg
>   Center, for planning and organizing all the
>   arrangements at the Center;
> Sandra Kilbourn for valuable assistance in planning;
> Barbara J. Korr for serving as unofficial hostess;
> Dean and Mrs. Myron S. Magen for their gracious
>   hospitality;
> Session Chairmen Murray Goldstein, Horace W. Magoun,
>   and Fred E. Samson;
> Discussion Initiators Harry Grundfest, Johan Sjöstrand,
>   and Marcus Singer.

Special thanks are due to Ethel H. Huntwork for her invaluable assistance in assembling and editing the invited papers and the discussion, and for preparing the entire camera-ready copy for publication.

Participants

Thomas Adams, Ph.D.: Professor, Department of Physiology, Michigan State University, East Lansing, Michigan

Otto Appenzeller, Ph.D.: Professor of Neurology and Medicine, University of New Mexico School of Medicine, Albuquerque, New Mexico

Martin Balaban, Ph.D.: Professor, Department of Zoology, Michigan State University, East Lansing, Michigan

David L. Beckman, Ph.D.: Professor of Physiology, School of Medicine, East Carolina University, Greenville, North Carolina

Stephen Brimijoin, Ph.D.: Department of Pharmacology, Mayo Graduate School of Medicine, Mayo Foundation, Rochester, Minnesota

A. A. Buerger, Ph.D.: Assistant Professor, Department of Medicine and Rehabilitation, California College of Medicine, University of California Irvine Medical Center, Orange, California

J. H. Coote, Ph.D.: Department of Physiology, The Medical School, University of Birmingham, Birmingham, England

James Cunningham, D.V.M., Ph.D.: Associate Professor, Department of Physiology and Small Animal Surgery and Medicine and African Studies Center, Michigan State University, East Lansing, Michigan

Ronald Gitelman, D.C., F.C.C.S.: Canadian Memorial Chiropractic College, Toronto, Ontario, Canada

C. M. Godfrey, M.D.: Professor, Department of Rehabilitative Medicine, University of Toronto, Toronto, Ontario, Canada

Murray Goldstein, D.O., M.P.H.: Director, Stroke and Trauma Program, National Institute of Neurological and Communicative Disorders and Stroke, National Institutes of Health, Bethesda, Maryland

Philip E. Greenman, D.O.: Associate Dean for Academic Affairs, College of Osteopathic Medicine, Michigan State University, East Lansing, Michigan

Harry Grundfest, Ph.D.: Professor Emeritus, Department of Neurology, Columbia University College of Physicians and Surgeons, New York, New York

Scott Haldeman, D.C., M.Sc., Ph.D., M.D.: Department of Neurology, University of California, Irvine, California

Doc. MUDr. Vladimír Janda, C.Sc.: Docent, Department of Rehabilitation, Charles University Hospital, Prague, Czechoslovakia

Martin E. Jenness, D.C., Ph.D.: Director of Research, Northwestern College of Chiropractic, St. Paul, Minnesota

Robert E. Kappler, D.O.: Professor, Department of Osteopathic Medicine, Chicago College of Osteopathic Medicine, Chicago, Illinois

Kiyomi Koizumi, M.D.: Professor, Department of Physiology, State University of New York, Downstate Medical Center, Brooklyn, New York

Irvin M. Korr, Ph.D.: Professor, Department of Biomechanics, College of Osteopathic Medicine, Michigan State University, East Lansing, Michigan

Doc. MUDr. Karel Lewit, Dr.Sc.: Docent, Department of Vertebrogenic Diseases, Central Railway Health Institute, Prague, Czechoslovakia

Myron S. Magen, D.O.: Dean, College of Osteopathic Medicine, Michigan State University, East Lansing, Michigan

Horace W. Magoun, Ph.D.: Professor Emeritus, Department of Psychiatry, School of Medicine, University of California at Los Angeles, Los Angeles, California

Alan J. McComas, M.D.: Professor and Director of Neurology, Department of Medicine, McMaster University Medical Centre, Hamilton, Ontario, Canada

P. W. Nathan, M.D., F.R.C.P.: The National Hospital for Nervous Diseases, London, England

Michael A. Nigro, D.O.: Glendale Neurological Associates, P.C., Osteopathic, Birmingham, Michigan

George W. Northup, D.O.: Editor in Chief, American Osteopathic Association, Chicago, Illinois

Sidney Ochs, Ph.D.: Professor, Department of Physiology, Indiana University School of Medicine, Indianapolis, Indiana

Michael M. Patterson, Ph.D.: Director of Research, College of Osteopathic Medicine, Ohio University, Athens, Ohio

Fred E. Samson, Ph.D.: Director, Kansas Center for Mental Retardation and Human Development, Ralph L. Smith Mental Retardation Research Center, Kansas City, Kansas

Marcus Singer, Ph.D.: Professor and Chairman, Department of Anatomy, School of Medicine, Case Western Reserve University, Cleveland, Ohio

Johan Sjöstrand, M.D., Ph.D.: Institute of Neurobiology, Faculty of Medicine, University of Göteborg, Göteborg, Sweden

Sir Sydney Sunderland, M.D.: Professor, Department of Experimental Neurology, University of Melbourne, Melbourne, Australia

Hans Thoenen, M.D.: Professor and Chairman, Department of Pharmacology, Biocenter of the University of Basel, Basel, Switzerland

Donald B. Tower, M.D., Ph.D.: Director, National Institute of Neurological and Communicative Disorders and Stroke, National Institutes of Health, Bethesda, Maryland

Charles D. Tweedle, Ph.D.: Associate Professor, Departments of Biomechanics and of Zoology, Michigan State University, East Lansing, Michigan

Lynne C. Weaver, D.V.M., Ph.D.: Associate Professor, Deparment of Physiology, Michigan State University, East Lansing, Michigan

Robert M. Worth, M.D.: Department of Neurological Surgery, Indiana University School of Medicine, Indianapolis, Indiana

Andrew A. Zalewski, M.D.: Department of Neurochemistry, National Institute of Neurological and Communicative Disorders and Stroke, National Institutes of Health, Bethesda, Maryland

Foreword

At the request of a Subcommittee of the United States Senate,
in February, 1975, the National Institute of Neurological Disorders
and Stroke (now the National Institute of Neurological and Communicative Disorders and Stroke) conducted a Workshop on the Research
Status of Spinal Manipulative Therapy. The Workshop was held in
response to the Senate Subcommittee's request for an "independent
unbiased study of the fundamentals of the chiropractic profession."
Since spinal manipulative therapy is a key tenet of chiropractic,
the Institute felt a research workshop focused on that issue would
provide a useful base upon which to examine the broad concept of
the role of biomechanical alterations of the spine in health and
disease. This would include the pathophysiologic and clinical
hypotheses formulated by medical and osteopathic physicians as
well as chiropractors.

Why the relatively sudden interest of the Senate Subcommittee
in chiropractic? There were probably many reasons for that interest,
but suffice to say anticipation of discussion on the role of chiropractic in any national system of health insurance could in itself
have provided adequate stimulus for the request. In any case, the
NINCDS was asked to review what was and what was not known about
the fundamentals of chiropractic. I stress "fundamentals" since
as a research organization, the NINCDS is not charged with reviewing matters such as clinical education, licensure or clinical practice. A small expert committee of scientific consultants helped the
Institute design the format and agenda for the Workshop. Fifty-eight
scientists and clinicians of international stature were invited to
participate. The agenda included a review of the history of manipulative therapy and presentations and discussion of the scientific
issues of spinal geometry and kinematics, the functional anatomy
of the intervertebral foramen, nerve root compression, nerve root
and peripheral nerve pain, the pathophysiology of back pain, and
clinical investigations relevant to palpatory and radiologic diagnosis and to manipulative therapy. Obviously, two and one-half days
to cover the breadth of the topic committed the Workshop organizers

to require specified papers which would provide adequate representation of the status of research in that area; this format in itself
limited the scope of discussion.

A paragraph from the NINCDS monograph summarizes the Workshop
Report:

> "The NINCDS Workshop on the Research Aspects of Spinal
> Manipulative Therapy and staff review and analysis of avail-
> able data clearly indicate that specific conclusions cannot
> be derived from the scientific literature for or against
> either the efficacy of spinal manipulative therapy or the
> pathophysiologic foundations from which it is derived. The
> efficacy of spinal manipulative therapy is based on a body
> of clinical experience in the 'hands' of specialized clini-
> cians. Chiropractors, osteopathic physicians, medical
> manipulative specialists and their patients all claim spinal
> manipulation provides relief from pain, particularly back
> pain, and sometimes cure; some medical physicians, particu-
> larly those not trained in manipulative techniques, claim it
> does not provide relief, does not cure, and may be danger-
> ous, particularly if used by nonphysicians. The available
> data do not clarify either view. However, most partici-
> pants in the Workshop felt that manipulative therapy was of
> clinical value in the treatment of back pain, a difference
> of opinion focusing on the issues of indications, contra-
> indications and the precise scientific basis for the re-
> sults obtained. No evidence was presented to substantiate
> the usefulness of manipulative therapy at this time in the
> treatment of visceral disorders."

What did the Workshop accomplish? It did several things.
First, it provided the Congress and specifically the Senate Subcommittee with the information it had requested: an analysis of
the status at that time of the research basic to the clinical use
of manipulative therapy. Second, it demonstrated that scientists
from several disciplines and clinicians from several professions
are able to communicate meaningfully on a research subject of
mutual interest, even when the scientific and clinical aspects of
that subject are as controversial as is this one. But perhaps of
most far-reaching importance, the Workshop documented that although there are a number of meaningful basic and clinical research
questions about manipulative therapy and vertebral biomechanics
that are amenable to investigation, there was relatively little
quantitative data either in support of or in opposition to the
several clinical hypotheses.

It was revealing to realize how much heat had been generated
in the past on scientific issues for which there were still only

subjective clinical impressions and at the best very preliminary
data either in support or in denial of these hypotheses. I suspect
the NINCDS Workshop cleared the air by demonstrating that there are
precise scientific issues relevant to manipulative therapy that deserve research attention. Clinicians and their patients are astute
people. They observe and experience biological phenomena in the
real world of the activities of daily living. As investigators we
have the opportunity of reviewing these phenomena and translating
them into meaningful formats for scientific investigation.

Since the NINCDS Workshop, there has been one other major
scientific Workshop concerned with manipulative therapy; it reviewed
the results of several clinical trials of manipulative therapy, a
few of which were randomized trials and others were case series.
However, the basic physiologic and pathologic mechanisms upon which
this therapy is supposedly based have not been further reviewed in
any depth.

Communication among clinicians and investigators has proven
to be an essential key in development of the rich body of information now available about health and disease. Within this framework,
the mechanism of the research workshop serves to review the status
of a research area, evaluate research results and stimulate focused
attention to the examination of promising hypotheses. The Research
Workshop on Neurobiologic Mechanisms in Manipulative Therapy sponsored and organized by the College of Osteopathic Medicine of
Michigan State University was designed to serve these purposes.
Because of this, the NINCDS-NIH felt it most appropriate to provide
financial assistance for the conduct of the MSU-COM Workshop.

A classical but as yet "unproven" approach to the maintenance
of health and the treatment of disease is that described under the
broad term manipulation or manipulative therapy. This clinical approach is more than a collection of techniques since it is said to
intervene in pathophysiologic processes. Specifically what those
processes are and in what ways manipulation might be efficacious
remain in the realm of hypothesis. However, fundamental research
in neurobiology offers the best promise for the solution of this
riddle.

The MSU-COM Research Workshop called on clinicians to recount
their experiences and clinical investigators to review the preliminary results of more recent controlled clinical trials. Neurobiologists described recently reported findings on mechanisms of
sensory input and on somato-autonomic pathways; they also provided
exciting descriptions of anterograde and retrograde axonal transport and its implications and of neurotrophic relations. The potential for meaningful hypothesis formulation and critical experiments were clearly delineated. The interaction between clinicians

and investigators provided a milieu for defining more precisely
research questions relevant to the ancient skill of manipulative
therapy.   This clinical area is one whose research "time has come";
the MSU—COM Workshop should certainly help keep the momentum going.

Murray Goldstein

OBJECTIVES AND HYPOTHESES IN THE DESIGN OF THE WORKSHOP

What Is Manipulative Therapy?

One of the unusual features of the Workshop was that few of the neuroscientists who convened to contribute their knowledge had had any prior contact with the area of medicine to which they were to make their contributions. Most of them arrived still uncertain of the relevance of their research, done for quite different purposes, to the subject of the Workshop. Because the Workshop setting was that of a forum rather than a clinic, they departed with a better perception of relevance, yet without a clear image of how manipulative therapy is performed or of its clinical value.

It seems likely that many readers, more interested in the nervous system than in manual medicine, will find themselves with similar uncertainties about the latter. To them, we recommend, as we did to the participants, the proceedings of an earlier workshop sponsored by the National Institute of Neurological and Communicative Disorders and Stroke,* and offer the following paragraphs.

Manipulative therapy involves the application of accurately determined and specifically directed manual forces to the body. Its objective is to improve mobility in areas that are restricted, whether the restrictions are within joints, in connective tissues or in skeletal muscles. The consequences may be the improvement of posture and locomotion, the relief of pain and discomfort, the improvement of function elsewhere in the body and enhancement of the sense of well-being.

Diagnosis, leading to the selection of body sites for manipulation and the mode of manipulation, is based on analysis of the

---

*NINCDS Monograph No. 15, *The Research Status of Spinal Manipulative Therapy*, edited by M. Goldstein. Bethesda, Maryland, 1976.

patient's history and complaints and on the evaluation of signs provided by palpation (tissue texture, muscular and fascial tension,
joint motion and compliance, skin temperature and moisture), by
visual observation (body contour, posture, locomotion, skin color),
and by radiographic and other instrumental means.

Manipulative procedures, even in the hands of the same practitioner, vary according to the findings and their changes in each
visit; they vary from practitioner to practitioner, from patient to
patient, and, for the same patient, from visit to visit. Manipulative therapy is no more a uniform therapeutic entity than is surgery,
psychiatry or pharmacotherapeutics. Clinical effects are thought to
be achieved through improvement in musculoskeletal biomechanics, in
dynamics of the body fluids (including blood circulation and lymphatic drainage) and in nervous function. It is on the last that
this Workshop was focused. Its concern, therefore, was with neither
the clinical efficacy of manipulation nor its evaluation, but with
its neural and neuronal mediation.

What are the Neurobiologic Mechanisms?

It has been clear for many decades that the nervous system is
a major mediator of the clinical effects of manipulative therapy,
yet the precise mechanisms are still, for the most part, obscure.
In view of the burgeoning of the neurosciences in recent years, it
seemed timely to convene a research workshop to examine to what extent that great mass of new knowledge might illuminate the neurobiologic mechanisms at work in manipulative therapy, while at the
same time to discern new and fundamental areas in the neurosciences
for exploration.

The objectives of the Workshop on which this volume is based
were:

1. To identify new fundamental questions in neurobiology
   which emerge from clinical observations in the practice
   of manipulative therapy.
2. To seek answers in research already accomplished.
3. To identify and project needed lines of research.

The design of the Workshop was based on the following assump-
tions and hypotheses. It seemed to the planners of the Workshop
that the musculoskeletal problems to which manipulative therapy is
addressed initiate their impairment of normal physiological processes in two primary ways:

1. Alterations in sensory input from the muscles, tendons,
   bones, joints, ligaments and other tissues which are
   involved in the musculoskeletal aberration.

2.   Direct insult to neurons, nerves and roots, and associated glial, connective-tissue and vascular structures.

According to our hypotheses, both the changes in afferent input and the trauma-induced changes in excitation and conduction of neural elements produce, in turn, changes in the central nervous system and in the periphery, reflected in aberrant sensory, motor and autonomic functions.   We chose to give emphasis to the impact on autonomic function and, therefore, to somato-autonomic interrelations.

The changes in afferent input (and the resultant changes in efferent output) and the nerve-trauma both affect, also, neuronal functions which are not based on excitation and conduction of impulses, much as they may be affected by impulses.   These functions are subsumed under such rubrics as axonal transport, transsynaptic influences, trophic function, neurotrophic relations, neuron-target-cell interactions, etc.   Hence, the Workshop was organized around two major themes, impulse-based and nonimpulse-based mechanisms, introduced by the *Fragestellung* implicit in reports by clinicians skilled in manipulative therapy as taught and practiced in three different professions.

It became clear in the course of discussions, not only between clinicians and scientists but between two groups of neuroscientists, that there is no clean separation between impulse-based and non-impulse-based mechanisms.   Each is involved in and influenced by the other, and disturbances in each potentially contribute to dysfunction elsewhere and are subject to manipulative amelioration. If barriers existed, they were in minds and methods, and not in the biological system; proving again that conceptual barriers, until identified and assaulted, are often much less permeable than cellular barriers.   Perhaps one byproduct of the Workshop, therefore, was a somewhat more coherent and unified view of nervous function and plasticity, incorporating both reflexes and neurotrophicity, both the instantaneous and the long-term phenomena.

An important feature in the design of the Workshop was the dialogue between clinician and scientist.   The clinicians were chosen not only for their clinical proficiency in the application of manipulative therapy, but for their concern, expressed in publications, about mechanism.   The neuroscientists were selected not only for the quality and importance of their research, but for the relevance of their work, as perceived by the planners, to manipulative therapy and to the problems with which it deals.   While no major answers have as yet emerged, the way has been opened for the formulation of new, approachable questions and testable hypotheses.

Irvin M. Korr

Contents

NONIMPULSE-BASED MECHANISMS
(Chairman: Fred E. Samson)

Clinical Observations and Emerging Questions

Chairman: Murray Goldstein

DR. MURRAY GOLDSTEIN: We begin the Workshop at the proper end of the scientific spectrum, namely the experiments which nature has provided us. As skilled observers, we have the opportunity to watch these natural experiments that usually occur in our patients and in the population as a whole, giving us insight and leads to biological phenomena for the study of which we can retreat to our laboratories, where we try to control all variables but one and to come out with meaningful data. Hence, we start with clinical observations and emerging questions and ask the skilled clinician to identify problems for us to explore.

THE CONTRIBUTION OF CLINICAL OBSERVATION TO NEUROBIOLOGICAL MECHANISMS IN MANIPULATIVE THERAPY

Karel Lewit

Central Railway Health Institute

Prague, Czechoslovakia

INTRODUCTION

Although both reflex mechanisms and direct nervous tissue involvement play a role in conditions amenable to manipulation, we believe that reflex mechanisms are the rule and mechanical nerve lesion the exception. Paradoxically, the neurosurgeon under the spell of disc herniation, and the chiropractor convinced of the subluxation theory are inclined to believe in mechanical root compression. Practice, however, teaches us that out of the millions who suffer from some vertebrogenic problem only a very few may profit from decompressive operation.

Physiological thinking helps us to understand why this must be so: The nervous system obtains information about all tissues through its receptors, processes this information and produces reflex responses. It is a system which produces signals. What would be the good of it acting upon the information gained from its receptors only when it is itself damaged? In fact, mere nerve compression usually produces not pain but numbness.

REFLEX MECHANISMS

Reflex mechanisms are widely accepted, as most of the current concepts about reactions in the spinal segment testify, e.g., segmental facilitation (Brügger, 1962; Figar et al., 1967; Gross, 1972; Korr et al., 1955; Lewit, 1975; Sautier, 1977). There is, however, particularly in the osteopathic literature, a very noticeable reticence about the actual cause of the reflexes. Yet, to put it

3

pointedly, a reflex without a stimulus is an absurdity.   Therefore, we should analyze first what we know about the effects of manipulation:

   1.   We know and teach that manipulation is effective only (a) if we find some passive movement restriction and (b) if we achieve normalization of mobility (Figar & Krausová, 1975).   That is why it is so essential for every student of manipulative therapy to learn the diagnosis of movement restriction.   If, for example, there is pain and normal or even exaggerated mobility, manipulation is futile or even harmful.   This in itself is good evidence that manipulation acts on joint mobility.

   2.   In the spinal column the "mobile segment" consists of both apophyseal joints and discs; indeed, quite a few authors believe that manipulation may act upon the disc (Cramer, 1967; Maigne, 1968; de Sèze, 1955; Stoddard, 1970).   I consider this most unlikely for the following reasons:

      (a)   Manipulation acts in exactly the same way in segments in which there is no disc (craniocervical junction, sacroiliac joints) as in those in which there are discs, - as well as in extremity joints.

      (b)   If manipulation acted on the disc and not upon the apophyseal joint all our manipulative techniques would be nonsensical.   They would be identical in each segment of the spinal column. As it is, they are carefully applied in each region of the spinal column so as to cause mainly gapping of joints.

      (c) The "click" as a sign of successful manipulation is a typical articular phenomenon, as is the restoration of joint play (Figure 1).

      (d)   There are typical radicular syndromes due to disc herniation without any movement restriction in the mobile segment of the spinal column.   We do not find them very frequently among patients in general, but they occur relatively frequently after successful joint manipulation.   In such cases, which we might call "pure disc syndrome", manipulation is absolutely futile.   Even the reverse is true: if a disc causes reflex antalgesic posture (kyphosis or scoliosis) we must not interfere with this position. One may say that it is possible to manipulate in spite of the disc, but not to manipulate the disc!

   3.   Some authors believe that movement restriction is rather due to muscle spasm and that manipulation somehow acts on the muscle (Cole, 1967; Cramer, 1967; Retzlaff et al., 1974).   It would be hard to understand how this could so regularly cause impaired

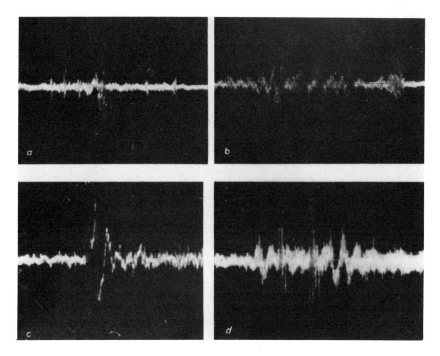

Figure 1. The "click" on a phonographic tape: (a) in normal joint, (b) in a blocked joint ("crack"), (c) and (d) a blocked joint treated twice in succession.

joint function including impaired joint play, springing of joints, etc. It is even more difficult to imagine how manipulation acts on the muscle. In most techniques muscle stretch is indeed minimal or absent. However, to refute this theory altogether we examined the cervical spine of patients who were prepared for operation. They were re-examined during general anesthesia with myorelaxants and intubation with artificial respiration. In 10 cases movement restriction remained unchanged and was even more readily recognizable during narcosis, as the patient was entirely relaxed! This again is evidence that the movement restriction is in the joint.

4. If manipulation has achieved its effect and we find normal mobility in the joint we have treated, we regularly can notice a marked and immediate reflex response. If before manipulation there was muscular hypertonus in the corresponding segment with increased resistance of the skin to folding, this gives way to hypotony and normalization of mechanical skin resistance. These changes can also be borne out by instrumental methods, e.g., plethysmography (Figure 2) (Figar & Krausová, 1975; Figar et al., 1967). This again

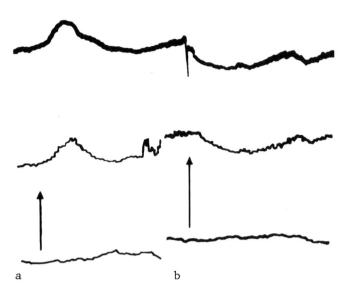

a   b

Figure 2. Electrocapacitance plethysmography done on patient suffering from a root lesion in upper extremity: (a) abnormal vasodilator reaction, (b) normal vasoconstrictor reaction immediately
following manipulation.

is strong evidence that the stimulus which caused the changes has
been removed. We would suggest that the reflex effect of manipulation is so intense (much more intense, for instance, than that of
massage and other procedures of physical therapy) because manipulation normalizes such an important function as joint mobility.

    5. The importance of the experiment in which we found that
blockage remained unaltered during narcosis with myorelaxants is
that it proved a mechanical obstacle in the joint. It was the
German pathologist, Emminger (1967; Zuckschwerdt et al., 1960) who
suggested that there are small meniscoids in all intervertebral and
most extremity joints which may get caught between the moving joint
facets. Indeed most joints have very incongruous facets and smooth
mobility is possible only if some additional tissue can fill the
redundant space. To do this the meniscoid must move freely between
the joint facets, and this may produce difficulties.

    Wolf and Kos (Kos, 1968; Kos & Wolf, 1972; Penning & Töndury,
1963; Wolf, 1974, 1975; Wolff, 1974) have further elaborated this
theory showing why this mechanism is easily disturbed: (a) the
meniscoid has a soft base and a hard edge, which cannot easily be

compressed; (b) joint cartilage is hard and elastic only if the force which acts on it does so rapidly. If, however, we put constant pressure on the cartilage, then it adapts to the material which exerts pressure as though it was fluid. If, therefore, the meniscoid is caught between the gliding surfaces of the joint facets the hard edge produces a cavity in the cartilage in which it is trapped.

    The implications for the theory of manipulation are obvious: if we separate the joint facets the meniscoid can slip out. Diagrams by Wolf illustrate how this may also be achieved by mobilization (Figure 3a-e).

    6. Most interesting evidence of the role of articular dysfunction and the effect of manipulation on the joints comes from observation and clinical experience with patients suffering from dizziness. Anyone with experience of manipulation knows that many patients (if not most) suffering from dizziness and vertigo profit from manipulation. The explanation most frequently put forward for this is interference with the vertebral artery which supplies both the labyrinths and the brainstem including the vestibular nuclei. That indeed the vertebral artery can be involved in lesions of the cervical spine is well established (Barré, 1952; Bärtschi-Rochaix, 1949; Gutmann, 1963; Lewit, 1969; Unterharnscheidt, 1956). There is, however, increasing evidence that not all cases of dizziness or vertigo of cervical origin are due to vertebral artery involvement and that afferent impulses from the upper cervical joints may be the cause:

        (a) Even if most cases of dizziness occur in age groups in whom some degree of arteriosclerosis may be expected, there are also quite young patients in whom this is most unlikely.

        (b) Although both the labyrinth and the cochlea are supplied by the vertebral artery, manipulative treatment is much more effective in improving dizziness than tinnitus or deafness.

        (c) On examining side deviation of the outstretched arms of the seated patient in various head positions (Hautant's test) we find that the position of the head which causes most deviation corresponds with the direction of blockage! On the other hand, the head position in which equilibrium is best corresponds with the free movement (Lewit, 1976) (Figure 4).

        (d) Norré, Stevens and Degeyter (1976), working with Greiner's swinging chair in which the head is fixed and the trunk rotates, showed that in many cases cervical nystagmus is provoked which changes its direction in the rhythm of the swinging chair (Figure 5). Now this rhythmic change could not possibly be due to

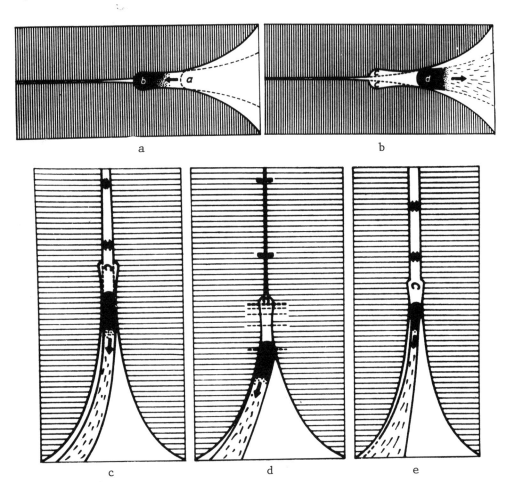

Figure 3. (a) Trapping of the tough inner edge of the meniscoid ("b") drawn in the direction of the arrow from its original normal position ("A") between the two joint cartilages; (b) the situation after the meniscoid is freed and has moved back in the direction of the arrow into its original position ("D"). The cavity caused by the trapped meniscoid still remains ("C") for several minutes. From the diagram it can be seen that the trapped edge of the meniscoid has only very slight resistance to overcome consisting of the two very shallow grooves which open smoothly (horizontal arrow) into the wedge-like space between the cartilages; (c) in manipulation the mechanism consists in a momentary separation of both joint cartilage surfaces (vertical arrows) enabling the inner edge of the meniscoid to slip out of the cavity ("c") back into the wedge-like space between the edges of the cartilage surfaces; (d) in "repetitive mobilization" a back-and-forth movement takes place meeting greater resistance in the direction of incarceration than that of liberation. After gradually   (Legend continued on next page)

(Figure 3 legend continued)   overcoming the last resistance the meniscoid slips back to its original position ("d"). The diagram also illustrates how resistance becomes less with each movement increasing the space between the dotted lines; (e) the probably mechanism of pressure mobilization using one-sided pressure: the change in position of the two joint cartilage surfaces producing a wedge-like opening of the trap ("c") in an outward direction is illustrated by the two vertical arrows. In this way the meniscoid can automatically slip back from "c" to "d" in the direction of the   · horizontal arrow.

the vertebral artery or its insufficiency, as in a vertebral artery lesion there is as a rule one pathogenic and one relief direction. Nor could a circulatory disturbance change in such a quick and rhythmical manner. This, however, can easily be explained by changes in joint afferent impulses. Sautier (1977) was able to show on the elctronystagmogram an effect of extreme head position similar to that of the swinging chair (Figure 6). Further evidence for the pure cervical origin of this nystagmus is that it appears in cases of labyrinth afunction (Simon & Moser, 1973; Simon et al., 1975).

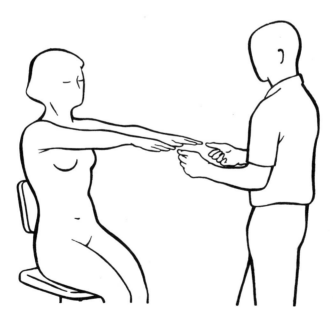

Figure 4.   Hautant's test for the examination of side-deviation.

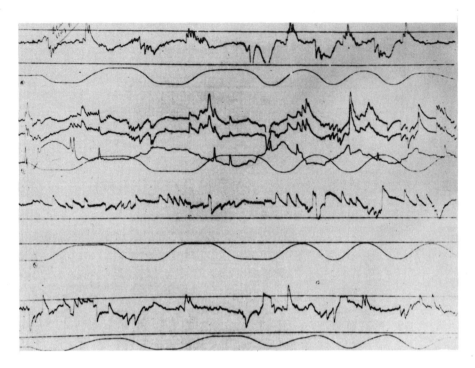

Figure 5. Electronystagmograms showing change in direction of
nystagmus with change in direction of rotation of the swinging
chair. Upward spikes correspond to right-sided, downward spikes
to left-sided nystagmus. Undulations indicate rotation of the
chair, upward to the right, downward to the left.

Obviously, the effect of head position on balance can only be
explained as owing to joint proprioception and not from the disc.
This has been shown by McCouch, Derring and Ling (1951) to stem
from the first three segments, i.e., precisely from the region
without discs (Moravec, 1962; Moritz, 1956-57; Moser et al, 1972).

REFLEX MECHANISMS IN VERTEBRO-VISCERAL RELATIONS

Other examples of pure reflex mechanisms are vertebro-visceral
or viscero-vertebral relations. In this type of segmental lesion
there are never signs of true root involvement. Moreover, the influence of spinal lesions on the viscera is largely hypothetical,
whereas there appears to be more evidence of the influence of visceral lesions on the mobile spinal segment (Gutzeit, 1951; Kunert,
1975; Metz, 1976; Schwarz, 1974; Walther, 1963).

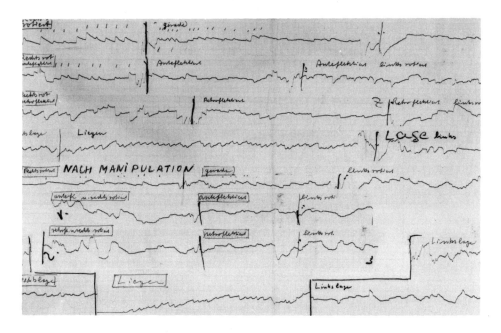

Figure 6. Electronystagmograms showing the influence of (extreme) head position on nystagmus. Line 1 - head erect; line 2 - head in anteflexion; line 3 - head in retroflexion; line 4 - patient supine and lying on left side. First section of lines 1 to 3 - head rotated to right; second section - head straight; third section - head rotated to left. The lower four lines show the corresponding lines after manipulation.

My collaborators and I were able to establish something like a "spinal pattern" for some visceral diseases, including peptic ulcer (Rychlíková & Lewit, 1976), gynecological affections (Lewit et al., 1970; Novotný & Dvorák, 1972; Novotný, 1973), and tonsillitis (Lewit & Abrahamovič, 1976).

The first of these patterns was established in adolescents with peptic ulcer: it consisted of a mid-thoracic lesion with maximum incidence in the segment Th 5/6 (68%), of sacroiliac displacement (in 87%!) and to a lesser degree of movement restriction in the craniocervical junction (58%), mainly between atlas and occiput (Figures 7 and 8).

The second pattern was established by Rychlikova (1975) in ischemic heart disease and myocardial infarction. Most frequently

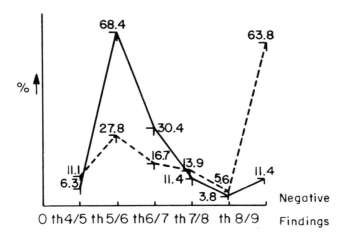

Figure 7. Blockages in the thoracic spine in peptic ulcer. Solid
line - patients (n = 79); interrupted line - controls (n = 36).
Negative findings shown on the right.

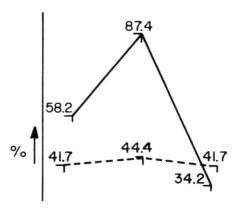

Figure 8. Blockages outside the thoracic spine in per cent. Left
to right: craniocervical junction, sacroiliac displacement and
"elsewhere". Solid line - patients; interrupted line - controls.

there is blockage in the segment Th 4/5, followed by blockage in the cervico-thoracic junction (Figure 9) and the 3rd and 4th ribs, mainly on the left (not shown).

In gynecological disturbances - especially in algomenorrhea - the typical lesion is lumbosacral and sacroiliac displacement with concomitant spasm of the iliac muscle (Figure 10).

Finally in chronic and relapsing tonsillitis there is blockage in the cranio-cervical junction, mainly in the atlanto-occipital segment (Figure 11; Table 1).

In these patterns it is likely that the spinal lesion is the result rather than the cause of visceral disease, in which case there can be no doubt of its reflex nature. Only in tonsillitis could we establish that blockage has an effect upon the tendency of tonsillitis to relapse, so that after manipulation about two-thirds of our patients no longer suffered relapses.

The nature of most of these reflex mechanisms is a response to nociceptive stimuli (Lewit, 1975). If, for example, there is blockage due to a mechanical obstacle in the joint, every movement in

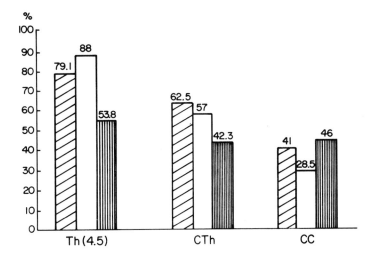

Figure 9. Incidence of blockage ("pattern") in cardiac involvement. Oblique stripes - myocardial infarction; no stripes - ischemic heart disease; vertical stripes - vertebrocardiac syndrome. Th(4,5) - thoracic segments 4-5; CTh - cervico-thoracic junction; CC - cranio-cervical junction.

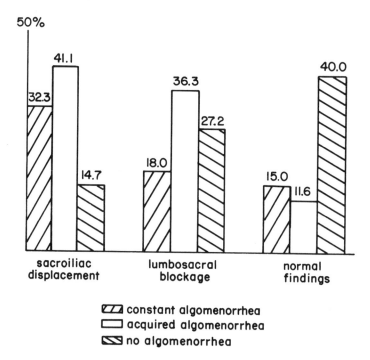

Figure 10. Incidence of algomenorrhea in a group of sacroiliac
displacement, lunbosacral blockage and in normal cases.

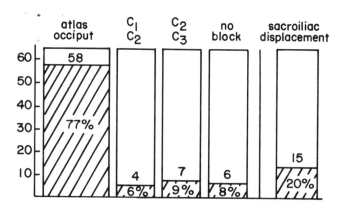

Figure 11. Blockage in 75 cases of chronic tonsillitis. Incidence:
69 cases (92%).

Table 1. Forty cases of chronic tonsillitis treated by manipulation only.

Year of First Treatment	Blockage a Tonsil-litis a	Blockage p Tonsil-litis a	Blockage a Tonsil-litis p	Blockage p Tonsil-litis p	Blockage a Tonsils Improved	No Control Examina-tion	Total
1972	1	2	0	0	1		4
1973	3	1	0	1 (TE)	0	1	6
1974	7	7	0	7 (3TE)	0		23
1975	2	3	2 (TE)	2 (1TE)	0		7
Total	13	13	2	10	1	1	40

a = absent

b = present

the direction of movement restriction produces pain. The pain
stimulus gives rise to reflex protective spasm, guarding the joint
against undue movement. It is easy to understand why this reflex
spasm disappears immediately after successful manipulation, as do
most of the reflex changes in the segment.

If, on the other hand, the nociceptive stimulus is of visceral
origin, we again have muscle spasm ("defense musculaire") usually
involving the segmental back muscles. This in turn acts on the
vertebrae and interferes with normal mobility of the intervertebral
joints, as spasm is superimposed upon muscle contraction produced
by normal movement. In this way faulty movement is produced,
jamming the joint of the involved segment and resulting in blockage.

                            NERVE LESIONS

In recent years there is increasing interest in what are now
called "entrapment syndromes". Formerly these clinical pictures
were attributed to neuritis; their mechanical origin has only recently been recognized. Amongst the best known are the extremely
frequent carpal tunnel syndrome, the syndrome of the thoracic outlet, ulnar tunnel, tarsal tunnel, etc. Even Bell's paralysis is
now explained as a compression syndrome in the Fallopian canal
(Richter, 1971).

For us it is of interest that many of these canals are formed
by a number of bones which are joined together by articulation.
This holds for the carpal tunnel and tarsal tunnels, and for the
thoracic outlet; it is, however, obviously not true for the Fallopian canal or the ulnar tunnel. Moreover, it is well known to
rheumatologists that patients with changes in their carpal joints
may suffer from carpal tunnel syndromes.

With this in view we started routine examination of the relative mobility of the carpal bones in patients suffering from the
carpal tunnel syndrome. This is done by trying to produce minimal
shifts between neighboring bony structures using the minimum force.
Under normal conditions it is almost impossible to avoid producing
some slight shift even on the slightest touch. In cases of carpal
tunnel syndromes we have invariably (17 cases) found increased resistance. The logical therapy was to establish normal mobility;
this was successful in 13 out of 17 cases. In one case in which
decreased conduction velocity was demonstrated these changes were
normalized. At the same time, in accordance with Upton and McComas
(1973), we found changes in the thoracic outlet which were also
treated.

From the physiological point of view it appears more logical to give treatment to the mobile structures which form the canal than to cut, for example, the more or less inert ligament. The theoretical implications are of no less interest. If we consider the carpal tunnel with its chain of relatively mobile bones we easily understand that nerve compression can hardly be due to narrowing and that such a purely morphological approach is inadequate. If, however, we think in terms of function, it is easy to see that if a nerve with its vascular supply passes through such a complicated and mobile structure as the carpal tunnel (or thoracic outlet) this structure must adapt itself to its contents under constantly changing conditions of movement, position and strain. Only under perfect conditions of mobility of all the parts forming such a tunnel can this be achieved. We should therefore consider such a nerve lesion to be due not so much to compression owing to lack of space but to impaired function interfering with the adaptability of the canal to its contents under varying conditions. Accordingly, the carpal tunnel syndrome invariably worsens after physical strain during the day, followed by symptoms during the night.

Having learned something about these mechanisms in entrapment syndromes and about the effects of manipulative therapy in such conditions, we may turn to the most frequent type of nerve compression, i.e., to radicular syndromes. There appears to be an important difference between radicular syndromes in the upper and lower extremity, inasmuch as radicular syndromes in the latter are most frequently caused by herniated discs which are much less common in the upper extremity. Therefore, the course of true radicular syndromes in the lower extremity is much more serious, conservative treatment including manipulation more frequently fails, so that surgery is required. Yet, even in typical discogenic radicular syndromes in the lower extremity there are cases which profit from manipulation, at times even dramatically, and I would like to offer an explanation on the basis of what has been said about entrapment syndromes. As I have already explained, it is difficult to see how manipulation could have any direct effect on a disc herniation. But it has an effect on articular blockage at the corresponding level. The intervertebral canal is then better able to adapt itself to what it encloses during the various movements and strains involved, if the joints can move than if they are blocked. True narrowing of the intervertebral canal owing to blockage has never been demonstrated, as far as we know.

There is another pathophysiological factor we were able to establish on the basis of x-ray findings during lumbar peridurography. There is a striking difference between the contrast picture in the upper and lower part of the lumbar spinal canal (Figure 12). Analysis of this difference suggested a difference in geometrical configuration, and this is indeed the case: the "typical" triangular

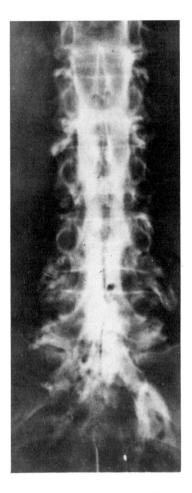

Figure 12. Normal peridurogram. Note difference in appearance in
the lower and upper part of the lumbar spine.

shape of the lumbar vertebral canal given in the textbooks of
anatomy applies only to the last two segments (Figures 13 and 14).
Now, it is precisely in these two segments that typical discogenic
root compression occurs, although disc herniation may occur in any
part of the lumbar spinal canal. The reason seems clear: whereas
in the round or oval-shaped parts of the spinal canal the root can
move back, away from the protruding disc, in the triangular lumbar
canal it gets trapped in the angle (Lewit, 1976; Lewit & Sereghy,
1975).

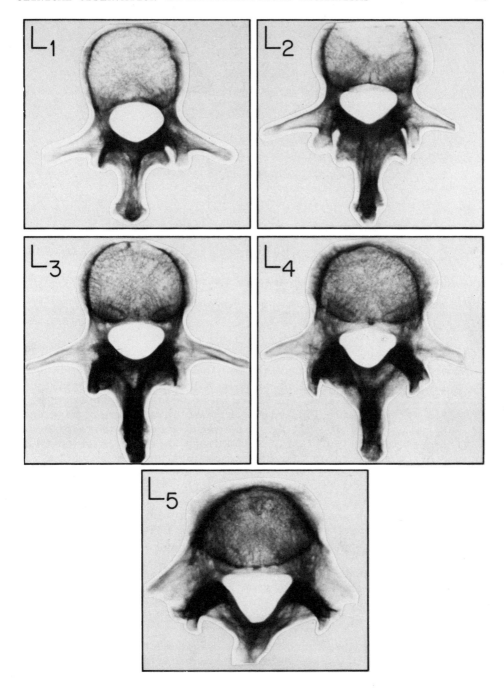

Figure 13.   Note the shape of the vertebral canal from L1   to L5.

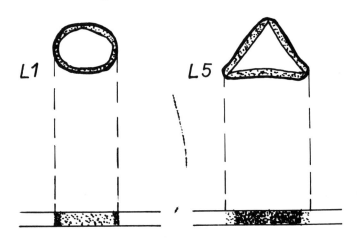

Figure 14.   Diagram explaining the appearance of the peridurogram –
Figure 12.

There is another important observation in root syndromes which
is important for the pathophysiology: usually in root syndromes
there is some degree of slight paresis which exact neurological
examination can establish.   In fact, we are reluctant to make the
diagnosis of true radicular lesion if there is absolutely no sign
of neurological deficit.   It is by no means exceptional to find,
after successful manipulation, an immediate increase in strength in
the paretic muscle and at times even some degree of restoration of
reflexes.

The electrophysiological investigations of Drechsler (1970)
showed that in root compression a decrease in conduction velocity
is an inconstant sign, found in the peroneus and not in the tibial
nerve, that there is more frequently a decrease in the H-reflex and
the tendon reflex, which, however, disappears under the influence
of facilitation maneuvers (Jendrassik, plantar flexion).   In this
way, it was shown that even in true radicular syndromes some of the
paretic signs are due to inhibition and only some to true nerve
lesion.

After this review of reflex and nervous mechanisms in vertebrogenic disorders established mainly on the basis of clinical investigations, I would like to express an opinion on the importance and
place of neurobiological mechanisms on both vertebrogenic lesions
in manipulative therapy.   Being a neurologist myself, these mechanisms were of the greatest interest to me.   Nevertheless, I feel

that vertebrogenic disorders are not a neurological disease in the proper sense of the word but a disease of the motor system and in particular of <u>motor function</u>. Manipulation, however important in view of its reflex effects and even with its possible effect on entrapment syndromes, is mainly a therapy of impaired joint function. It is therefore an important tool by which we normalize the function of the motor system. I would see the importance also of neurobiological mechanisms in that they subserve mobility, motor function and its normalization being the final goal of our endeavors. The motor system is the effector by which the personality establishes itself in the outside world. It is precisely in this field that lie our greatest assets: manipulative therapy with its diagnosis of impaired joint function has become increasingly the branch of medicine which is pioneering on the virgin soil of what we might call the "Functional Pathology of the Motor System" (Lewit, 1975).

REFERENCES

BARRÉ, J. A. Sur un trouble serieux à l'anxiété vestibulaire. *Rev. Neurol.* 86:242, 1952.

BÄRTSCHI-ROCHAIX, W. *Migrain cervicale.* Bern: Medizin. Verl. Huber, 1949.

BRÜGGER, A. Über vertebrale radiculäre und pseudoradiculäre Syndrome. *Acta Rheumatol.* Documenta Geigy No. 18, 1960; No. 19, 1962.

COLE, W. V. Die klinischen Aspekteder Gelenksblockierung. *Therapie über das Nervensystem*, Bd. 7 (Chirotherapie-manuelle Therapie). Stuttgart: Hippokrates, 1967, p. 225-240.

CRAMER, A. Zur Chirotherapie des Zervikalsyndroms. *Physikal, Med. u. Rehab.* 8:63, 1967.

CYRIAX, J. *Textbook of Orthopaedic Medicine.* London: Cassel, 1965.

DRECHSLER, B. Spinale Muskelsteuerung und Wurzelkompression. *Man. Med. und ihre wiss.* Heidelberg: Grundlagen. Physical, Med., 1970, p. 92-105.

EMMINGER, E. Die Anatomie und Pathologie des blockierten Wirbelgelenks. *Therapie über das Nervensystem*, Bd. 7 (Chirotherapie-Manuelle Ther.). Stuttgart: Hippokrates, 1967, p. 117-140.

FIGAR, Š., and L. KRAUSOVÁ. Measurement of degree of resistance in
    vertebral segments. In: *Functional Pathology of the Motor
    System*, Suppl. 10-11 (Rehabilitácia). Bratislava: Orbis
    Publ., 1975, p. 60-63.

FIGAR, Š., L. KRAUSOVÁ, and K. LEWIT. Plethysmographische
    Untersuchungen bei manueller Behandlung vertebragener
    Störungen. *Acta Neuroveg.* 29:618-623, 1967.

GROSS, D. *Therapeutische Lokalanästhesie.* Stuttgart: Hippokrates,
    1972.

GUTMANN, G. *Die Chiropraktik als rationelle ärztliche Therapie,*
    28. Stuttgart: Hippokrates, 1957.

GUTMANN, G. Das cervico-diencephale Syndrom mit sykopaler Tendenz
    und seine Behandling. *Wirbelsäule in Forschung u. Praxis,* 26.
    Stuttgart: Hippokrates, 1963, p. 138-155.

GUTZEIT, K. Wirbelsäule als Krankheitsfaktor. *Dtsch. Med. Wschr.*
    76:1/2, 1951.

KORR, I. M., P. E. THOMAS, and H. M. WRIGHT. Symposium on the
    functional implications of segmental facilitation. *J. Am.
    Osteop. Assoc.* 54:265-282, 1955.

KOS, J. Contribution à l'étude de l'anatomie et de la vasculariza-
    tion des articulations intervertebrales. *Bull. de l'Assoc. des
    Anatomists 53,* Congrès, Tours, 1968, No. 142, p. 1088-1105.

KOS, J., and J. WOLF. Die "Menisci" der Zwischenwirbelgelenkes
    und ihre mögliche Rolle bei Wirbelblockierung. *Man. Med.*
    10:195-214, 1972.

KUNERT, W. *Wirbelsäule und innere Medizin.* Stuttgart: F. Enke,
    1975.

LEWIT, K. Beitrag zur reversiblen Gelenksblockierung. *Z. Orthop.*
    105:150-158, 1968.

LEWIT, K. Vertebral artery insufficiency and the cervical spine.
    Brit. J. Geriatr. Practice 6:37-44, 1969.

LEWIT, K. Functional pathology of the motor system. In: *Functional
    Pathology of the Motor System,* Suppl. 10-11 (Rehabilitácia).
    Bratislava: Orbis Publ., 1975, p. 25-28.

LEWIT, K. *Manuelle Medizin.* Leipzig: J. A. Barth, 1976.

LEWIT, K.   The contribution of peridurography to the anatomy of the
lumbosacral spinal canal. *Folia Morphol*. 24:289-295, 1976.

LEWIT, K., and M. ABRAHAMOVIC.   Kopfgelenksblockierungen und
chronische Tonsillitis. *Man. Med*. 14:106-109, 1976.

LEWIT, K., V. KNOBLOCKH, and Z. FAKTOROVÁ.   Vertebragene Störungen
und Entbindungsschmerz. 8:79-85, 1970.

LEWIT, K., and T. SEREGHY.   Lumbar peridurography with special
regard to the anatomy of the lumbar peridural space. *Neuro-
radiology* 8:233-240, 1975.

MAIGNE, R.   *Douleurs d'origine vertébrale et tratments par manipulations*. Paris: Expansion Scientifique, 1968.

McCOUCH, G. P., I. D. DEERING, and T. H. LING.   Location of receptors
for tonic neck reflexes. *J. Neurophysiol*. 14:191-195, 1951.

METZ, E. G.   Manuelle Therapie in der Inneren Medizin. *Zschr.
Physiother*. 28:83-94, 1976.

MORAVEC, I.   Vertigo cervicalis. *Cas. lék. Ces*. 101:20-25, 1962.

MORITZ, W.   Zerviko-kephale Wirbelsäulensyndrome und ihre Behandlung.
Therapiewoche 7:292, 1956-57.

MOSER, M., C. CONRAUX, and G. GREINER.   Der Nystagmus zervikalen
Ursprungs und seine statische Bewertung. *Ohrenheilk. u.
Laryngo-Rhinol*. 106:259-273, 1972.

NORRÉ, M., A. STEVENS, and P. DEGEYTER.   Der Zervikal-Nystagmus und
die Gelenkblockierung. *Man. Med*. 14:45-51, 1976.

NOVOTNÝ, A.   Theoretische Erwägungen zur Klinik und Therapie der
Wirbelsäulenstörungen in der Frauenheilkunde. *Man. Med*. 11:
1-6, 1973.

NOVOTNÝ, A., and V. DVORÁK.   Funktionsstörungen der Wirbelsäule in
der gynäkologischen Praxis. *Man. Med*. 10:84-88, 1972.

PENNING, W. L., and G. TÖNDURY.   Entstehung, Bau and Funktion der
meniskoiden Strukturen in den Halswirbelgelenken. *Z. Orthop*.
98:1-14, 1963.

RETZLAFF, E. W., A. H. BERRY, H. S. HAIGHT, P. A. PARENTE, H. A.
LICHTY, D. M. TURNER, A. A. YEZBICK, J. S. LAPCEVIK, and D. J.
NOWLAND.   The piriformis muscle syndrome. *J. Am. Osteop.
Assoc*. 73:1-9, June, 1974.

RICHTER, R. Die Bedeutung der "entrapment neuropathy" für die
    Differential-diagnose der vertebragenen Schmerzzustände. *Man.*
    Med. 9:101-111, 1971.

RYCHLÍKOVÁ, E. Vertebragene funktionelle Störungen dei chronischer
    ischämischer Herzkrankheit. *Münch. Med. Wschr.* 117:127-130,
    1975.

RYCHLÍKOVÁ, E., and K. LEWIT. Vertebrogenní funkční poruchy a
    reflexní změny při vředové nemoci mladistvých (Disturbances of
    spinal function and reflex changes in peptic ulcer in adoles-
    cents). *Vnitř. lék.* 22:326-335, 1976.

SAUTIER, P. HNO, HWS und Chirotherapie. *Ärztl. Praxis* 29:320-
    323, 1977.

SCHWARZ, E. Manuelle Therapie und innere Medizin. *Schweiz. Rdsch.*
    Med. (Praxis) 63:837-841, 1974.

SÈZE, de, S., et al. Les manipulations vertébrales. *Sem. Hop.*
    Paris 39:2313-2322, 1955.

SIMON, H., and H. MOSER. Manuelle Medizin und Oto-Rhino-
    Laryngologie. *Man. Med.* 11:49-51, 1973.

SIMON, H., M. MOSER, and M. HOLZER. Der Cervical-Nystagmus – ein
    Weg zur Objektivierung von cervikalem Schwindel und von chiro-
    therapeutischen Eingriffen an der Halswirbelsäule. In:
    Functional Pathology of the Motor System, Suppl. 10-11
    (Rehabilitácia). Bratislava: Orbis Publ., 1975, p. 132-138.

STARÝ, O. Some problems of the pathogenesis of the disc disease.
    Státní Zdravotnické Nakladatelství. Praha, 1959.

STODDARD, A. Cervical spondylosis and cervical osteoarthrosis.
    Man. Med. 8:133-139, 1970.

UNTERHARNSCHEIDT, F. Das synkopale cervicale Vertebralsyndrom.
    Nervenarzt 27:481, 1956.

UPTON, A.R.M., and A. J. McCOMAS. The double crush in nerve entrap-
    ment syndromes. *Lancet II* (August, 7825:359-361, 1973.

WALTHER, G. Halswirbelsäule und Herz. *Therapiewoche* 13:469-473,
    1963.

WOLF, J. The reversible deformation of the joint cartilage surface
    and its possible role in joint blockage. *4th Congress of the*
    FIMM, Prague, 9-12th October, 1974.

WOLF, J.   The reversible deformation of the joint cartilage surface
    and its possible role in joint blockage.   In: *Functional
    Pathology of the Motor System,* Suppl. 10-11 (Rehabilitácia).
    Bratislava: Orbis Publ., 1975, p. 30-35.

WOLFF, H. D.   Wandlungen theoretischer Vorstellungen über die
    Manuelle Medizin. *Man. Med.*   12:121-129, 1974.

ZUCKSCHWERDT, L., F. BIEDERMANN, E. EMMINGER, and H. ZETTEL.
    Wirbelgelenk und Bandscheibe. Stuttgart: Hippokrates,
    2. Aufl., 1960.

MUSCLES, CENTRAL NERVOUS MOTOR REGULATION AND BACK PROBLEMS

Vladimír Janda*

Department of Rehabilitation Medicine, Postgraduate

Medical Institute, Prague, Czechoslovakia

The purpose of this paper is not so much to bring some new data about the function of the motor system, as to present problems concerning muscle function and back pain which the clinician has to face and solve. Not only do these problems need to be explained from the viewpoint of basic research, but their importance in explanation of pathogenesis should be recognized as well. We would like to express some ideas and problems which we think to be important for the functional pathology of the motor system, especially of muscles. Special emphasis will be given to analysis of our therapeutic failures.

The functional pathology of the motor system is a rather new concept and the importance of functional changes within the motor system has not yet been satisfactorily recognized. It should be emphasized, however, that these changes play an important role in the pathogenesis of various pathological conditions of the motor system; to neglect them unfavourably influences the results of the entire rehabilitation process. This is especially true of painful conditions. For these reasons the main subject of the 1974 Congress of the International Federation of Manual Medicine (FIMM) in Prague was devoted in particular to the functional pathology of the motor system.

According to Lewit (1974), under the term "functional pathology of the motor system" we understand the vast field comprising functional impairment of the motor system and its interactions with the whole organism, mainly of a reflex nature. The reflex changes and

---

*Dr. Janda could not attend the workshop and, on the Editor's invitation, submitted this paper for inclusion in the proceedings.

the functional impairment constitute an entity which not only may
result in clinical manifestations of pain arising from functional
lesions of the motor system but may influence the results of the
whole process of motor re-education. To what extent these lesions
of the motor system play a role in functional, reflex disturbances
of our viscera is still largely conjectural.

The concept of a functional lesion must be understood, however,
in a broad but nevertheless precise sense. The symptomatology
especially must be well defined and an appropriate technique used
in order to be able not only to discover but to define these changes,
and to understand their significance and relationship to other
lesions, either within the motor system or apart from it. We have
to keep in mind that the motor system functions as an entity and
that it is in principle a wrong approach to try to understand im-
pairments of different parts of the motor system separately, without
understanding the function of the motor system as a whole.

There are, indeed, many indications showing that a local lesion
or, better said, dysfunction may be a secondary one due to a lesion
which may be quite remote and at first sight with no obvious relationship to the lesion which provokes the symptoms for which the
patient is seeking help. Many of these examples are known. Let us
mention only some types of cervical headaches due to altered function of the muscle-joint complex of the pelvis and hip. It is
evident, of course, that such a relationship may seem doubtful to
those who are accustomed to think in terms of localisation as is
usual in structural changes. On the other hand, many good clinicians who have noticed a relationship between signs which might be
described as "far distant symptoms" did not understand the chain of
reflex reactions resulting in the clinical picture. As a matter of
fact, considering all known facts, we think we are right to maintain
that any local lesion within the motor system provokes more or less
evident changes of function of the whole motor system. In other
words, this means that a local lesion produces a chain of reflexes
which involve the whole motor system, and vice versa. This is more
and more understandable with our increasing knowledge of principles
of function of the nervous system.

The joint dysfunctions are more or less known and are the basis
of manual medicine. However, it should be emphasized that these
joint dysfunctions are only one expression of impairment of motor
system as a whole, i.e., of both neuromuscular as well as osteoarticular systems.

Changes of muscle function are less well known and even less
understood, in spite of the fact that they evidently play at least
as important a role in the pathogenesis of various syndromes as
does joint dysfunction in some painful conditions.

Perhaps even less appreciated is dysfunction at the central nervous level, mainly cortical. Therefore, we would like to devote more time to this problem and to stress its importance for better understanding of various pathological conditions. Many syndromes are still being considered as strictly localised in the periphery of the motor system, i.e., in joints, as typically low back pain syndrome. Central motor nervous influence is too often ignored as an integral part of the motor system.

After these few introductory remarks (which we consider necessary, however), let us come back to our main topics and raise several important questions, limiting ourselves to those which relate to muscle and joint correlations and which may explain some common pathological conditions.

As we have shown in previous papers (Janda, 1969a, 1969b, 1971, 1974; Janda & Stará, 1970, 1971), changes in muscle function play an important role in the pathogenesis of many painful conditions of the motor system and constitute an integral part of postural defects in general.

There are sufficient observations that some muscles usually respond to a given situation (e.g., to pain) by tightness, while others react by inhibition, atrophy and weakness. This fact can be demonstrated in different examples, as in hip or knee affections. Various back and neck syndromes are typical. It is known that tightness of hamstrings or trunk erectors frequently develops in these and similar postural defects, whereas abdominal and gluteal muscles show signs of weakness. A similar "distribution" can be found in the upper part of the body, where mainly tightness of the upper trapezius, levator scapulae and pectoralis is found; on the other hand, the deep neck flexors and lower stabilizers of the scapula react by weakness.

The tendency of some muscles to get tight or weak is known. However, such responses have been considered to be more or less random. Detailed, careful clinical analysis of different pathological conditions of the motor system, however, reveals that such responses follow some typical rules. We are convinced, therefore, that we may speak about a typical nuscle pattern of changes of function in various pathological conditions. Just as we have, e.g., a capsular pattern (Cyriax, 1975), so may we have a typical muscle pattern.

If we accept that there exists a typical response of certain muscles under different pathological conditions, the question of explaining these reactions remains. Unfortunately, histological, histochemical and physiological studies up to now do not give the necessary data. It should be emphasized that these results are,

for a clinician, rather confusing, and in many ways even discour-
aging. In other words, existing data do not explain clinical observations.

  ✗   Thus up to now the clinical symptomatology remains open to
discussion in many respects and we may ask: (1) Does muscle tightness develop only because, from the biomechanical point of view,
some muscles are strong in comparison to those which respond by
weakness? (2) Does imbalance between these two muscle systems develop as a mechanical response only to a change in the centre of
gravity in faulty posture, or to reflex relationships between various muscles within movement patterns? (3) Is there any difference
of innervation between the two systems? This is a valid question
if we consider the fact that muscles which respond by tightness are
those more commonly subject to spasticity and contracture in spastic
syndromes of cerebral (especially capsular) origin. (4) Are muscle
changes and postural defects evidence of a common motor dysfunction
or do they develop independently? To what extent do they influence
each other?

     Certainly, other questions may be raised, such as comparisons
of spurt and shunt muscles (MacConaill & Basmajian, 1969) and of
one- and two-joint muscles; or whether there exists some correlation
between muscles with a tendency to tighten and those participating
mainly in flexor reflexes; and correlation between muscles with a
tendency to weakness and those participating mainly in extensor
reflexes.

  ✗   As has already been said, histological data are still confusing. The fact that it is not possible histologically to differentiate convincingly among different types of muscles in man is not
decisive from the clinical point of view.

     However, on the other hand, there is some other evidence of
differences between two systems of muscles respectively. Thus it
is evident, if we study the electric threshold to stimulation –
and these observations are today almost 100 years old (Bourgignon)
– that muscles with a tendency to get tight have shorter chronaxy
compared to muscles with a tendency to get weak.

     As we have said, many experimental results do not explain
clinical problems. It is difficult to understand why most skeletal
muscles are so homogeneously mixed in man. According to Saltin and
co-workers (1976), one explanation might be that although some
muscles may have special functions demanding a special fibre type,
all muscles are also involved in other activities, so that the
characteristics of all the different fibre types are required.

On the other hand, again according to findings of Saltin and
co-workers (1976), the size and some histochemical qualities of
some muscle fibres may change due to overwork. Thus physiological
properties of muscles may differ considerably, ranging from subjects
doing only sedentary work to athletes. Surprisingly enough, however, the changes are not substantially different in athletes in
different types of sports, such as long-distance runners vs. sprint-
ers. Saltin offers several explanations, all of which, however,
have to face the same difficulties as we have in our clinical
problems.

However, one fact concerning clinical problems should be
pointed out here. As we have shown in our previous papers (Janda,
1969a, 1969b, 1971, 1974; Janda & Stará, 1970, 1971), society in
developed countries suffers not only from insufficient movement,
but also from lack of variety of movement. Thus, we activate relatively more muscles which show a tendency to get tight and shortened, and neglect muscles which are getting weak. To some extent
tight muscles appear to behave similarly to those muscles which are
well trained or even overtrained in athletes. But as we have said,
all these suggestions are only hypotheses, which, however, seek explanations relating more to the functional than to the morphological
quality of a given muscle.

We should not forget, either, that in man who moves mostly in
the upright position, the muscular response or reaction will always
be due to a combination of at least two factors, namely, the physiological properties of a muscle itself (and in this respect we should
not ignore phylogenetic aspects as well), and the adaptation of the
human erect posture to the influence of gravity and other mechanical
factors. In brief, a clinically developed imbalance between different muscle groups will probably be a result of a combination of both
reflex and mechanical mechanisms. Whatever the physiological basis
for these changes of muscle function, the clinical fact remains that
a developed muscle imbalance should be treated and that muscles in
which we find a predominantly static or postural function and which
show a tendency to get tight are activated in various movement patterns relatively more than muscles with a predominantly dynamic,
phasic function, which show a tendency to get weak.

The importance of a tight and shortened muscle can be demonstrated fairly well by the following example: A woman aged 48 suffered for many years from low back pain without radicular symptoms.
For changes in intervertebral joint function she had been repeatedly
treated by manipulation with only a temporary effect. A detailed
kinesiological analysis showed a typical general imbalance between
the postural and phasic systems; the abdominals especially were weak
and the trunk extensors tight, so that the forward-bending test
(Thomayer-Neri test) showed 32 cm between finger-tips and the floor.

Strengthening exercises for the weakened abdominal muscles, among
others, were recommended. After this exercise programme, however,
the patient's condition became even worse. EMG examination revealed
that she activated the trunk extensors in all movements of the trunk
and even in those in which they should be inactive, such as slowly
curling up from the supine position. Thus all exercises for strengthening the abdominal muscles resulted in strengthening of the trunk
extensors. The imbalance between weak abdominal and tight back
muscles became more and more pronounced. It should be emphasized
that in this patient the trunk extensors were activated even in
those movements in which they should be silent. Their activation
even produced a kind of "functional" ankylosis, blocking the normal
and necessary movements in the lumbar segments of the vertebral
spine. Of course, it cannot be said that because trunk extensors
were activated during a sitting-up movement they are able to perform
such a movement, i.e., that trunk extensors would produce trunk
flexion. But we can say that in this particular patient the activation of the trunk extensors, e.g., during trunk flexion, is an
inseparable part of the trunk-flexion patterns. This knowledge is
of course of paramount importance in understanding this case. This
realisation, followed by stretching and inhibition of the extensors,
resulted not only in normalisation of ventral and dorsal trunk
muscle interplay, but improved the patient's condition substantially.
From the therapeutic point of view, balanced muscle coordination is
perhaps the best protection of our osteoarticular system.

Figures 1 and 2 illustrate the importance of tight muscles.
There are today enough clinical and physiological considerations
which support the idea that, in pathogenesis as well as in treatment of muscle imbalance and back problems, tight muscles play a
more important and perhaps even a primary role in comparison to
weak muscles. Clinical experience and especially therapeutic results support the assumption that (according to Sherrington's law
of reciprocal innervation) tight muscles act in an inhibitory way
on their antagonists. Therefore, it does not seem reasonable to
start with strengthening of the weakened muscles as most exercise
programmes do. It has been clinically proved that it is better to
stretch the tight muscles first, thus inhibiting the weakened, inhibited antagonists. It is not exceptional that, after stretching
of the tight muscle, the strength of the inhibited, weakened
antagonist improves spontaneously, sometimes immediately, sometimes
within a few days, without any additional treatment. By stretching
it is sometimes possible to inhibit the tight muscle and to avoid
undesirable overactivation during different movement patterns.
This may be of great value in further exercise programmes. Figure 2
is a good example of such a situation. During an attempt to curl up
with tight trunk extensors, these muscles were overactive. After
stretching, their activation during this movement decreased almost
to zero; simultaneously, the activity of the abdominal muscles

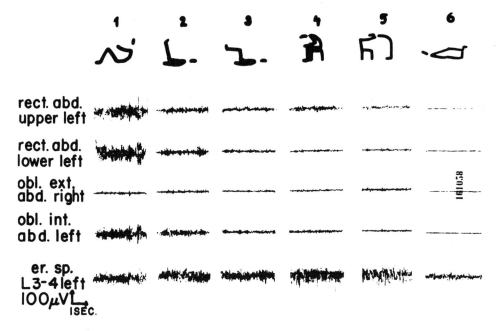

Figure 1. Electromyographic activity of selected trunk muscles in postures shown by line drawings. Muscles: rect. abd. - rectus abdominis; obl. ext. abd. - obliquus externus abdominis; obl. int. abd. - obliquus internus abdominis; er. sp. - erector spine.

increased. In this case after stretching, curling up may be considered as a good exercise not only to improve the abdominal muscles, but especially to improve the balance necessary between abdominal and dorsal muscles. The same exercise performed with tight trunk extensors strengthened these muscles and enhanced the undesirable imbalance.

Let us switch now to another question, namely, to the problem of the central nervous regulation of motor functions, especially with regard to vertebrogenic diseases and motor re-education.

There is no doubt that fine muscle coordination is needed to prevent damage of a joint, especially during a fast movement. It is well known that, at the end of a fast movement, the active inhibition of the antagonist switches into rapid facilitation and contraction in order to slow down the movement and prevent injury. If this reciprocal interplay is altered, great danger for the joint occurs. This reciprocal reflex mechanism is evidently based at spinal level.

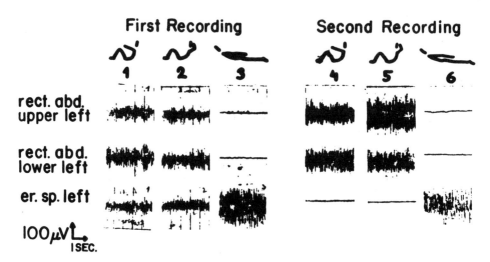

Figure 2. Electromyographic activity before and after stretching tight muscles. See text for further explanation.

For smaller, finer and slower movements, however, fine muscle coordination is also needed. As has been shown (Starý, 1959), good coordination at least between abdominal and dorsal muscles is necessary to protect the joints of the vertebral column. Such coordination is based on the working out of stable, but at the same time adaptable, movement patterns. The quality of working out of a movement pattern depends primarily on the functional efficiency of the cerebral cortex and, later on, of other central nervous structures and their functional connections. In other words, good movement habits depend to a large extent on the functional efficiency of the central nervous system.

As we have shown in several previous papers (Janda, 1969a, 1969b, 1971, 1974; Janda & Stará, 1970, 1971), incorrect, basic and important movement patterns appear in conjunction with joint dysfunctions. In any event, a bad movement pattern alters the distribution of pressures on the most important segments not only during various movements, but during statics as well. The position of a joint in statics and movements no longer corresponds to the lines of bone structures; the result of this must then be overstrain and the acceleration of degenerative processes. We have demonstrated this situation on movement patterns in the pelvic region (Janda, 1969a, 1969b, 1971, 1974; Janda & Stará, 1970, 1971).

Thus, the importance of altered movement patterns for the pathogenesis of functional and later on degenerative joint diseases seems to be evident. We may presume, therefore, that an inability to work out good movement patterns may set up conditions for earlier joint dysfunction or may influence therapeutic results.

As it seems that we can often learn more from therapeutic failures, we have analyzed 100 patients who were either suffering from painful vertebrogenic conditions at various sites since early adulthood, with poor therapeutic results, or who had been admitted to our rehabilitation clinic after injury and in whom the therapeutic results were unsatisfactory. All patients were evaluated very thoroughly, especially with respect to motor regulation, the motor system in general and psychological state.

A detailed analysis of these patients will be the subject of another study. Here we would like to present a survey and take up several specific points, ignoring the local pathological findings. The patients with vertebrogenic disorders were from 17 to 61 years old, the average age being 40. In most cases the painful troubles started without any evident cause between 20 to 25 years of age, occasionally even earlier. The intensity of back pain varied but was almost constant despite long treatment. Therapeutic relief was in general only very brief. In cases of traumatic etiology, the final motor syndrome resulted in a general impairment of function of the motor system and the response to motor re-education was unexpectedly poor despite the fact that in most cases the injury was uncomplicated, with a generally good prognosis.

In the analysis of reasons for such therapeutic failure, three striking findings emerged: neurological examination, evaluation of the ability to work out movement patterns, and psychological evaluation. All three findings, however, were in general agreement.

In the neurological examination, the symptomatology was mostly slight yet quite evident to an experienced neurologist who is familiar especially with the evaluation of motor functions. The symptomatology may be divided roughly into three groups, although it is impossible to maintain a strict distinction among them as the symptoms are frequently combined.

The first group might be described as a clinical picture of microspasticity: increased muscle tonus, tendon reflexes, usually asymmetrical, slight paretic signs, a decreased threshold for provocation of spastic phenomena, as of the Babinski sign, very often small developmental asymmetries, etc. In summary, slight hemiparesis, or quadriparesis, was found.

The second group showed some hypotonia, usually asymmetrical, irregular tendon reflexes, mostly decreased, an evident instability in static functions as in the Mingazzini sign and/or lack of coordination in the manner of a slight adiadochokinesis. During mental concentration some involuntary movements, especially of fingers, could be noticed. In summary, the picture was very similar to that of a slight choreoathetotic syndrome.

In the third group slight changes of proprioception could be observed. The patients failed in examinations in which greater demands on the quality of afferent pathways were made, as in standing on one leg, especially with eyes closed. In most of these cases, slight changes in sensitivity, especially in discrimination, were found.

The evaluation of movement patterns was done clinically, in most cases by means of multichannel electromyography. In principle, almost all patients showed some alterations in the ability to work out a finely adjusted coordination so that they activated many more muscles than one would expect. Often, they were unable to activate one side of the body only, so that a tendency to mirror movements could be electromyographically observed.

In psychological examination, besides the usual personality characteristics, we tried to evaluate perceptuomotor coordination, visual and space orientation and motor memory and learning. For this we used, apart from the usual methods (Wechsler, Raven, Eysenck, etc.), the "Copying of geometrical designs", a rather simple test similar to that used in developmental assessment, then "Drawing of a human figure", similar to the "Draw a Person Test" (DAPT, Goodenough) and the "Number Square", popular in our country for detection of learning disabilities, especially in concentration power, learning curve, memory and visual field mastery.

In drawing, fine motor coordination was found to be poor in more than two-thirds of the cases, with frequent tremor, uncertain timing and joining of the lines and overshooting the mark. Visual analysis of the designs was conspicuously poor in estimation of length and distance, and two parts of an interrupted line (e.g., where the middle part was not visible) were often not perceived as a whole. The more complex designs were pieced together from small parts with no understanding of the general structure. Fine motor coordination was equally poor in the representation of the human figure, which was frequently primitive, distorted and even incomplete.

In the "Number Square", the learning curve was irregular and jerky and in many subjects did not improve. In normal subjects,

the so-called "motor memory" is a help in remembering the respective
positions of the numbers, but many of the group simply "could not
find their way around", with numerous superfluous movements ,
"blocks" or stops in the performance and overlooking the correct
target.

Some, mostly patients with college education, complained of
poor sustained attention, though this was not always confirmed by
psychological assessment. Many reported real trouble in concentration at school age but seemed to have arrived at a satisfactory
level at present. In a few, forced responsiveness to stimuli was
observed; surprising, though rare, was the phenomenon of difficult
distribution of attention to two more activities (e.g., clumsy
treading on an old sewing machine at the occupational therapy department when sewing, or difficulty in taking out a purse while
walking). This of course is consistent with slow automation of
movements as well.

In intellectual performance, no general impairment was found;
many of the subjects had had a college education or were even of
high scientific standing. Yet difficulties in changing over from
one type of working method to another, and in abstracting from
simple sensory ideas, were marked in some.

In addition to the motor and perceptuomotor dysfunctions, at
the detection of which our assessment was aimed, two other characteristics stood out.

Wide individual variations in the general activation level
were found, and a higher activation level with medium or poor control was apparent, e.g., in superfluous strokes by the pencil when
drawing, in stamping feet or tapping fingers when solving a problem,
in numerous superfluous movements in the "Number Square", in the
patient's social interrelations in the clinical setting, sometimes
reported as frequent accidents or many types of sports attempted,
or even as a personal complaint of interference with the patient's
work while studying. Another group of patients was evidently
slower than the general population, with delayed reactions, long
reaction times, slow in pace, in language, although this might not
have been true for their work.

As the last striking trait, more than half the patients seemed
to be affected by their low tolerance to stress; they appeared to
live in high tension, worrying over trifles, unable to cope with
the problems of daily life or managing this only with undue strain.
Some appeared as neurotics, but the cause of their trouble seemed
to be out of proportion to the severity of strain experienced.
Some might be said even to produce these stresses by their own
"over-reactivity", "over-excitability".

Only in very few persons (3 out of 82) did the psychological evaluation not reveal at least some of these (motor, perceptuo-motor, intellectual or basic neuropsychologic) dysfunctions, despite evident somatic findings.

The psychologist's impression of the group is that of a general lack of coordination of behavior at all levels and in all areas of mental functioning, from motor, sensory, to intellectual, and from control of activation to general tolerance and adaptability to stress.

Considering the results of the psychological examination, it may be concluded that in our patients symptoms could be found which indicate an organic lesion of the central system. This is quite important, as on superficial estimation, many symptoms might be explained as due to a neurotic reaction. As a matter of fact, most patients of the studied group were regarded as neurotics and were suspected of exaggeration. The treatment was then largely psychiatric, which was completely inappropriate.

It is important to mention that with a few exceptions the results of the neurological and psychological examination and the evaluation of patterning ability were in complete agreement. It was a real exception if the psychologist did not find the typical pathology in a case in which somatic examination showed disturbances in central nervous motor regulations.

We can thus summarize that in the great majority of patients with difficult problems of the motor system, a symptomatology was found which shows that these patients are unable to adjust or adapt themselves adequately to altered physiological conditions. In pathological situations this maladaptation is even more evident. Such difficulties in adaptation can be demonstrated not only within the motor system but in various psychological reactions as well. While these difficulties may lead finally to a neurotic overlay, all these reactions have an evident organic basis. As far as the motor system is concerned, there is an evident over-activation even of those muscles which should not be activated during a given movement. The motor coordination is poor, the movements are not ideally smooth, but rough and somewhat jerky, with a tendency to mass movements. All these signs show that the patterning abilities are decreased, resulting in poor movement control. This, then, forms an ideal basis for the development and fixation of a general dysfunction of the motor system. This does not occur only on the cortical level, but eventually involves all parts of the motor system, especially those in which vulnerability and demand for adaptation are the greatest, as in muscles and joints.

Another problem is that of explaining the etiology of such a central nervous dysfunction. We do not want to go into details here, but different symptoms reveal that most, if not all, of these changes are inborn or emerge soon after the birth of the subject.

Here we would like to mention a new clinical entity, minimal brain dysfunction. This syndrome is now fairly well recognized in children, it has been estimated that about 10 to 15 percent of the child population suffers from at least some signs of this syndrome. It is believed that due to maturation of the central nervous system and development of new reflex mechanisms the symptoms more or less disappear in adolescents and adults. It is believed that if some of the symptoms should persist until adulthood, these appear as sensory and communicative defects; motor symptomatology is completely overlooked.

The anamnestic data and especially the developmental history and social maladaptation together with the motor and psychologic evaluation allow us to be sure that all these pictures are due to minimal brain dysfunction. As, however, this syndrome is practically unknown in adults, it would be helpful to give a brief description of it as it occurs in children.

Perhaps the most useful analysis of the minimal brain dysfunction syndrome was made by Paine (1962). He divided dysfunctions due to organic lesions of the brain into four main syndromes: dysfunction of the motor system, dysfunction of the sensory system, psychic dysfunctions, and disturbances of consciousness. Each may be involved separately or in combination. The alteration of a certain function may be so slight that it will be discovered only by special examination; or the dysfunction may be evident, with significant functional capacity remaining in the involved system; or in the most severe cases the function may be virtually abolished. Especially in cases of a minimal dysfunction, the final clinical picture may be substantially influenced by many other factors, even educational.

As far as motor dysfunction is concerned, symptomatology very similar to that described above can be seen in children. Perhaps clumsiness, instability and some involuntary movements are a little more pronounced but in general the clinical picture does not differ greatly. Usually, the motor patterning process is poor and labile, and there is inability to adapt to new motor conditions. Thus the lack of central nervous regulation of movements influences the function of the peripheral part of the motor system, especially of muscles and joints. No wonder that in such a situation functional impairment of joints develops earlier and to a more generalized extent. In these cases, manipulation is relatively contraindicated, as its effect may be only temporary. In this respect the state may be compared to another, better-known condition, that of Parkinson's syndrome.

In the literature we have found only one paper which deals even partly with this problem. Huffmann (1974) observed that it is difficult to evaluate the working capacity of subjects suspected of this syndrome, that they have problems during the rehabilitation process and that after reaching 40 years of age they age much faster than normal subjects.

From the practical point of view, then, it means that in cases where back problems developed early and resist treatment, we must search for joint-muscle dysfunction in other parts of the motor system. In our present experience, altered central nervous motor regulation based on minimal brain dysfunction is one of the most common causes.

REFERENCES

CYRIAX, J. *Textbook of Orthopaedic Medicine*. London: Balière and Tindall, 1975.

HUFFMANN, G. Der leichte frühkindliche Hirnschaden bei Jugendlichen und Erwachsenen. *Deutsch Med. Wochenschr.* 99/51:2620-2622, 1974.

JANDA, V. Muskelfunction in Beziehung zur Entwicklung vertebrogener Storungen. In: *Manuelle Med. (Kongressband d.2., Kongress der Internat. Gesellschaft f. manuelle Med., Salzburg, 1968).* Heidelberg: Verlag phys. Med., 1969a, pp. 127-130.

JANDA, V. Postural and phasic muscles in the pathogenesis of low back pain. In: *Proc. XIth Congress of the Intern. Soc. Rehabil. Disabled*, Dublin, 1969b, pp. 553-554.

JANDA, V. Zur Muskelfunktion am Achsenorgan des Rumpfes - Funktionelle Pathologie u. Klinik der Wirbelsäule. In: *Die Wirbelsäule in Forschung u. Praxis*. Stuttgart: Hippokrates Verlag, 1971, Band 52, pp. 30-38.

JANDA, V. Muscle and joint correlations. In: *Proc. IVth Congr. Intern. Fed. Man. Med.* Prague, 1974.

JANDA, V., and V. STARÁ. Zur Bedeutung der posturalen Muskeln in Entwicklung der Motorik. In: *Symp. Entwicklungsneurologie des Kindes, Beiheft z. Z. Psychiat., Neurol. u. med. Psychol.* 13/14:71-74, 1970.

JANDA, V., and V. STARÁ. Comparison of movement in healthy and
    spastic children. In: *Proc. 2nd Intern. Symp. Cerebral
    Palsy, Praha, 1967.* Praha: Balnea, 1971, pp. 119-122.

LEWIT, K. Functional pathology of the motor system. In: *Proc.
    IVth Congr. Intern. Fed. Man. Med.* Prague, 1974.

MacCONAILL, M. A., and J. V. BASMAJIAN. *Muscles and Movements.*
    Baltimore: Williams and Wilkins Co., 1969.

PAINE, R. S. Minimal chronic brain syndromes in children. *Devel.
    Med. Child Neurol.* 4:21, 1962.

SALTIN, B., K. NAZAR, D. L. COSTILL, D. STEIN, D. JANSSON, B.
    ESSEN, and D. GOLLNICK. The nature of the training response:
    Peripheral and central adaptations to one-legged exercise.
    Acta Physiol. Scand. 96:289-305, 1976.

STARÝ, O. Some problems of the pathogenesis of the disc disease.
    Státní Zdravotnické Nakladatelství. Praha, 1959.

MANIPULATIVE THERAPY IN RELATION TO TOTAL HEALTH CARE

Philip E. Greenman

College of Osteopathic Medicine

Michigan State University, East Lansing, Michigan

INTRODUCTION

The history of manipulation is as old as the history of medicine itself (Cyria & Schiotz, 1975). Hippocrates, the acknowledged
father of medicine, apparently used manipulative therapy in patient
care. His disciples, and subsequent physicians throughout the
ages, have applied manual therapy to the human body. A study of
the history of manipulative therapy or manual medicine leads one
to two basic conclusions. In the first instance, most manipulative
therapy was utilized for the treatment of "structural" problems.
Treatment was designed to restore altered structure to a more
"normal" condition. The treatment of kyphosis, lordosis, and
scoliosis, by varying means of traction, compression, and other
manual forces, was apparently to restore structural form. In the
second instance, much of the therapy was on the basis of empirical
result, rather than upon the basis of "scientific" research and
study. If the therapy was effective, it was utilized.

By further study of the history of medicine (Northup, 1966),
one is impressed with the ebb and flow of the healing art between
two emphases: on the patient, and on the disease. Hippocrates and
his disciples are generally acknowledged as the founders of the
patient-oriented school of the healing arts, whose main concern was
the patient and his response to the environment resulting in some
departure from health leading to a "diseased" state. The conflicting school of the healing art appeared to be more interested in the
disease which had entered the body of the patient. For centuries,
physicians have utilized varying treatments for their patients' ills
because the treatment was effective, even though the scientific basis

43

had not been identified. Manipulative therapy has likewise been
utilized for treatment of multiple conditions based upon some evidence of its effectiveness. We continue to explore its scientific
mechanisms.

The osteopathic profession has made its contribution to the
evolution of the healing art (Hoag et al., 1969; Northup, 1966;
Still, 1899). Founded in the tradition of Hippocrates, as a patient-
oriented school of practice, it has extensively used structural
diagnosis and manipulative therapy as part of its philosophy and
practice of medicine. It has utilized structural diagnosis and
manipulative therapy in total patient care, not confining it to
painful conditions of the musculoskeletal system. The structural
and functional inseparability of the total human organism is
fundamental to osteopathic philosophy and practice.

TERMINOLOGY

In discussing structural diagnosis and manipulative therapy,
I feel it most important that we define the terminology. Previous
conferences and workshops (Buerger & Tobis, 1977; Goldstein, 1975)
dealing with this subject, as well as much of the diverse literature available, use a variety of terms for the pathology of the
musculoskeletal system identified by the examining physician, and
the therapeutic modality utilized by the therapist. In the area
of diagnosis, we speak of the chiropractic subluxation, the osteopathic lesion, the joint lock, and most recently the term somatic
dysfunction. In the therapeutic realm we talk of mobilization,
manipulation, manipulative treatment, physiotherapy, rehabilitative
therapy, and a variety of terms such as massage, effleurage, etc.
Until general agreement on terminology is achieved, much confusion
about structural diagnosis and manipulative therapy will continue.
We must abandon jargon and rely on anatomical and physiological
terminology. Too much time and effort have been expended defending
and justifying terms which have little, if any, anatomical and
physiological basis. Resolution of the issue of terminology can
lead to better understanding in the field.

For the purpose of this discussion, we will utilize the term
somatic dysfunction. The definition of the term is

"An area of impaired function of related components of
the musculoskeletal system (muscle, bone, fascia, ligament)
and its associated or related parts of the vascular,
lymphatic, and nervous systems." (Rumney, 1975)

Attention is called to the role of neural elements, since this
workshop focuses on neurologic mechanisms. The neurological elements

involved include those relating to the motor system, and those of
the autonomic nervous system relating to visceral and vascular
function. Finding abnormality of neural elements related to the
motor system and the autonomic nervous system is important to the
practicing clinician in diagnosis, prognosis and therapy.

DIAGNOSIS, PROGNOSIS, THERAPY

The musculoskeletal system is not only the largest organ system of the body but it is an integral part of the total body economy.
It responds to, and participates in, the rapid moment-to-moment
changes of the body's internal and external environment.

The three diagnostic findings of somatic dysfunction are
(1) asymmetry, (2) restricted motion, and (3) tissue texture abnormality (Walton, 1977). Asymmetry is utilized to describe abnormality of the structural and functional relationships of the
right to left half of the body. Asymmetry also connotes dispro-
portion between the anterior/posterior, and superior/inferior
halves of the body from a structural and functional perspective.
Restricted motion is reduction in range of mobility within the
anatomical and physiological limits of a joint. This can apply to
a single joint (e.g., interphalangeal joint), or an anatomical part
involving multiple joints (e.g., a vertebral segment involving two
superior arthrodial joints, two inferior arthrodial joints, a superior and inferior invertebral disc, and, in the thoracic area, two
costovertebral joints). Restriction of motion can be in any one or
combination of the three planes of motion of flexion-extension,
rotation or sidebending. The exact cause of restriction of motion
has been a subject of much debate. The theory of Kos and Wolf
(Kos & Wolf, 1972; Pointon, 1976) on the role of meniscoids between
the joint surfaces may well be one explanation. Further investigation to substantiate this theory, or provide other explanations,
seems indicated. Tissue texture abnormality is a clinical phenomenon observable by inspection and palpation. It has been described
by many as having change in consistency, such as doughy, boggy;
changes in temperature, described as hot or cold; changes in color,
such as the cutaneous red response. These phenomena of somatic
dysfunction appear to be due to alterations of sympathetic nervous
activity affecting vascular and secretomotor activity in the somatic
structures. Many research questions can be raised about these phenomena of tissue texture abnormality. What is the origin of this
stimulus of abnormal vascular and secretomotor activity? How is it
mediated? How is it maintained? What factors influence its
perpetuation?

To this point attention has been drawn to the diagnostic
criteria of this entity we have called somatic dysfunction. An

additional point must be made, namely, that this is not an isolated
entity but one which participates in, and may well be a significant
and contributing factor to, the ongoing process of the total human
organism. Not only is "somatic dysfunction" an entity organized by
the nervous system, but it may also be an entity which contributes
to disorganization within the nervous system. What is the role of
somatic dysfunction in the patient's total disease process?

The role of manipulative therapy in the treatment of the human
body is to restore physiological motion of dysfunctional areas of
body function. By improving function of the musculoskeletal system
there is expectation of improved function of all of those parts of
the body interrelated with the musculoskeletal system, through the
communicating systems of the body. Manipulative therapy is not
utilized just to treat a specific disease, but rather to maximize
the structural-functional integrity of the total human organism to
cope with its internal and external environmental stresses which
have resulted in the patient's dis-ease. Legitimate research questions can be raised on manipulative therapy within this context.
Does manipulative therapy alter restricted ranges of joint motion?
How is this accomplished? Does it change the position of a meniscoid? Does it alter the congruence of opposing joint surfaces?
Does it alter muscular tone between the agonist and antagonist of
joint motion? Does manipulative therapy alter the tissue texture
abnormalities of somatic dysfunction? Does it influence sympathetic
nervous system activity affecting vascular and secretomotor tone?
How is this mediated?

Many practitioners of the manual medicine art speak of the diagnostic value of structural examination (Walton, 1977) and therapeutic
usefulness of manipulative therapy. Few have spoken of the value of
structural evaluation of the musculoskeletal system as a prognostic
tool. I have been impressed with the prognostic value of serial
structural evaluation to ascertain effectiveness of therapy applied,
whether it be manipulative therapy, medication, or surgery. Clues
to the progress of the patient are reflected in the musculoskeletal
system, both as to improvement and lack of it. What are the
mechanisms at work? How are they mediated?

NEURAL MECHANISMS

Many authors have described changes within the musculoskeletal
system related to disease of the internal organs (Judovitch & Bates,
1946; Pottenger, 1930; Speransky, 1944). Pain and rigidity of musculature in the lower right quadrant with appendicitis, anterior
chest pain radiating to the left arm in coronary heart disease,
right upper quadrant muscle splinting and pain with radiation to
the right shoulder tip in acute gall bladder disease, are all

examples. Some form of neural mechanism is operative in each instance. Referred pain in remote areas of the musculoskeletal system
from stimulus to trigger zones, described by many authors, appears
to have some form of neural mechanism operative, as yet undefined.
External stimulation to the musculoskeletal system, e.g., acupuncture (Nemerof, 1974), acupressure, moxibustion, Chapman's reflexes
(Owens, 1937), injection of trigger zone (Travell & Rinzler, 1952),
manipulative therapy (Hoag et al., 1969), seems to influence referred
pain and alterations in visceral function. The mechanisms continue
to be obscure, but the clinical effectiveness of these therapies
seems to justify their inclusion in the armamentarium of the physician until scientific identification of the mechanisms is available.

Reference has been made previously not only to the relationship
of tissue texture abnormalities in the diagnosis of somatic dysfunction, but also to their relationship to aberrant autonomic nervous
system activity affecting vasomotor and secretomotor tone. Although
the reference has been to vascular and glandular activity in the
musculoskeletal system, it is reasonable to assume that aberrant
autonomic nervous system activity might alter vasomotor and secretomotor activity of visceral organs (Hix, 1976). Abnormal autonomic
nervous system activity might well be in a form of both impulse
and nonimpulse neural transmission. Previous studies (Thomas, 1974)
have demonstrated that a rise in autonomic nervous system activity
can increase atherosclerotic change of innervated vessels. If
somatic dysfunction is a process which contributes to disturbed
neural activity, particularly in the autonomic nervous system, is
it not reasonable to look to its relationship to the genesis of
diseases of vascular origin?

ILLUSTRATIVE CLINICAL EXPERIENCE

The following are some clinical examples of diagnostic, prognostic, and therapeutic experience which are similar to those of
others engaged in the practice of manual medicine. These conditions
have been chosen because they are more difficult to explain concep-
tually than those conditions of the musculoskeletal system which
are related to the finding of somatic dysfunction. They raise
interesting clinical research questions.

1. Acute and Chronic Coronary Artery Disease

The finding of restricted extension (backward bending), left
side bending, and right rotation of the upper thoracic spine has
been described by several authors (Burchett, 1976; Frymann, 1949;
Koch, 1957, 1961; Patriquin, 1957; Wilson, 1947, 1956) and corrobo-
rated in my clinical experience. The paravertebral tissues in the

upper thoracic spine from T1 to T5 (Rychlikova, 1975) usually show
some of the tissue texture abnormalities described above. The level
of acuteness or chronicity of the tissue texture changes is a valuable prognostic sign. In my experience, the response of the tissue
texture findings while under therapy, either improvement or continued aggravation, is as reliable a predictor of the patient's
outcome as are serial electrocardiographic or serum enzyme changes.
Appropriate manipulative therapy to the involved segments has
assisted in pain control and management of arrhythmias of the patient. A number of research questions can be raised from these
clinical observations (Holmes & Creamer, 1960). What are the neural
mechanisms available that explain the relationship of the somatic
dysfunction of the thoracic spine and the heart? Can the finding of
somatic dysfunction of this typical pattern in asymptomatic patients
be statistically significant as a potential risk factor in coronary
artery disease? Does appropriate therapy to the somatic dysfunction
alter the mortality and morbidity of patients with acute myocardial
infarction?

2.   Acute Chest Pain, Diagnosis Undetermined

One of the enigmas with which the clinician deals is the patient with acute chest pain (Stiles, 1977). The differential between acute cardiac or pulmonary pathology, and pain involving the
chest wall, is one with which every experienced clinician has dealt.
One finding that has been of assistance to the author in making this
difficult differential diagnosis has been the severity of tissue
texture changes of the upper- and mid-thoracic spine and the localization on one side or the other. If the condition is localized and
more severe on the left side, acute pathology involving the heart
is given higher consideration. If the finding is more acute on the
right side or symmetrical, pulmonary or aortic pathology has been
found to be more likely. Again the mechanisms for explanations are
obscure, but are worthy of additional clinical research.

3.   Peptic Ulcer Disease

Almost without exception, patients with peptic ulcer disease,
of either the stomach or the postpyloric cap, have had somatic dysfunction in the mid-thoracic spine at T5, T6, and occasionally T7
(Magoun, 1962), with the most usual finding being a single vertebral
segmental restriction of flexion (forward bending), right side bending, and right rotation. This finding in patients with upper abdominal distress, even in the absence of x-ray evidence of peptic ulcer,
raises a high index of suspicion of ulcer pathology in the stomach
or postpyloric cap and duodenum. The acuteness of the findings,
of both motion restriction and tissue texture abnormality, appears

correlate well with the acuteness of the visceral pathology. The
therapeutic response of the ulcer pathology also appears to reflect
itself in positive or negative response in the motion restriction
and tissue texture abnormalities of the involved vertebral segments.
Patients who have undergone subtotal gastrectomy with removal of the
ulcerated portion of the stomach, and who periodically have upper
abdominal distress, will manifest correlative acute changes of the
T5 to T7 area of the thoracic spine. What are the neural mechanisms operative between the T5 to T7 area of the spine and the
stomach, postpyloric cap, and duodenum? Does somatic dysfunction
of T5 to T7 increase or decrease the autonomic nervous system activity to the stomach, postpyloric cap, and duodenum? Is there a
long-term effect mediated through nonimpulse transmission of trophic
substances?

4. Gallbladder and Biliary Tract Disease

The findings of somatic dysfunction in the lower thoracic
spine from T6 to T10, and the attached lower right ribs, are common
in patients with gallbladder disease (Conley, 1944). The possibility
of relationship of the somatic changes to autonomic nervous system
outflow to the viscera can be postulated, but needs much further
substantiation by clinical research. A not infrequent occurrence
in patients following cholecystectomy is the return of flatulence,
fatty food intolerance, and various forms of dyspepsia. These
patients, with the so-called postcholecystectomy syndrome, frequently exhibit acute exacerbation of the somatic dysfunction findings in the lower thoracic spine and associated right lower ribs.
A diseased gallbladder has been removed, but the disease continues
within the patient. Manipulative therapy directed toward the somatic
dysfunction is frequently of great value in management of these patients. What is the nature of the neural mechanism interrelating
the somatic structure, the spinal cord, the liver, the residual
ductal structures in this process? Is this a phenomenon of spinal
reflex habituation (Patterson, 1976), and sensitization, as
postulated by some?

5. Colon Disease

Patients presenting with functional disturbances of the colon
frequently appear in clinical practice. The symptoms are variably
described as "irritable bowel syndrome", "colitis", and "functional
bowel syndrome". A frequent physical finding in these patients is
nonspecific somatic dysfunction of the mid- and lower-thoracic spine
and the upper-lumbar spine (Alexander, 1950). Management of these
patients is frequently assisted by appropriate manipulative therapy
to the involved areas of somatic dysfunction (English, 1976). It

can be postulated that there is a relationship of the somatic
changes to the autonomic nervous system outflow to the viscera
through the superior, middle, and inferior mesenteric ganglia. The
diagnostic and therapeutic implications of this clinically observed
phenomenon would be another fruitful area of clinical research.

DISCUSSION AND CONCLUSIONS

This presentation has been developed to focus upon a conceptual
framework for the discussion of neurobiologic mechanisms and manipulative therapy. It is the author's opinion that we must focus on a
more global look at the mechanisms underlying structural diagnosis
and manipulative therapy. Attention needs to be directed, not only
to complaints referrable to the musculoskeletal system, and to
specific disease entities, but rather to the role of abnormalities
of the musculoskeletal system affecting the total response of the
human organism in the maintenance of health and the genesis of
disease. The musculoskeletal system must be viewed as a participant in the response of the total body to the stresses placed upon
it by the internal and external environment. Attention has been
directed towards the diagnostic, prognostic and therapeutic implications of the musculoskeletal system in this ongoing process. It
appears imperative that appropriate anatomical and physiological
terminology be utilized in the discussion of the abnormalities of
the musculoskeletal system described in this presentation as somatic
dysfunction. An attempt has been made to provide illustrative cases
which focus on the role of somatic dysfunction of the musculoskeletal
system in conditions of acute health care of the "nonstructural"
type. Simplistic questions concerning the possible neural mechanisms present in these conditions have been raised. No attempt has
been made to postulate the answers. However, the clinical experience described indicates the vast number of research questions
calling for further study.

REFERENCES

ALEXANDER, D. D. The role of the osteopathic lesion in functional
        and organic gastrointestinal pathology. *J. Am. Osteop. Assoc.*
        50:25-27, 1950.

BUERGER, A. A., and J. S. Tobis. *Approaches to the Validation of
        Manipulation Therapy.* Springfield: Charles C. Thomas, 1977.

BURCHETT, G. D. Somatic manifestations of ischemic heart disease.
        Osteop. Ann. 4:373-375, 1976.

CONLEY, G. J. The role of the spinal joint lesion in gall bladder
        disease. *J. Am. Osteop. Assoc.* 44:121-123, 1944.

CYRIA, J., and E. H. SCHIOTZ. *Manipulation Past and Present.* London: William Heineman Ltd., 1975.

ENGLISH, W. The somatic component of colon disease. *Osteop. Ann.* 4:150-157, 1976.

FRYMANN, V. M. The role of the osteopathic lesion in the production of cardiac pathology. *J. Am. Osteop. Assoc.* 48:246-248, 1949.

GOLDSTEIN, M., editor. *The Research Status of Spinal Manipulative Therapy.* NINCDS Monograph No. 15, 1975.

HIX, E. L. Reflex viscero-somatic reference phenomena. *Osteop. Ann.* 4:496-503, 1976.

HOAG, J. M., W. V. COLE, and S. G. BRADFORD, editors. *Osteopathic Medicine.* New York: McGraw-Hill, 1969.

HOLMES, J. A., and G. F. CREAMER. Clinical research combining medical and special osteopathic therapy for angina pectoris and coronary heart disease. *Yearbook Acad. Appl. Osteop.,* 1960, pp. 63-66.

JUDOVITCH, B., and W. BATES. *Segmental Neuralgia in Painful Syndromes.* Philadelphia: F. A. Davis, 1946.

KOCH, R. S. A somatic component in heart disease. *J. Am. Osteop. Assoc.* 60:735-740, 1961.

KOCH, R. S. The spinal component in heart disease. *Yearbook Acad. Appl. Osteop.,* 1957, pp. 67-70.

KOS, J., and J. WOLF. Die "Menisci" der Zwischenwirbelgelenkes und ihre Mögliche Rolle bei Wirbeblockierung. *Man. Med.* 10:195-214, 1972.

MAGOUN, H. I. Gastroduodenal ulcers from the osteopathic viewpoint. *Yearbook Acad. Appl. Osteop.,* 1962, pp. 117-120.

NEMEROF, H. Medical acupuncture, 1974. *Osteop. Ann.* 2:18-26, 1974.

NORTHUP, G. W. *Osteopathic Medicine: An American Reformation.* Chicago: American Osteopathic Association, 1966.

OWENS, C. *An Endocrine Interpretation of Chapman's Reflexes.* Chattanooga, Tenn.: Chattanooga Printing & Engraving Co. (date unknown)

PATRIQUIN, D. A. Osteopathic management of coronary disease. *Yearbook Acad. Appl. Osteop.*, 1957, pp. 75-80.

PATTERSON, M. M. The reflex connection: History of a middleman. *Osteop. Ann.* 4:358-367, 1976.

POINTON, R. A possible cause of acute osteopathic lesions. *Brit. Osteop. J.* 8:10-19, 1976.

POTTENGER, F. M. *Symptoms of Visceral Disease.* St. Louis: C. V. Mosby, 1930.

RUMNEY, I. The relevance of somatic dysfunction. *J. Am. Osteop. Assoc.* 74:723-725, 1975.

RYCHLIKOVA, E. Reflex changes and vertebrogenic disorders in ischemic heart disease (IHD) - Their importance in therapy. *Rehabilitacia* 8:109-114, 1975.

SPERANSKY, A. D. *A Basis for the Theory of Medicine.* New York: International, 1944.

STILES, E. G. Osteopathic approach to the patient with chest pain. *Osteop. Med.* 2:93-95, 1977.

STILL, A. T. *Philosophy of Osteopathy.* Kirksville, MO: A. T. Still, 1899.

THOMAS, P. E. The role of the autonomic nervous system in arteriosclerosis. *Osteop. Ann.* 2:12-20, 1974.

TRAVELL, J., and S. RINZLER. The myofascial genesis of pain. *Postgrad. Med.* 2:425-434, 1952.

WALTON, F. C. Palpation and motion testing in acute and chronic disease. *Osteop. Med.* 2:81-86, 1977.

WILSON, P. T. Angina pectoris. *Yearbook Acad. Appl. Osteop.*, 1947, pp. 176-177.

WILSON, P. T. Osteopathic cardiology. *Yearbook Acad. Appl. Osteop.*, 1956, pp. 27-32.

THE CLINICAL BASIS FOR DISCUSSION OF MECHANISMS

OF MANIPULATIVE THERAPY

Scott Haldeman

Department of Neurology

University of California, Irvine

"There is no scientific basis for manipulative therapy," has been the most commonly stated and the most damaging criticism levied against practitioners of manipulation (Crelin, 1973; Farfan, 1973). Many noted physicians and scientists, after reviewing the available literature and research, have come to the conclusion that "there is no justification for the use of manipulative therapy" (Nachemson, 1975; Pearce & Moll, 1967; Sham, 1974). On the other hand, practitioners of manipulation feel that their clinical results are indisputable (Gitelman, 1975; Maitland, 1973; Mennell, 1960), and that there is ample experimental evidence to support their theories on how manipulation works (Cyriax, 1975; Homewood, 1963; Janse, Houser & Wells, 1947; Maigne, 1972). One reason for this dichotomy of opinion is the fact that certain basic criteria requisite for the evaluation of the rationale for any treatment have been frequently neglected.

Most of the papers which are to be presented at this conference are on research in the field of neurobiology which was conducted with no aim of investigating the mechanisms of action of manipulative therapy. Nonetheless, such research is widely quoted as a rationale for this approach to patient care. In order to place this research into perspective in the overall evaluation of the scientific basis for manipulative therapy, it would perhaps be of value to restate the basic criteria on which a proposed neurobiological mechanism of manipulative therapy will be judged.

CRITERION I: A specific manipulative procedure must be demonstrated to have consistent clinical results under controlled conditions in the treatment of a specific pathological process, organ dysfunction or symptom complex.

CRITERION II: The specific manipulative procedure must be demonstrated to have a specific effect on the musculoskeletal system to which it is applied.

CRITERION III: The musculoskeletal effect caused by the manipulation must be shown to have a specific influence on the nervous system.

CRITERION IV: This influence on the nervous system must be demonstrated to have a beneficial influence on the abnormal function of an organ, tissue pathology or symptom complex under study.

Figure 1 illustrates the four areas of research which must be considered in order to satisfy these criteria for a proposed neurobiological mechanism of manipulative therapy. The remainder of this paper will discuss these criteria. The greatest emphasis will be placed on a review of the type of clinical research which has been conducted to satisfy Criteria I and II. This may help to set the stage for the more intense discussion, later in the conference, of the neurobiological research on which Criteria III and IV rest.

CRITERION I - THE EFFECT OF MANIPULATIVE THERAPY ON SPECIFIC SYMPTOM COMPLEXES, ORGAN DYSFUNCTION AND TISSUE PATHOLOGY

If one searches the literature and includes a review of pamphlets, lay books and advertisements of practitioners of manipulative therapy, it is possible to find someone, somewhere, who has made a claim of successful treatment through manipulation of almost every ailment which afflicts man. It is impossible at this time to discuss every claim made by practitioners of manipulation. A number of these claims border on the absurd and have served to discredit the field as a whole. There are, however, several conditions for which manipulative therapy is currently being prescribed by licensed practitioners and which continue to be described in textbooks on manipulation and in professional journals. They can be broken down into groups based on the neurobiological mechanisms through which manipulation supposedly works in each case. To save time, only one or two examples from each of these groups will be discussed. In each case the example which has been subjected to the greatest amount of clinical research has been chosen.

1. The Somatic Pain Syndromes

By far the greatest number of manipulations given today are for the treatment of somatic pain, specifically back and neck pain (Breen, 1977; Vear, 1972). This is also the area of clinical research which has received the most attention and many practitioners

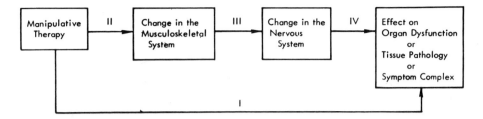

Figure 1.   The four areas of research required to confirm a proposed neurobiological mechanism of action of manipulative therapy.

of manipulative therapy limit their practice exclusively to the management of pain of musculoskeletal origin (Cyriax, 1975; Maitland, 1973).

Despite this intense interest and wide usage, the documented evidence that spinal manipulation is of benefit in low back pain is not great.   There have been a number of reports in the literature on the results of uncontrolled trials of patients with back pain undergoing manipulative therapy.   As can be seen from Table 1, all observers demonstrate a high percentage of patients with back pain who improve while under this form of therapy.   Nachemson (1975) and others, however, have repeatedly pointed out that back pain is to a large extent a self-limiting disorder, and that one can expect 70 to 80% of such patients to improve no matter what type of treatment is offered.   It is for this reason that the results have served to convince few physicians that manipulation deserves a major role in the treatment of patients with low back pain.   The results of the two or three research programs in which manipulation has been compared to other forms of treatment for low back pain have not helped to clear up the controversy.   Coyer and Curwen (1955) compared the effectiveness of spinal manipulation to bed rest and analgesia in 152 patients suffering from acute back pain.   They found that 50% of those patients who underwent manipulation were symptom-free within one week compared to 27% in the non-manipulated group.   At three weeks 87% of the manipulated group were symptom-free compared to 60% of the non-manipulated group.   This study has been criticized on the basis that statistical analysis was not carried out to determine the significance of these results (Nachemson, 1975).   Doran and Newell (1975) compared manipulation to treatment with physiotherapy, corsets and analgesia.   They found a slightly higher number of patients improved under manipulation after three weeks as compared with other therapeutic approaches.   However, this difference was not statistically significant and disappeared after six weeks of treatment.   Glover and co-workers (1974, 1977) have completed the

Table 1. Reports from uncontrolled trials of manipulation in low
back pain.

Number of patients in trial	Improved	Worse	Author
68	(50) 74%	0	Henderson (1952)
72	80%	0	Mensor (1955)
133	71%	0	Mensor (1955)
39	(25) 64%		Bechgaard (1966)
378	(339) 90%		Fisk (1971)
92	(65) 71%	(10) 11%	Doran & Newell (1975)
26	(24) 94%	0	Bosshard (1961)
39	(20) 51%	0	Chrisman et al. (1964)
100	85%		Hutton (1967)*
500	63%	0	Warr et al. (1972)

*Manipulation and epidural injections.

only single blind controlled study in this field. They compared the
results of a single rotatory spinal manipulation with detuned ultrasound which acted as a placebo. They were able to show significant
immediate improvement following manipulation in patients who had
suffered from back pain for less than seven days, but this significance disappeared by the next day and could not be demonstrated in
patients with more chronic back pain. The results of these, and
similar research projects which show widely varying results, have
brought up the question of how great a part training, experience
and technical skill in manipulation may play in the results one
could expect from manipulation (Haldeman, 1977). It is obvious
that a great deal of research has yet to be carried out before this
question is answered. Hopefully, blind controlled studies such as
those currently being undertaken at the University of Toronto (Drum
& Godfrey, 1976) and the University of California at Irvine (Buerger,
1976) will help to throw some light on this subject.

In most textbooks and articles on manipulative therapy, as
much emphasis is placed on the management of pain originating from
the dorsal and cervical spine (Cyriax, 1975; Maigne, 1972; Maitland,
1973; Mennell, 1960) as on the lumbar spine. However, the amount
of clinical reporting on the results of manipulation in these conditions is considerably less than for low back pain, and there are
no reports where spinal manipulation is compared to other treatment

procedures, or to no treatment at all. A number of clinicians
recommend manipulation for cervical pain syndrome and radiculitis
in conjunction with other conservative therapies, such as exercise
or traction (Mettier & Capp, 1941; Robertson, 1968). Boake (1972)
has expressed the opinion that 70% of his patients with cervical
headaches respond to manipulation and Bechgaard (1966), in a letter
to the editor of the *British Medical Journal*, stated that 78% of
23 patients with posttraumatic headache and 64% of 309 patients
with cervical problems responded dramatically to manipulative
therapy.

These opinions and statistics are difficult to interpret since
a large percentage of these patients are likely to recover spontaneously. It will require prospective controlled and comparative
trials to determine the value of manipulation in these syndromes.
Unfortunately such trials do not appear to be forthcoming at this
time.

2. Nerve Compression Syndromes

One of the most commonly debated mechanisms of action of
spinal manipulation is the relief of nerve compression (Crelin,
1973; Gayral & Neuwirth, 1954; Janse, Houser & Wells, 1947; Palmer,
1910). It could be expected therefore that clinical reporting on
the effect of manipulation on known compression syndromes such as
those found in the cervical and lumbar spine is widespread. This
in fact is not the case. Most studies on the effect of manipulation in cervical and lumbar pain have specifically screened out
those patients with neurological signs of root compression (Doran
& Newell, 1975; Glover, Morris & Khosla, 1974, 1977). Admittedly,
many of these studies did include patients with radicular pain
which may have been due to nerve root compression. In the patients
with back pain and sciatica described by Bosshard (1961) there were
at least six with absent reflexes or sensory deficit in the legs.
Unfortunately, he does not state whether these signs improved along
with the relief of pain symptoms following manipulative therapy.

Fisk (1975) has demonstrated that there is an improvement in
the straight leg raising test in patients with low back pain and
this has been confirmed by the team of investigators at the University of California-Irvine College of Medicine in a single blind
trial (1977). In the series quoted by Fisk none of the patients
with signs of frank disc herniation and neurological deficit showed
any improvement. For this and other reasons (Fisk, 1975; King,
1977; Manipulation Project, 1977), there is a growing feeling that
sciatic pain and limited straight leg raising may not be an indi-
cator of root compression, but instead may be due to muscle spasm
in paraspinal muscles or referred pain from the posterior joints

or paraspinal ligaments. It is therefore probably not valid to
equate relief of radicular pain with reduction in nerve compression.
This assumption is supported by the observation that the injection
of hypertonic saline into paraspinal muscles can mimic most of the
radicular pain syndromes (Feinstein et al., 1954). It remains to
be demonstrated clinically that manipulation has any effect on
nerve compression syndromes at the spinal level.

3. Functional Disorders of Visceral Organs

Perhaps the most commonly quoted neurobiological theory for
manipulative therapy in modern times is the concept of "structure-
governs-function", "the facilitated reflex", or "abnormal somatovisceral reflexes" (Homewood, 1963; Korr, 1976). Under these
varying headings it is assumed that manipulation of the musculoskeletal system will change the sensory feedback to the central
nervous system, alter the "central excitatory state" in the cord
and cause abnormal discharges in the sympathetic nervous system.
This, in turn, is assumed to cause changes in function in those
visceral organs under sympathetic influence.

Once again the clinical evidence that manipulation may influence internal organ function is sketchy and based primarily on
anecdotal reporting or opinion originating from individual experience together with the occasional uncontrolled trial. The most
widely discussed systems which are assumed to be influenced by
manipulation are the respiratory and cardiovascular systems.

There are a number of reports in the literature where manipulative therapy is assumed to be beneficial to patients with respiratory diseases. In a 1975 Forum of the *Journal of the American
Osteopathic Association*, 60   practicing osteopaths described
their management of hayfever (Forum, 1975). Of these, 28 stated
that manipulation of the cervical and dorsal spine or facial bones
was of value in the treatment of hayfever. A letter in the *Medical
Journal of Australia* by Swan (1968) presented a patient who had
suffered from asthma and bronchitis for over two years. This patient apparently became asymptomatic after two cervical manipulations. Miller (1975) claimed that 92% of 23 patients with chronic
obstructive pulmonary disease described subjective improvement of
their respiratory symptoms after spinal manipulative therapy. In
order to determine which respiratory factors were influenced by
manipulative therapy, he examined these patients from a neuromuscular and pulmonary point of view and compared the results with
21 controls. He found that patients with C.O.P.D. had an increased
incidence of neuromuscular findings such as hypermobility, costovertebral dysfunction and alteration of side bending and rotation
of the spine. He then compared blood gases and basic pulmonary

function between a control group who did not receive any manipulative therapy and those who underwent manipulation. He was unable to find any statistical difference in the parameters measured between the two groups, despite the subjective feeling of improvement experienced by these patients. This inability to document significant change in organ function following manipulative therapy suggests that the subjective reports of improved symptoms may be psychological in origin.

A single case report by Howell and Kappler (1973) on a patient with C.O.P.D. and cor pulmonale who was treated with osteopathic manipulation and diuretics resulted in similar conclusions. The patient improved symptomatically over 18 months while his pulmonary function continued to decline. The only report where manipulation was assumed to influence lung function was by Howell et al. (1975) who followed 17 patients with C.O.P.D. who were being treated with manipulation combined with conventional medical management including bronchodilators, expectorants and corticosteroids. They demonstrated a significant improvement in a number of lung functions after nine months of treatment and commented that thoracic mobility improved following manipulation. However, the authors admit that in the absence of blinded controls, it was impossible to say how much of this improvement was due to manipulative therapy and how much was due to the drug therapy.

Spinal manipulative therapy has been advocated in the management of such cardiovascular disorders as congestive heart failure (Howell & Kappler, 1973), coronary artery disease (Rogers & Rogers, 1976) and hypertension (Celander, Koenig & Celander, 1968; Hood, 1974). These claims have encouraged a number of researchers to investigate the effects of spinal manipulative therapy on a few simple parameters of cardiovascular function. The most widely utilized measurement has been blood pressure (Clymer, Levin & Sculthorpe, 1972; Fichera & Celander, 1969; Norris, 1964; Tran & Kirby, 1977). Norris (1964) reported on the effects of the manipulation on the blood pressure of 317 students and used 118 students as controls. He found that 2 h after the manipulation, 48% of those students with pressures above 125 mmHg showed a lowering of this pressure by greater than 5 mmHg compared to only 26% of the nonmanipulated group. On the other hand, 30% of the students with blood pressure below 115 mmHg showed an increase in blood pressure 2 h after manipulation compared to 0% in the nonmanipulated group. He came to the conclusion that the effect of the manipulation was to normalize blood pressure. Tran and Kirby (1977) did similar blood pressure recordings in 20 students with similar results, but did not use controls. The interesting point of this report is that actual blood pressures are listed rather than simple statistics. From these tables, the results of the manipulation appear far less convincing. Fichera and Celander (1969) give one of the few reports

on the effect of manipulation on the blood pressure of patients who
are clearly hypertensive. They found that 73% of these patients
showed a drop in systolic blood pressure of greater than 3 mmHg and
41% showed a similar drop in diastolic blood pressure 30 min after
manipulation of the cervical and dorsal paraspinal muscles.

There are many obvious criticisms of this type of research
which make any conclusion no more than speculation. Firstly, there
was no effort to blind the examiners in any of these trials and
since many of the readings were taken by students or faculty with
a specific interest in manipulative therapy, it is impossible to
rule out an unintentional bias of 3 to 5 mmHg in the measurement
of blood pressure. Secondly, the effects noted were generally quite
small and all recordings were taken either 30 min or 2 h after
manipulation. It is impossible to say whether these effects, if
they exist, would be likely to last for any prolonged period of
time, and therefore be of any therapeutic value. As in other fields
where manipulation is said to be effective, there are isolated case
reports of patients with hypertension which have improved dramatically for prolonged periods following manipulative therapy (Blood,
1964). However, these reports cannot serve any purpose beyond
whetting the appetite for properly controlled research.

Similar reports and trials have suggested that manipulation may
alter heart rate (Fichera & Celander, 1969), pulsatile blood volume
(Busch, Danelius & Drost, 1974; Clymer, Levin & Sculthorpe, 1972),
fibrinolytic activity (Celander, Koenig & Celander, 1968; Fichera
& Celander, 1969), and hematocrit (Fichera & Celander, 1969). These
results are subject to the same type of criticisms mentioned above
for blood pressure. As most of the authors of these papers have
stated, these results should be used as a basis for further, more
intensive, investigation rather than as a justification for the
treatment of patients with disorders of these functions by manipulative therapy. The same statement can be made for most of the
visceral organ dysfunctions which are said to respond to manipulative
therapy.

4. The Posterior Cervical Syndrome

Maigne, who has published one of the most widely read textbooks on manipulative therapy (1972), devotes an entire chapter to
the manipulative management of the posterior cervical syndrome of
Barré and Lieou. This syndrome usually occurs following neck trauma
and includes cervical pain, headaches, vertigo, positional nystagmus,
tinnitis, hoarseness, vasomotor disturbances and occasionally
psychic disturbances. These symptoms are generally considered to
be due to vertebrobasilar insufficiency (Lindsay & Hemenway, 1956;
Tissington-Tatlow & Bammer, 1957). However, there have been

suggestions that many such symptoms may be due to irritation of the
sympathetic nervous system (Barré, 1926; Gayral & Neuwirth, 1954).
Maigne (1972) claims that these symptoms respond extremely well to
manipulative therapy and provides three case reports with nystagmographs from patients before and after manipulative therapy. These
nystagmographs are reported to be markedly abnormal prior to the
manipulation and to improve along with symptomatology following
manipulation. Lewit (1961) agrees with this point of view and has
presented the results of 124 cases with either posterior cervical
syndrome, Meniere's disease or Barré-Lieou syndrome. He states that
79% of the cases with Meniere's disease and 90% of the cases with
Barré-Lieou syndrome had either excellent results or improved significantly after treatment with cervical traction and manipulation.

    Despite this enthusiasm for the use of manipulation in these
syndromes by practitioners of manipulation in Europe, North American
clinicians have avoided many of these cases. The major reason is the
fact that the most devastating side effects which have occurred following manipulative therapy have been directly related to interruption of the vertebrobasilar blood supply to the brainstem (Lyness &
Wagman, 1974; Pratt-Thomas & Berger, 1947). For this reason, most
practitioners of manipulation in North America, while treating
cervical pain syndromes and suboccipital headaches, consider any
symptoms suggesting of compromised blood supply to the brainstem, a
contraindication to cervical manipulation. There is, however, some
recent literature to suggest that this approach may be too cautious.
Chrisman and Gervais (1962) followed 62 patients diagnosed as having
the posterior cervical syndrome. These patients were treated with
conventional orthopedic protocols of cervical collars, ultrasound,
traction and exercises. They found that 57 of these patients improved significantly following such treatment. Figar, Krausova
and Lewit (1967) conducted plethysmographic studies in the hands
of 30 patients with cervical spine problems and found abnormalities
or asymmetric readings in 27 of them. These abnormalities improved
in 18 patients simultaneously with improved symptoms, following
cervical spine manipulation. These reports suggest that there may
well be some degree of sympathetic disturbance which accompanies
cervical spine injuries. It may be necessary for clinicians in
North America to re-evaluate their approach to this problem provided that some accurate method of ruling out a compromised vertebral artery can be worked out.

                5. Psycho-Somato-Psychic Syndromes

    The close interaction between various psychological disturb-
ances and somatic symptoms such as neck and back pain, muscle spasm,
trigger areas, etc., has been repeatedly noted (Meltzer, 1973;
Rimon, Stenback & Huckman, 1966; Sternbach et al., 1973). The most

widely held opinion is that these problems originate with psychological disturbance and the somatic manifestations are secondary. There are, however, practitioners of manipulation who believe that somatic lesions may aggravate existing psychological illnesses (Bradford, 1965; Dunn, 1950; Quigley, 1973). These practitioners recommend manipulative therapy as part of the overall treatment of the mentally ill patient.

This is one of the most difficult areas in which to conduct clinical trials and an almost impossible field in which to evaluate published clinical results. Quigley (1973) has reported on 72 psychotic patients who received manipulation within a mental health sanitorium. He states that 70% of the schizophrenic patients and 33% of the patients diagnosed as having affective disorders and so-called "brain syndromes" were released and socially restored following treatment. Hartzman and Schwartz (1973) conducted a survey by means of a questionnaire mailed to practitioners of manipulation to determine the effectiveness of manipulation in mentally ill patients. The answers they received suggested that 85% of patients with a wide variety of ill-defined psychological problems treated by these practitioners were either "cured" or much improved following manipulation. Both these reports leave much to be desired from a research point of view and by the authors' own admission do not help to shed any light on the problem. Interpretation of this type of result is further complicated by the fact that those practitioners of manipulation who make it a point to treat patients with mental illnesses have a specific interest in such patients and have often become quite skilled in psychological counseling. This factor, rather than any specific effect of manipulative therapy, may explain the reported improvement noted in patients in their care.

Psychodynamics, however, are of importance in any discussions of the mechanism of action of manipulative therapy. Many of the conditions for which manipulative therapy is prescribed, including back pain, neck pain, headaches, hypertension, asthma, etc., have strong psychological components. If it could be demonstrated that manipulative therapy was of value in reducing stress, tension or any other psychological factor important in the genesis of these ailments, then the use of manipulative therapy could be justified on this basis alone. Any other neurobiological mechanism of action which might be demonstrated to exist would be an added bonus.

CRITERION II - THE DIRECT EFFECT OF MANIPULATIVE THERAPY
ON THE MUSCULOSKELETAL SYSTEM

Each professional group which practices manipulative therapy, many of the numerous schools of thought within these professions, and most authors on the technique or principles of manipulation

Table 2.   A few of the proposed mechanisms of action of manipulative therapy with one author who has supported each theory.

	Theory	Author
1.	Restore vertebrae to normal position	Galen (1958)
2.	Straighten the spine	Pare (1958)
3.	Relieve interference with blood flow	Still (1899)
4.	Relieve nerve compression	Palmer (1910)
5.	Relieve irritation of sympathetic chain	Kunert (1965)
6.	Mobilize fixated vertebral units	Gillet (1968)
7.	Shift of a fragment of inter-vertebral disc	Cyriax (1975)
8.	Mobilize posterior joints	Mennell (1960)
9.	Remove interference with cerebro-spinal fluid circulation	De Jarnette (1967)
10.	Stretch contracted muscles causing relaxation	Perl (1975)
11.	Correct abnormal somatovisceral reflexes	Homewood (1963)
12.	Remove "irritable" spinal lesions	Korr (1976)
13.	Stretching or tearing of adhesions around the nerve root	Chrisman et al. (1964)
14.	Reduce distortion of the annulae	Farfan (1973)

have a separate and distinct concept or opinion on what the primary effect of manipulation is. These concepts are often rigidly adhered to and on occasion great effort is made by the originators of one idea to ridicule or discredit the theories of colleagues who also practice manipulative therapy. The unfortunate part of this ongoing argument is that very little objective research has been done to verify any of these theories.

Table 2 lists a few of the more commonly proposed mechanisms of manipulative therapy with at least one author who has supported each theory. Two points become very clear when one reviews these theories: (a) many of the theories are vague and nonspecific; and (b) for almost every proposed mechanism of spinal dysfunction someone has suggested that manipulation will correct it.

There are a few points which can be stated about the actual
process of delivering a spinal manipulation.

(1) The first maneuver in any manipulation is the laying on
of hands. This process has only one basic effect and that is the
distortion of cutaneous and subcutaneous tissues. It has been well
demonstrated that this in turn will cause stimulation of a variety
of skin receptors which in turn send impulses to the central nervous
system (Adrian, 1926; Perl & Whitlock, 1961). This in turn may have
psychological effects (Dunn, 1950), influence pain from deeper
structures (Melzack & Wall, 1965) or bring about reflex changes in
somatic or sympathetic effectors (Norman & Whitman, 1973; Sato &
Schmidt, 1973). The discussion of these changes falls under
Criteria III and IV.

(2) The second maneuver in a manipulation is the movement of a
joint. This, once again, has been demonstrated to cause direct
stimulation of a number of receptors in tissues surrounding the
joint (Gardner, 1950). The question which must be asked is whether
there is an additional permanent change in the function of the joint.
It has been suggested that the spinal manipulation will correct abnormal fixation or joint locking and presumably thereby increase
the range of motion (Gillet & Liekens, 1968; Mennell, 1960). The
number of experiments which have been conducted to demonstrate any
change in joint mobility following manipulative therapy are again
very sparse. Hviid (1971) recorded the rotational mobility before
and after cervical manipulation on 92 patients. He found that
91.3% of the patients showed some increased rotation of the head
following manipulation. These increases averaged 14.1 degrees or
9% of the premanipulative range of motion. Other changes which have
been thought to occur as a result of moving a joint, such as increasing the size of the intervertebral foramen or decreasing the curva-
ture in scolioses, have yet to be investigated.

(3) Reduction in the amount of paraspinal muscle spasm has
been considered a major part of the initial effect of the spinal
manipulation. England and Deibert (1972) and Grice (1974) have attempted to record change in paraspinal muscle spasm following manipulative therapy by means of the electromyograph. They were able
to record spontaneous localized motor unit activity in the area of
palpable paraspinal muscle rigidity in the majority of patients
tested. Following active mobilization of the spinal segments adjacent to the electrode needles there was an immediate increase in
the interference pattern and cessation of spontaneous potentials in
these muscles. It would be nice to see these experiments repeated
using larger numbers of patients and better controls as well as
some attempt at statistical analysis.

(4) Cyriax (1975) and Maigne (1972) place great emphasis on the theory that the primary goal of spinal manipulation is to reduce disc protrusions. The paper which is most often quoted to support this thesis is a preliminary communication by Matthews and Yates (1969). This paper consists of two case reports of patients with acute low back pain in whom minor concavities in the area of the lumbar discs were demonstrated on x-rays following epidural injection of contrast medium. These concavities were noted to disappear or decrease in size following spinal manipulation. In contradiction to this report, Chrisman et al. (1964) failed to demonstrate any reduction in the size of disc protrusions following manipulation in 26 patients with myelographic abnormalities. In this study, patients with low back pain and normal myelograms were more responsive to manipulative therapy than those patients with documented disc protusions. Siehl et al. (1971) came to similar conclusions using electromyography to diagnose disc protrusions. They felt that there is a greater chance of improvement following manipulation in patients with low back pain and normal electromyograms, and that any improvement noted is more likely to be long lasting in the former group compared to patients with positive electromyographic evidence of disc protrusion. It is possible that manipulation affects only small disc protrusions, but this remains to be demonstrated in an adequate manner.

CRITERION III - THE EFFECT ON THE NERVOUS SYSTEM AS A RESULT OF MUSCULOSKELETAL CHANGES BROUGHT ON BY THE MANIPULATION

As has been mentioned before, a number of neurophysiological theories have been proposed to explain the results of manipulative therapy. Many of the proponents of these theories start with the evidence which supports Criteria III and IV of the schema on which this paper was based. The temptation of starting and often ending at this level of discussion is evident in other papers in this volume. Since these theories incorporate one or more established neurophysiological processes, there is a great deal of research available which describes these processes and their relationship to other physiological functions. It has been very tempting in the past to quote basic-science research on a neurophysiological process in an attempt to give the appearance of scientific respectability to a specific theory of manipulation.

The major neurophysiological processes which are invoked to satisfy Criterion III are (1) pain physiology, (2) nerve compression and axoplasmic flow, and (3) basic reflex physiology. As these processes are to be discussed in depth in other papers, this discussion will be limited to a simple statement of how they are utilized by practitioners of manipulation.

Since the relief of pain is the prime goal of a great percentage of manipulations, research which has been done on pain
physiology has been the center of much of the discussion of the
mechanism of action of manipulative therapy and other forms of
treatment for back pain (Haldeman, 1975; Nachemson, 1975; Perl,
1975). In the attempt to understand what is happening in the spine
and paraspinal tissues of a patient with back pain, it has become
necessary to understand such physiological processes as the
nature of the chemical mediators of pain (Nachemson, 1969), the
innervation of muscles, joints, ligaments, etc. (King, 1977),
the central connections, inhibitory and excitatory neuronal interactions (Melzack & Wall, 1965; Perl, 1975), referred pain (Feinstein et al., 1954), psychological factors (Meltzer, 1973) and
descending inhibitory systems (Haldeman, 1975; Melzack & Wall,
1965). Since the exact nature of the lesion which produces back
pain is not known, any attempt to attribute the relief of this pain
following manipulative therapy to a specific mechanism of action
remains speculation.

Nerve compression is one of the oldest and most controversial
theories of manipulation. Much of the controversy has ranged
around the effect of compression on the conduction of neuronal impulses. More recently, axoplasmic and endoneurial flow along the
nerve, which may have a trophic influence on innervated structures,
has been demonstrated (Droz & LeBlond, 1962; Weiss, 1943). The fact
that this flow can be interrupted by constriction of the nerve
(Haldeman & Meyer, 1970; Weiss & Hiscoe, 1948) has caused increased
interest in nerve compression among practitioners of manipulative
therapy. Once again, however, it is necessary to keep in mind that
manipulation has not been demonstrated to relieve nerve compression.

The ability of manipulative therapy to influence reflex activity in the central nervous system holds perhaps the greatest
interest for those individuals who are trying to establish a role
for manipulative therapy which extends beyond the management of
pain syndromes. The suggestion is that sensory input to one part
of the nervous system can influence almost any function of the
nervous system (Homewood, 1963; Korr, 1976). Although many of these
reflex connections have been documented from somatic and visceral
nerve stimulation (Coote, Downman & Weber, 1969; Sato & Schmidt,
1973), the evidence that manipulation per se has these specific
reflex influences remains minimal.

CRITERION IV - THE EFFECT OF THE NEURONAL CHANGES BROUGHT
ABOUT BY MANIPULATIVE THERAPY ON THE ABNORMAL FUNCTION OF
AN ORGAN, TISSUE PATHOLOGY OR SYMPTOM COMPLEXES

Abuse of Criterion IV has led to some of the most blatantly
excessive claims for manipulative therapy. It is not uncommon to
note that when the nervous system has been implicated in a particular disease state, a practitioner will make the claim that manipulative therapy is likely to be of benefit in the management of
that disease. It is possible to find some experimental evidence
implicating the nervous system in the control of almost any body
function, including glucose metabolism (Nijima & Fukuda, 1973),
blood clotting (Ruxin, Bidder & Angle, 1972), and immunogenesis
(Gordienko, 1958), as well as in the genesis of such unlikely disease states as cystic fibrosis (Bolande & Towler, 1973) and cancer
(Stein-Werblowsky, 1974). Although these findings are of importance
in the understanding of physiology and the pathogenesis of disease,
it is an abuse of science to suggest that manipulative therapy is
of value in the treatment of cystic fibrosis, cancer, diabetes,
etc., based on isolated experiments alone. Criterion IV remains
an important part of the overall evaluation of the neurobiological
mechanism of manipulative therapy. However, in the absence of firm
evidence supporting the other three criteria, it forms the least
justification for offering manipulative therapy in a specific
disease state.

CONCLUSION

In this review of the clinical basis for discussing the neurobiological mechanisms of manipulative therapy, it is perhaps wise
to conclude on a cautious note. In the deliberations of this conference and in future research, neurobiologists must be careful
that, in the search for some clinical significance for their experimental research, they do not form elaborate theories for
clinical procedures which have not yet proved to be effective. At
the same time, clinicians who practice spinal manipulation must
avoid using the results of research in the neurosciences to justify
their therapeutic approach to patients in the absence of adequate
clinical research. It is essential that there be cooperation and
open discussion between clinicians and neurobiologists who may then
work together to determine whether a proposed neurobiological
mechanism of manipulation satisfies the criteria on which it will
be judged.

REFERENCES

ADRIAN, E. D., and Y. ZOTTERMAN. The impulses produced by sensory nerve endings. *J. Physiol.* 61:151-171, 1926.

BARRÉ, M. Sur un syndrome sympathique cervical posterieur et sa cause fréquente l'arthrite cervicale. *Rev. Neurol.* 33:1246-1248, 1926.

BECHGAARD, P. Late post-traumatic headache and manipulation. *Corres. Brit. Med. J.,* June 4:1419, 1966.

BLOOD, H. A. Manipulative management of hypertension. *Acad. Appl. Osteopath. Yearbook,* pp. 189-195, 1964.

BOAKE, H. K. Cervical headache. *Canadian Family Physician* May: 75-78, 1972.

BOLANDE, R. P., and W. F. TOWLER. Terminal autonomic nervous system in cystic fibrosis. *Arch. Pathol.* 95:172-181, 1973.

BOSSHARD, R. The treatment of acute lumbago and sciatica. *Ann. Swiss Chirop. Assoc.,* pp. 50-61, 1961.

BRADFORD, S. G. Role of osteopathic manipulative therapy in emotional disorders: A physiologic hypothesis. *J. Am. Osteop. Assoc.* 64:484-493, 1965.

BREEN, A. C. Chiropractors and the treatment of back pain. *Rheumatol. Rehabil.* 16:46-53, 1977.

BUERGER, A. A. Clinical trials of manipulation therapy. In: *Approaches to the Validation of Manipulation Therapy,* edited by A. A. Buerger and J. S. Tobis. Springfield, Ill.: Charles C. Thomas, 1976, pp. 315-321.

BUSCH, B. W., B. D. DANELIUS, and S. F. DROST. Cardiovascular changes after chiropractic. *Am. Chiropractic Assoc. J.* 8: s-33-38, 1974.

CELANDER, E., A. J. KOENIG, and D. R. CELANDER. Effect of osteopathic manipulative therapy on autonomic tone as evidenced by blood pressure changes and activity of the fibrinolytic system. *J. Am. Osteop. Assoc.* 67:1037-1038, 1968.

CHRISMAN, O. D., and R. F. GERVAIS. Otologic manifestations of the cervical syndrome. *Clin. Orthop.* 24:34-39, 1962.

CHRISMAN, O. D., A. MITTNACHT, and G. A. SNOOK. A study of the results following rotatory manipulation in the lumbar intervertebral disc syndrome. *J. Bone Joint Surg.* 46A:517-524, 1964.

CLYMER, D., F. L. LEVIN, and R. H. SCULTHORPE. Effects of osteopathic manipulations on several different physiologic functions. *J. Am. Osteop. Assoc.* 72:204-207, 1972.

COOTE, J. H., C.B.B. DOWNMAN, and W. V. WEBER. Reflex discharges into thoracic white rami elicited by somatic and visceral afferent excitation. *J. Physiol.* 202:147-159, 1969.

COYER, A. B., and I.H.M. CURWEN. Low back pain treated by manipulation: A controlled series. *Brit. Med. J.* 1:705-707, 1955.

CRELIN, E. S. A scientific test of chiropractic theory. *Am. Scientist* 61:574-580, 1973.

CYRIAX, R. *Textbook of Orthopedic Medicine.* Vol. 1, *Diagnosis of Soft Tissue Lesions.* 6th ed. London: Baillierc Tindall, 1975.

DeJARNETTE, B. *The Philosophy, Art and Science of Sacro-Occipital Technique.* Nebraska City: B. DeJarnette, 1967.

DORAN, D.M.L., and D. J. NEWELL. Manipulation in treatment of low back pain: A multicenter study. *Brit. Med. J.* 2:161-164, 1975.

DROZ, B., and C. P. LeBLOND. Migration of proteins along the axon of the sciatic nerve. *Science* 137:1047-1048, 1962.

DRUM, D. C., and C. M. GODFREY. Personal communication and presentation to the North American Academy of Manipulative Medicine annual meeting, October 1976.

DUNN, F. E. Osteopathic concepts in psychiatry. *J. Am. Osteop. Assoc.* 49:354-357, 1950.

ENGLAND, R., and P. DEIBERT. Electromyographic studies. Part I: Consideration in the evaluation of osteopathic therapy. *J. Am. Osteop. Assoc.* 72:162-169, 1972.

FARFAN, H. F. *Mechanical Disorders of the Low Back.* Philadelphia: Lea & Febiger, 1973.

FEINSTEIN, B., J.N.K. LANGTON, R. M. JAMESON, and F. SCHILLER. Experiments on pain referred from deep somatic tissues. *J. Bone Joint Surg.* 36A:981-997, 1954.

FICHERA, A. P., and D. R. CELANDER. Effect of osteopathic manipulative therapy on autonomic tone as evidenced by blood pressure
change and activity of the fibrinolytic system. *J. Am. Osteop.
Assoc.* 68:1036-1038, 1969.

FIGAR, S., L. KRAUSOVÁ, and K. LEWIT. Plethysmographische Untersuchungen bei manuelle behandlung vertebragener Störungen.
Acta Neuroveg. 29:618-623, 1967.

FISK, J. W. Manipulation in general practice. *New Zealand Med. J.*
74:172-175, 1971.

FISK, J. W. The straight leg raising test: Its relevance to possible disc pathology. *New Zealand Med. J.* 81:557-560, 1975.

FORUM. Diagnosis and treatment of uncomplicated hayfever. *J. Am.
Osteop. Assoc.* 74:588-595, 1975.

GALENUS. Opera Bd. IV Venetia 1625, quoted by E. H. Schiotz.
Manipulation treatment of the spinal column from the medical-
historical viewpoint (NIH Library Trans.). *Tidsskr. Nor.
Laegeforn* 78:359-372, 1968.

GARDNER, E. Physiology of movable joints. *Physiol. Rev.* 30:127-
176, 1950.

GAYRAL, L., and E. NEUWIRTH. Oto-neuro-ophthalmologic manifestations of cervical origin. *New York J. Med.* 54:1920-1926,
1954.

GILLET, H., and M. LIEKENS. *Belgian Chiropractic Research Notes.*
7th ed. Brussels: Gillet and Liekens, 1968.

GITELMAN, R. The treatment of pain by spinal manipulation. In:
The Research Status of Spinal Manipulative Therapy, edited by
M. Goldstein. NINCDS Monograph #15, DHEW Publ. No. NIH 76-998,
1975, pp. 277-285.

GLOVER, J. R., J. G. MORRIS, and T. KHOSLA. Back pain: A randomized clinical trial of rotational manipulation of the trunk.
Brit. J. Ind. Med. 31:59-64, 1974.

GLOVER, J. R., J. G. MORRIS, and T. KHOSLA. A randomized clinical
trial of rotational manipulation of the trunk. In: *Approaches
to the Validation of Manipulation Therapy,* edited by A. A.
Buerger and J. S. Tobis. Springfield, Ill.: Charles C.
Thomas, 1977, pp. 271-283.

GORDIENKO, A. N.   Changes in bioelectric potentials of afferent
    nerves in immunized animal as antigen action skin receptors.
    Control of Immunogenesis by the Nervous System.   Publication
    U.S. Dept. of Commerce, TT 60-51069:53-57, 1958.

GRICE, A. A.   Muscle tonus changes following manipulation.   *J. Can.
    Chiropractic Assoc.*   19:29-31, 1974.

HALDEMAN, S.   What is meant by manipulation?   In: *Approaches to
    the Validation of Manipulative Therapy*, edited by A. A.
    Buerger and J. S. Tobis.   Springfield, Ill.:   Charles C.
    Thomas, 1977, pp. 299-302.

HALDEMAN, S.   Why one cause of back pain?   In: *Approaches to the
    Validation of Manipulative Therapy*, edited by A. A. Buerger
    and J. S. Tobis.   Springfield, Ill.:   Charles C. Thomas, 1975,
    pp. 187-197.

HALDEMAN, S., and B. S. MEYER.   The effect of experimental con-
    striction on the structure of the sciatic nerve.   *South
    African Med. J.*   44:888-892, 1970.

HARTZMAN, G. W., and H. S. SCHWARTZ.   An analysis of 350 emotionally
    maladjusted individuals under chiropractic care.   Chapter 16
    in: *Mental Health and Chiropractic*, edited by H. S. Swartz.
    New York: Sessions Publisher, 1973.

HENDERSON, R. S.   The treatment of lumbar intervertebral disc pro-
    trusion.   *Brit. Med. J.*   2:597-598, 1952.

HOMEWOOD, A. E.   *The neurodynamics of the vertebral subluxation*.
    Willowdale, Ont.:   Chiropractic Publishers, 1963.

HOOD, R. P.   Blood pressure.   *Digest Chiropractic Econ.*   16:36-38,
    1974.

HOWELL, R. K., and R. E. KAPPLER.   The influence of osteopathic
    manipulative therapy on a patient with advanced cardiopulmonary
    disease.   *J. Am. Osteopath. Assoc.*   73:322-327, 1973.

HOWELL, R. K., T. W. ALLEN, and R. E. KAPPLER.   The influence of
    osteopathic manipulative therapy in the management of patients
    with chronic obstructive lung disease.   *J. Am. Osteop. Assoc.*
    74:757-760, 1975.

HUTTON, S. R.   Combination of traction and manipulation for the
    lumbar disc syndrome.   *Med. J. Australia*   54-1:1196, 1967.

HVIID, H. The influence of chiropractic treatment on the rotary
    mobility of the cervical spine - a kinesiometric and statis-
    tical study. *Ann. Swiss Chiropractic Assoc.* 5:31-44, 1971.

JANSE, J., R. H. HOUSER, and B. F. WELLS. *Chiropractic Principles
    and Technique.* Lombard, Ill.: National College of Chiro-
    practic, 1947.

KING, J. S. Randomized trial of the Rees and Shealy methods for
    the treatment of low back pain. Chapter 4 in: *Approaches to
    the Validation of Manipulative Therapy,* edited by A. A. Buerger
    and J. S. Tobis. Springfield, Ill.: Charles C. Thomas, 1977.

KORR, I. M. The spinal cord as organizer of disease processes:
    Some preliminary perspectives. *J. Am. Osteop. Assoc.* 76:
    89-99, 1976.

KUNERT, W. Functional disorders of internal organs due to vertebral
    lesions. *Ciba Symposium* 13-3, 1965.

LEWIT, K. Meniere's disease and the cervical spine. *Rev. Czecho-
    slovak Med.* 2:129-139, 1961.

LINDSAY, J. R., and W. G. HEMENWAY. Postural vertigo due to un-
    limited sudden partial loss of vestibular function. *Ann. Otol.*
    65:692-706, 1956.

LYNESS, S. S., and A. WAGMAN. Neurological deficit following
    cervical manipulation. *Surg. Neurol.* 2:121-124, 1974.

MAIGNE, R. *Orthopedic Medicine - A New Approach to Vertebral
    Manipulations,* translated and edited by W. T. Liberson.
    Springfield, Ill.: Charles C. Thomas, 1972.

MAITLAND, G. D. *Peripheral Manipulation,* 3rd ed., 1970. London:
    Butterworths, 1973.

MATTHEWS, J. A., and D.A.H. YATES. Reduction of lumbar disc pro-
    lapse by manipulation. *Brit. Med. J.* 20:696-699, 1969.

MELTZER, H. Y. Skeletal muscle abnormalities in patients with
    affective disorders. *J. Psychiat. Res.* 10:43-57, 1973.

MELZACK, R., and P. D. WALL. Pain mechanisms: A new theory.
    Science 150:971-979, 1965.

MENNELL, J. McM. *Back Pain - Diagnosis and Treatment Using Manipu-
    lative Therapy.* Boston, Toronto: Little, Brown & Co., 1960.

MENSOR, M. C. Non-operative treatment, including manipulation, for lumbar intervertebral disc syndrome. *J. Bone Joint Surg.* 37A: 925-936, 1955.

METTIER, S., and C. CAPP. Neurological symptoms and clinical findings in patients with cervical degenerative arthritis. *Ann. Int. Med.* 14:1315-1322, 1941.

MILLER, W. D. Treatment of visceral disorders by manipulative therapy. In: *The Research Status of Spinal Manipulative Therapy,* edited by M. Goldstein. NINCDS Monograph No. 15, DHEW Publication No. NIH 76-998, 1975, pp. 295-301.

NACHEMSON, A. Intradiscal measurements of pH in patients with rhizopathies. *Acta Orthop. Scand.* 40:23-33, 1969.

NACHEMSON, A. A critical look at the treatment for low back pain. In: *The Research Status of Spinal Manipulative Therapy,* edited by M. Goldstein. NINCDS Monograph No. 15, DHEW Publication No. NIH 76-998, 1975, pp. 287-293.

NIJIMA, A., and A. FUKUDA. Release of glucose from perfused liver preparation in response to stimulation of the splanchnic nerves in the toad. *Japan. J. Physiol.* 23:497-508, 1973.

NORMAN, J., and J. G. WHITMAN. The vagal contribution to changes in heart rate evoked by stimulation of cutaneous nerves in the dog. *J. Physiol., London* 234:89P-90P, 1973.

NORRIS, T. A study of the effect of manipulation on blood pressure. *Acad. Appl. Osteopath. Yearbook*:184-188, 1964.

PALMER, D. D. *The Science, Art and Philosophy of Chiropractic.* Portland, Ore.: Portland Printing House Co., 1910.

PARE, A. Opera, Liber XV, S. 440-440, Paris, 1582, quoted by E. H. Schiotz. Manipulation treatment of the spinal column from the medical-historical viewpoint (NIH Library translation). *Tidsskr. Nor. Laegeforn* 78:359-372, 1958.

PEARCE, J., and J.M.H. Moll. Conservative treatment and natural history of acute disc lesions. *J. Neurol. Neurosurg. Psychiat.* 30:13-17, 1967.

PERL, E. R. Pain: spinal and peripheral factors. In: *The Research Status of Spinal Manipulative Therapy,* edited by M. Goldstein. NINCDS Monograph No. 15, DHEW Publication No. NIH 76-998, 1975, pp. 173-182.

PERL, E. R., and D. G. WHITLOCK. Somatic stimuli exciting spino-
thalamic projections to thalamic neurons in cat and monkey.
Exp. Neurol. 3:356-396, 1961.

PRATT-THOMAS, H. R., and K. E. BERGER. Cerebellar and spinal injuries after chiropractic manipulation. *J. Am. Med. Assoc.*
133:600-603, 1947.

QUIGLEY, W. H. Physiological psychology of chiropractic in mental
disorders. Chapter 10 in: *Mental Health and Chiropractic -
A Multidisciplinary Approach,* edited by H. S. Schwartz. New
York: Sessions Publishers, 1973.

RIMON, R., A. STENBACK, and E. HUCKMAN. Electromyographic findings
in depression patients. *J. Psychosom. Res.* 10:159-170, 1966.

ROBERTSON, A.H.M. Manipulation in cervical syndrome. *The Practitioner* 200:396-402, 1968.

ROGERS, J. T., and J. C. ROGERS. The role of osteopathic manipulative therapy in the treatment of coronary artery disease. *J.
Am. Osteop. Assoc.* 76:71-81, 1976.

RUXIN, R. L., T. G. BIDDER, and D. P. ANGLE. The influence of
autonomic arousal on blood clotting time in patients receiving
electroconvulsive treatments. *J. Psychosom. Res.* 16:185-192,
1972.

SATO, A., and R. F. SCHMIDT. Somatosympathetic reflexes: afferent
fibers, central pathways, discharge characteristics. *Physiol.
Rev.* 53:916-947, 1973.

SHAM, S. M. Manipulation of the lumbosacral spine. *Clin. Orthop.
Related Res.* 101:146-150, 1974.

SIEHL, D., D. R. OLSON, H. E. ROSS, and E. E. ROCKWOOD. Manipulation of the lumbar spine with the patient under general anesthesia: Evaluation by electromyograph and clinical-neurologic
examination of its use for lumbar root compression syndrome.
J. Am. Osteop. Assoc. 70:433-437, 1971.

STERNBACH, R. A., S. R. WOLF, R. W. MURPHY, and W. H. AKESON.
Traits of pain patients: the low-back "loser". *Psychosomatics*
14:226-229, 1973.

STEIN-WERBLOWSKY, R. The sympathetic nervous system and cancer.
Exp. Neurol. 42:97-100, 1974.

STILES, E. G.   Osteopathic manipulation in a hospital environment.
    J. Am. Osteop. Assoc.   76:243-258, 1976.

STILL, A. T.   *Philosophy of Osteopathy*.   Kirksville: A. T. Still
    Publisher, 1899.

SWAN, B.   Cervical manipulation.   *Med. J. Australia*   2:811, 1968.

THE MANIPULATION PROJECT.   California College of Medicine, Univer-
    sity of California, Irvine.   Preliminary Report: Effect of
    rotational manipulation of the pelvis and lumbosacral spine
    on straight leg raising.   Submitted for publication, 1977.

TISSINGTON-TATLOW, W. F., and H. G. BAMMER.   Syndrome of vertebral
    artery compression.   *Neurology*   7:331-340, 1957.

TRAN, T. A., and J. D. KIRBY.   The effects of upper cervical adjust-
    ment upon the normal physiology of the heart.   *Am. Chiropractic
    Assoc. J.*   11:S-58-62, 1977.

VEAR, H. J.   A study into the complaints of patients seeking
    chiropractic care.   *J. Canad. Chiropractic Assoc.*   Oct.:9-13,
    1972.

WARR, A. C., J. A. WILKINSON, J.M.B. BURN, and L. LANGDON.   Chronic
    lumbosciatic syndrome treated by epidural injection and manip-
    ulation.   *The Practitioner*   209:53-59, 1972.

WEISS, P.   Endoneurial edema in constricted nerve.   *Anat. Rec.*
    86:491-522, 1943.

WEISS, P., and H. B. HISCOE.   Experiments on the mechanism of nerve
    growth.   *J. Exptl. Zool.*   107:315-395, 1948.

DISCUSSION OF CLINICAL OBSERVATIONS AND EMERGING QUESTIONS

Murray Goldstein, Chairman

[Editor's note: At this point Dr. A. A. Buerger and Dr. C. M. Godfrey were invited to discuss briefly the clinical trials being conducted under their direction at the University of California-Irvine and at the University of Toronto, respectively, on the efficacy of manipulative therapy in the relief of back pain. Their presentations were followed by an extended exchange of comments with respect to pain, manipulative procedures, criteria for selection of patients for study, evaluation of efficacy, placebos and other aspects of the design of clinical trials.

Since clinical efficacy and its evaluation are not directly related to the theme and objectives of the Workshop, the presentations and much of the discussion have been omitted from these proceedings. Only those comments have been retained which, in the opinion of the editor and his consultants, have a direct bearing on neurobiologic mechanisms.]

DR. GOLDSTEIN: These two presentations seem to revolve around a single phenomenon: the end point of pain. The issue seems to be whether the manipulative approach diagnostically or therapeutically ameliorates or in some way eliminates the phenomenon of pain—again, a central nervous system phenomenon. Physiologically, whether we are talking about restriction of motion or what have we, we seem constantly to come back to the issue of pain, whether or not we learn anything about what pain is or how manipulation affects the phenomenon.

I wonder, Dr. Grundfest, as one of the senior citizens in this area, whether you have any comments about the phenomenon of pain as it may relate to this issue.

DR. HARRY GRUNDFEST: One question I have is in connection with our own experience with measurements of pain and of analgesia in laboratory-induced pain. I have been impressed by the chaos in the field of pain measurements and of analgesic effectiveness. I

can refer, for example, to Henry Beecher's book on subjective
responses. I am sure most of you are familiar with it.

Now it is a chaotic situation, I think, because somewhere between 30 and 40% of subjects who have pain are what we call placebo
reactors, and this is a common experience. And in order to overcome the problems of placebo reactors, Beecher, for example, used
very elaborate statistical techniques in mass studies on clinical
pain. He rejected, for example, laboratory measurements of
laboratory-induced pain. Towards the end of his life, however, he
came over to the side of measuring pain and of reducing pain in
the laboratory. I think it was still not very good technique.

Now, it seems to me that if you assume that Dr. Buerger's 25
pairs of patients are a normal population of whom, say, 35% are
placebo reactors, I don't know whether your data are specifically
significant or can be statistically significant, although the tests
might indicate that they may be.

There are possibilities, however, at least in our own kind of
work. We found, purely by accident, that we could avoid placebo
reactors, or eliminate placebo reactors, from our sample population.
And the result was that we could have all-or-none answers. I wonder
whether some techniques for eliminating placebo reactors or detect-
ing placebo reactors should not be used in studies of this kind.

Furthermore,--I don't know the clinical feasibility of this--
but could you run, for example, alternate tests on these patients?
One with the manipulative technique and one with your placebo techniques? In this way you might be able to tell from one day to every
five days, as you said, whether some groups of people have general
reactions of this kind.

I think that is about as much as I can say at the moment, because I really don't know what causes these kinds of extreme pains.

DR. GOLDSTEIN: Dr. Ochs, it has been proposed in the presentation that we have a dynamic compression, perhaps of nerve
root, leading to pain. Does continuing pressure on a nerve, say
a sensory nerve, lead to pain?

DR. SIDNEY OCHS: I can't answer that particular question from
my personal experience, but I have heard it said that pressure per
se does not cause pain. However, it seems to me possible that in
some of the smaller fibers, pressure may lead indirectly to pain,
if they become sensitized to ions, ionic changes in the milieu,
possibly acetylcholine. So, I must defer to my colleagues on that
particular question.

I did want to say something with regard to Dr. Grundfest's comments, which intrigued me very much. Years ago, we had some small experience in the use of the Hardy-Wolff-Goodell technique. We applied it to the fingernail instead of the blackened forehead spot used in the original technique. With the blackened fingernail we get a very sharp endpoint, a bright pain, when a threshold is reached. And I just wondered, going along with Harry's excellent suggestion, if the same patients who are undergoing these particular trials could also be tested by the Hardy-Wolff-Goodell technique and be given a placebo, to see if they are placebo-reacting people, and match them against the others.

DR. GOLDSTEIN: What you are suggesting is essentially a parallel evaluation of the patients in terms of their response to pain and to placebos.

DR. GODFREY: That is very difficult. A reactor to one placebo may not have the same response to another placebo. You are complicating the whole thing. We have enough problems with a simple experiment like this without compounding them with some other thing added on top. I would be interested in knowing how Dr. Grundfest would rule out the placebo reactors. I would want those people in the study, because when I get back 30% or better, I know I am being honest. What I am looking for is the 30 to 60%; that percentage would tell me whether manipulation effective or not.

DR. GRUNDFEST: One trouble with that kind of arithmetic is that the placebo reactor reacts in either direction. He can go plus or he can go minus, so that you really don't know what you have got at the end.

Now I think we have a very valid and important statement that the placebo reactors react in a different manner to different kinds of placebos, or in different kinds of pain situations. I think it would be an excellent idea if we developed methods for investigating placebo reactors in different kinds of situations.

For example, Dr. Ochs referred to the Hardy - Wolff - Goodell test. He used the fingernail test, which in my opinion is probably an appropriate way of applying that particular test. Some pain tests are not useful because they result in a mixed sensation. I am sure many of you have exposed yourselves to the tourniquet block -- the Lewis-Pochin experiment which blocks the large fibers and thus leaves only the small fibers, that is, the slow pain system, in operation.

The sensation is very, very different when you apply a stimulus to the finger after you have blocked the A-fibers, and have only the C-fibers left. It is a very different sensation from the normal type. These masking phenomena, of course, are very important, and I think this is the reason why the Hardy-Wolff-Goodell test got into disrepute, because it didn't apply to an appropriate kind of test object. The forehead is a bad place to study pain - to elicit pain, pure pain.

DR. IRWIN KORR: To return to the question of the effects of continuous pressure on a nerve: I think most will agree that the application of pressure to an axon may, at the moment of application, initiate an impulse, but that after that there is no continuation of impulses. I would like to remind you, however, that in the living body, there is no steady pressure. It is a living, breathing, pulsating, moving environment in which the pressure-stimulus would be a fluctuating stimulus that may very well generate continual trains of impulses, or at least intermittent trains of impulses. Wouldn't you agree?

DR. OCHS: Yes, but I think it is a different situation, as Dr. Sunderland has pointed out many times, when you are dealing with the nerve trunk as compared with situations where you have very small fascicles or very small numbers of fibers, and in an environment which is definitely different. I think you have to differentiate between the protected nerve trunk and the relatively unprotected smaller fibers.

DR. SCOTT HALDEMAN: There may in fact be a single impulse discharge each time the pressure goes on and off. This is unlikely to cause pain, any prolonged pain, and definitely not the pain one experiences in back pain. The point is that we know the pressure from a disc, for example, does cause inflammation. And any surgeon who goes in and looks at a compressed nerve finds the nerve surrounded by inflammatory tissue; it is red, it is hyperemic, and this inflammation, caused by pressure, does in fact cause pain. It does everywhere else. There is no reason to believe it wouldn't do so in that region.

DR. GOLDSTEIN: Dr. Sunderland, in your studies, have you seen much evidence of inflammation?

DR. SYDNEY SUNDERLAND: Unquestionably. This is a factor, but there are a number of questions I would like to ask at this stage, if I may. With reference to Dr. Buerger's valuable analysis of this situation and other discussions, it would appear that with the procedure we are treating a symptom. In other words, it would seem that manipulation is not used to treat a lesion other, perhaps, than a hypothetical one at this stage, which is nerve root compression. Am I correct in following it to that particular point? Because I think we are on dangerous ground if we infer that the basis of the symptomatology in these cases is nerve root compression. I think that point was brought out by earlier speakers, Dr. Lewit and others. Nerve root compression is not necessarily the basis of the pain in the condition to which we refer.

Now in general, what I call pure compression as a mechanical deformation is not painful. I will come back to that point again in my paper, but we have many examples of that. The sleep palsy which gives you a conduction block of the radial nerve is painless. The compression palsy of the lateral popliteal that follows a badly applied plaster to the lower extremity is painless. I can now, in my advanced years, without any difficulty, send my ulnar nerve to sleep. And it is always painless. And one could go on multiplying these examples.

Normal nerve fibers will tolerate considerable degrees of deformation before they will begin to complain and usually it is not a complaint, it is a failure of conduction. However, when nerve fibers become abnormal as they can after trauma, and you are now dealing with a sensitive area, or if the nutrition or oxygen supply of that nerve fiber is being depleted, or it is damaged in an inflammatory situation, then that nerve will complain and that lesion is a painful one.

So that in the case of the intervertebral foramen, I believe that nerve root compression is an unusual cause of the pain. But more commonly, it is due to other factors; one is the involvement of the spinal nerve in a disc which creates an inflammatory situation. Not from pressure, but from a friction fibrosis, because with almost every movement we make, the spinal nerves are moving in and out of the intervertebral foramen. And if you have the development of osteophytes or any pathological change which modifies the smooth contour of the foramen, you are going to get into difficulty if there has been any precipitating lesion.

There is another possible circumstance in which pain may be associated with traumatized nerves. I think it is possible, with severe traction, and traction lesions do occur in the sciatic nerve roots, you can in fact rupture nerve fibers. When this occurs, again there is an inflammatory reaction in the vicinity and the disc can be a source of pain.

So I think in Dr. Buerger's study, the manipulation is being performed to relieve the pain, but we do not know what the specific lesion is, either in the nerve or at the vertebral column.

DR. KAREL LEWIT: I would like to make a few statements about pain and nerve lesions. First, when I spoke about the possibility of mobile compression in the carpal tunnel syndrome, I did not mean pain, because the prevailing symptom is numbness. Second, if there is compression of a spinal nerve, I would suggest that pain is most likely due to impact on the nerve sheath, because the sheaths are full of receptors. And the third, and most important, the evaluation of our success in manipulation should not center so much on pain, because by manipulation we do not treat pain but we treat impaired mobility. You can't do anything else.

Therefore, the evaluation before and after manipulation should be in regard to (a) whether there was impaired mobility, and (b) the presence or absence of such reflex phenomena as spasm, hyperalgesic zones, etc. If after manipulation, movement restriction is abolished and there is no hyperalgesic zone, then manipulation has done what it can have done. If pain then goes on, then it is because there are different reasons, and there is exactly in this, the difficulty of controlled trials of the type which are frequently presented. "We have a group of patients with back pain." That is no diagnosis. Back pain is no indication for manipulation. Indication for manipulation is only if you find the specific lesion which can be treated by manipulation. Very often in pain clinics, you find low back pain due to so many different reasons that to compare the results is a comparison between apples and potatoes.

Every patient is so individual that we incur the great danger of being dismissed as anecdotal, but any patient, if really assessed in a very special way, becomes an individual anecdote. That is the great difficulty. Take the patient with back pain because he has a muscular imbalance, a ligamentous problem, and an articular problem. Once I have solved the articular problem by manipulation, he may still have pain because of muscle imbalance, and it is absolutely nonsensical to go on manipulating him.

I want to just point out these very few things. We should assess any matter by its specific impact --massage impact on muscles, manipulation on joint mobility, and it is difficult to get around that.

DR. GOLDSTEIN: Dr. Lewit, you have made a very interesting sociological comment also. Apparently in central Europe, inept investigators mix apples and potatoes. In this country, it is apples and oranges.

DR. FRED E. SAMSON: I got the impression from Dr. Greenman's presentation that different practitioners may use different procedures, and indeed that he uses different procedures for different patients. I would like to ask what is this range and to what extent

is there a common element? What are we talking about when we are
talking about manipulative therapy?

DR. PHILIP GREENMAN: I would respond that regardless of the
type of therapeutic procedure that I use of a manipulative nature,
its design is to effectuate as appropriately as I can, normalization of motion of the dysfunctional joint or series of joints.
Sometimes the type of procedure will vary considerably, but the end
point, to my way of thinking, is always the same, and that is restoration of physiological motion within the normal constraints of
that joint. To restore it to its maximum efficiency of range of
motion.

There are various ways of doing that, all with the same
objective, the same common "bottom line". And this is precisely
the problem with clinical trials that purport to evaluate the efficacy of manipulative therapy and which use a standardized manipulative procedure on all of the patients. That is totally unrealistic.
If you are going to evaluate manipulative therapy, then you ought to
test it as practiced. Every patient that I see--even the patients
with the common complaint of back pain--I treat differently. Each
patient is different, with a different kind of musculoskeletal
problem, requiring an appropriate manipulative approach. I would
never use the same treatment on a series of patients, because my
experience tells me that it would be at least as frequently
inappropriate as appropriate.

This brings me to another point about clinical trials of
manipulative therapy, and that is the efforts to develop, for
double-blinding purposes, a sham kind of manipulative procedure
which would "not have manipulative results", to correspond to the
placebo in more conventional clinical trials. Again, my clinical
experience tells me that we are not going to be able to develop a
sham type of manipulative procedure. Because anything that you do
to the musculoskeletal system affects it, as those of us who attempt to teach the manipulative art to students repeatedly find.
By the time one or more students have examined the patient, the
situation has changed, and the findings are different. Why? Because just the procedure of putting the musculoskeletal system
through a series of diagnostic tests will often cause therapeutic
things to happen. These are the kinds of things we have to be
aware of when we deal with structural diagnosis and manipulative
therapy.

There is a wide and varying range of techniques that now fall
under the term manipulation, or spinal manipulotherapy, and if one
picks up various textbooks on the subject, one notes whole different systems. They vary from mild mobilization or from very slight
movements to various forms of massage, to gross nonspecific movement using femurs and shoulders and so on, to minute specific kinds

of adjusting techniques which put a specific contact on either a
transverse or a spinous process and give a very short, sharp
thrust. So there is great variation in techniques by people who
claim to be spinal manipulators, and a generalization can never
be made from a single qualified practitioner to the entire field
of manipulation. Nevertheless, all of manipulative therapy is
often dismissed on the basis of one technique.

One may offer the counter-criticism that if any single trial
comes out negative, showing no significant effect, then it's because the manipulator in the trial doesn't know how to do it;
another, more skilled, would do it so much better. These are the
kinds of problems which we are going to have to come to grips with
in trials of manipulative therapy and structural diagnosis.

DR. ALAN J. McCOMAS: I would like to add a personal note. I
acknowledge the importance of the sort of controlled study which
is presently being conducted by Dr. Buerger and Dr. Godfrey. However, equally impressive for any physician are the observations
which he is able to make upon himself, and I would like to bet that
amongst us sitting around these tables, about one-third will have
suffered from low back pain of some kind or other.

I am also prepared to speculate that at least half of those
will have found that they could, at one time, during the start of
these symptoms, get rid of their pain simply by adjusting their
position, bending themselves in a certain way, and perhaps applying
pressure to their back. This is certainly true in my own case,
and one does have the sensation of something clicking into place.
I think it is also important to recognize the possibility that those
patients in the controlled study who were not having manipulation
may nevertheless themselves have unconsciously manipulated themselves during their rest procedure, and this has to be taken into
account.

May I also make a comment on the effects of nerve stretch and
nerve compression. Sir Sydney Sunderland referred to the fact that
in stretch injuries to nerves, nerve roots, it is possible that
there may be a herniation of the epineurium, of the nerve sheath.
And this reminds one of work which was carried out by Denny-Brown
and his collaborators in the 1940's, where they stretched cat
nerves by hand and showed that they could produce a tear in the
nerve sheath, with a herniation of nerve fibers, and that these
fibers appear to be pinched off at the base. I would find it very
difficult to conceive of any sort of manipulation which could deal
with that sort of injury.

The last point I wanted to make was about nerve compression
as a cause of pain. Sir Sydney's remarks are very apposite, and I

don't think it can cause pain. But it can, under certain circumstances, produce a very intense discomfort, and I think the most obvious example of this is when we are sitting on a hard edge and we compress our sciatic nerve, and then we get up and start walking about. I think it would be everyone's experience that those first few paces we take are intensely uncomfortable.

Now analyzing this phenomenon, the receptors which are stimulated every time we place our foot on the ground, are the mechanoreceptors which we would normally be stimulating. But what seems to happen is that the temporal and spatial pattern of impulses coming into the spinal cord has been disrupted, and this is interpreted by the central nervous system as being at least uncomfortable, if not actually painful.

DR. DONALD B. TOWER: I may be a little naive, but it seems to me that everyone is tending to focus in on the nerve lesion, and I wonder if we aren't falling into the trap of oversimplification. Neural factors may be our concern, but on the other hand, there are a great many clinically apparent muscular lesions which don't involve the nerve root and the spine, and I am concerned that in this discussion we really haven't considered them. I would like to hear some discussion of that aspect of it because I am sure in the patient population at large one would find the figure nearer to two-thirds rather than Dr. McComas' estimate of one-third. Don't we have to assume muscular lesions in a lot of those even though this rather complicates rather than simplifies the issue?

DR. OTTO APPENZELLER: I would like to return to a notion which I think has been introduced by Dr. Grundfest, that we actually don't feel the pain in our back, but we feel it with some other structures higher up. I think it is important to distinguish patients who have chronic pain from those who don't. The presence of pain changes the capacity of the nociceptive system in the brain to perceive pain, and patients with chronic pain may, in fact, have l o w e r thresholds to pain than controls who don't have a chronic painful state. I think a case in point was a paper that Dr. Nathan, I think, wrote some time ago when reporting a test of transcutaneous nerve stimulation in patients with postherpetic neuralgia. He found that this was effective in reducing pain in such patients, but when he used this modality on normal controls who did not have a chronic painful state, their pain thresholds were not altered by this transcutaneous nerve stimulation.

So I think that, in the studies that were reported here, it might be important to assess both in the controls and in the other group, this state of receptiveness of the nociceptive system by other modalities rather than just their response to manipulation.

DR. GOLDSTEIN: I think this was the point also that Dr. Grundfest was alluding to in terms of sensitivity of the system and its
fine tuning.

DR. BUERGER: I would like to go on and say that my biggest
concern with the trial that we are carrying out is that the bulk
of the data we are generating is in the form of answers to multiple-
choice questions, and we really are not producing objective physical measurements which are susceptible to careful statistical
analysis.

There is some evidence that was originally introduced by James
Fisk, M.D., a physician in New Zealand, suggesting that rotational
manipulation of the osteopathic kind had some positive effects on
straight leg raising tests. We followed that up in a prospective
single-blind study, and he seems to be right. But I am very concerned that it seems difficult at the present time to generate
numbers which reflect the effects of treatment, and I think one
thing that must happen before this subject is finally laid to rest
is that someone is going to have to find a way of generating those
numbers, and I frankly don't know one.

DR. HALDEMAN: There have been attempts reported in the literature to generate just such numbers. Two or three of the parameters which can be measured (and there is a tendency by many people
in manipulation to believe they cannot be measured) are the degrees
of joint fixation alluded to by Dr. Lewit. One group has radio-
graphically measured movements between individual segments of
vertebrae on side bending or forward and backward flexion. They
have been able to show decreased or aberrant movement between segments suggesting there is something wrong with the function of the
joint.

The other thing that can be measured is the electromyographic
changes in the spinal musculature. This is what Dr. Tower is
alluding to, I think. Part of at least an osteopathic and a
chiropractic evaluation of the manipulable lesion, whatever it
happens to be, is an evaluation of joint mobility, muscle spasm,
and areas of tenderness. There have even been attempts to evaluate
the areas of tenderness by Glover at Welsh National Hospital. We
had a pressure measuring machine which we applied to tender points
to see how much pressure was required to create pain or tenderness
in this area. So one could use this type of technique for measuring tenderness, electromyography to measure spasm, motion X-rays
to measure joint fixation, straight leg raising to measure the
degree of irritation. I think it is possible to get a reasonable
evaluation of what a manipulator is really looking at when he makes
an evaluation of a patient.

DR. GODFREY: I disagree very highly. Are you going to tell me that you can put an EMG needle in the paraspinal muscle, sample the "spasm", do a manipulation, then resample, and find there has been a change? I would like to see the technique.

DR. HALDEMAN: I certainly say attempts have been made.

DR. GODFREY: The straight leg raising? Fine. That very nicely shows what is going on with the S_1 root. But you haven't delineated that we are looking at S_1 roots. You are talking about back pain. Once again, lack of specificity. Sir Sydney said we were treating symptoms. No, we are not. We are treating a dysfunction. We have found a reduction of movement. The manipulation, by hypothesis, reduces the reduction of movement. Whether that reduces the pain or not is another matter that we are trying to determine. I agree with Dr. Grundfest on the difficulty of assessing pain. Very difficult. But I think if we could just show that as a result of manipulation there has been an increase of movement, we would be one step along the road, without getting into any of the other parameters.

DR. TOWER: Dr. Godfrey, haven't you got it a bit the wrong way around? It seems to me in most of the cases that it is the pain that reduces the movement, and not the other way.

DR. GODFREY: If the back is examined properly, you can do it painlessly, and still find a reduction of movement. I think that is where chiropractors and osteopathic physicians have it over us, the allopathic physicians, because they do have a technique with which they can examine painlessly, putting the patient's joints through that passive range of movement without causing pain, even though the patient has his pain back again after being examined.

DR. TOWER: You must never have had a disc, Dr. Godfrey.

DR. GODFREY: I am not talking about discs. I am talking about a joint block that causes the pain.

DR. LEWIT: This is really so. If you know the technique, you will find movement restrictions without pain. The movement restriction due to a radicular pain is due to overall muscle spasm, not joint blockage--something completely different.

DR. TOWER: You are arguing with the wrong man. I am with you.

DR. P. W. NATHAN: I have two comments. One is in regard to what Dr. Grundfest says about positive placebo reactors. They are the ordinary placebo reactors, whose pain is stopped by drugs and placebos. There is another kind of patient whose attitude is:

"Whatever you do, you will not stop my pain." I found these when
I was first testing analgesic drugs many years ago. Their pain just
stayed up at maximum all the time on large doses of morphine or
anything. This is one group which investigators somehow forget.

Now on quite a different subject. Many years ago there was
an interesting paper from Scandinavia by Frykholm and three colleagues. One was an American who had discs operated on under
local anesthetic. The exposed roots were then stimulated. As
Sydney Sunderland was saying, the roots which were clearly inflamed were painful, including anterior roots, when they stimulated
them. Neighboring roots which were not inflamed were not painful.

DR. KIYOMI KOIZUMI: I would like clinicians to explain to me
what is really involved in manipulative therapy. What is involved
in it physiologically, when you apply manipulative therapy? If you
try to create the same situation in experimental conditions, what
changes would be observed? Would they be local or do some other
widespread changes occur in the body?

DR. GOLDSTEIN: I think that that is the "sixty-four dollar
question". That, I would guess, is perhaps what the final summary
of the conference would begin to address as a question. I know
Dr. Sunderland has some discussion on this in his paper. I don't
want to cut off the discussion, but I think that since this is
essentially what the whole conference is about, we should defer
further discussion until later.

As I understand the ground rules, Dr. Koizumi, we are focusing
on one aspect of your question. Namely, what are the neurobiologic
mechanisms which may be involved, and just that. As our chairman
has instructed us, we are supposed to be addressing that issue, and
not the several other issues which probably would occupy another
conference.

DR. KOIZUMI: I want to know simply what is the physical
action. Is it massage, or pressure or what?

DR. GOLDSTEIN: I think Dr. Koizumi is asking the question
from a pathophysiologic viewpoint. Does anybody wish to try to
offer a pathophysiological answer?

DR. RONALD GITELMAN: I think the way I have always attempted
to explain it is simply to state that we attempt to locate disturbed biomechanics of the spine and pelvis primarily, and to restore normal biomechanics by manually applying force to that spine
or pelvis. This is a physical application of a well directed
specific artistic force to the body.

DR. SUNDERLAND: I think that what the nonclinician wants to
know really, is what the clinician is doing. What does he actually
do to the patient? These are the simple, obvious things that are
so familiar to the clinician, that it never occurs to him that the
nonclinician doesn't understand what he is doing. I think the
question was, as I interpret it, what in fact does the manipulation
really involve?

DR. LYNNE WEAVER: I believe I would like to express
Dr. Koizumi's question a little differently. Is it necessarily
an orthopedic readjustment or can it be merely related to some soft
tissue alignment of some sort? Is it necessarily orthopedic?

DR. LEWIT: Even at the danger of oversimplification, I would
put it this way: that with any technique we apply a force which
frees a joint.

DR. GOLDSTEIN: Would it be fair to say that in the same way
that one discusses surgical therapy that is a generalization of an
approach to a whole range of disorders, and that certainly surgery
in terms of technology, say, on brain, is somewhat different from
the surgical technology as it applies to a specific disorder in
another part of the body. One has exactly the same thing with
pharmacological agents and biological agents which occur in a large
variety of classes, from which selections are made relatively specific to the clinical situation. I suspect that in our discussion
of manipulative therapy, we have a tendency to address it as if it
were a single procedure used in a single way to accomplish a single
purpose, and I wonder if the analogy with pharmacological agents
and other approaches to therapy may help us. It is a very broad
scope of activity of that type.

Impulse-Based   Mechanisms

Chairman: Horace W. Magoun

SOMATIC SOURCES OF AFFERENT INPUT AS FACTORS IN ABERRANT

AUTONOMIC, SENSORY AND MOTOR FUNCTION

J. H. Coote

Department of Physiology, The Medical School

University of Birmingham, England

The control of autonomic effectors and the influence of afferent input on them has received a great deal of attention in the
last fifteen years and has been the subject of a number of reviews
(Janig, 1975; Koizumi & Brooks, 1972; Sato, 1971, 1975; Sato &
Schmidt, 1973; Schmidt, 1974). Many parts of the brain are involved
in this control but directly or indirectly they ultimately influence
the brainstem and spinal cord wherein lie the cells, the preganglionic motoneurones, whose axons pass out of the central nervous system
to synapse with postganglionic neurones in the peripheral ganglia.
The preganglionic motoneurone is probably the last site at which any
major integration of central and peripheral input occurs. Therefore, to gain a perspective on the influence of somatic afferent
inputs I think we can best start by examining the synaptic organisation of the motor nuclei that form the final common pathway out
of the central nervous system. In the hope of preventing confusion
and for the sake of brevity, I will confine this review to the
sympathetic nervous system about which much more is known anyway.

THE SYMPATHETIC PREGANGLIONIC MOTOR NUCLEI

The sympathetic preganglionic neurones lie in the zona inter-
media of the thoracic-lumbar cord concentrated in a triangular
region on the lateral border of the gray matter between the dorsal
and ventral horn (the intermediolateral cell column). Scattered
cells are also found in the adjacent white matter of the lateral
funiculus and in the medial gray matter (nucleus intercalatus,
Figure 1). The location and organisation of these neurones appears
to be very similar in the several species so far studied, rat, cat,

91

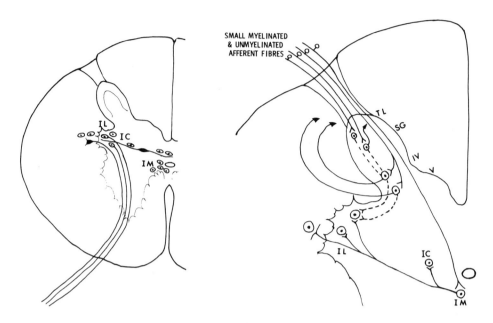

Figure 1. Two drawings which attempt to summarise the location in
the thoraco-lumbar cord of the sympathetic preganglionic neurones
and the principal afferent connections to them. Broken lines indicate pathways on which there is no firm evidence. IL, intermediolateral nucleus; IM, intermediomedial nucleus; IC, nucleus intercalatus; TL, tract of Lissauer; SG, substantia gelatinosa. Modified
from Petras and Cummings (1972).

dog, monkey and man (Bok, 1928; Gagel, 1932; Henry & Calaresu, 1972;
Petras & Cummings, 1972; Pick, 1970; Poljack, 1924; Rethelyi, 1972,
1974). In the cat the intermediolateral nucleus and associated cell
groups extend from T_1 to L_4 segments of the spinal cord with the
highest concentration of neurones in segments T_1-T_2 and L_3-L_4 (Henry
& Calaresu, 1972). The cell bodies are smaller (15 to 40 μm) on
average than somatic neurones of the ventral horn but larger than
cells of the dorsal horn, and may be round or elongated with dendrites orientated in the longitudinal direction unlike cells in the
surrounding gray matter (Chung et al., 1975; Petras & Cummings,
1972; Rethelyi, 1972, 1974). The axons pass out ventrally with no
sign of collateral branching (Petras & Cummings, 1972; Rethelyi,
1972) which is consistent with the electrophysiological evidence
that there is no sign of recurrent inhibition in the sympathetic
preganglionic neurones (Mannard et al., 1977; Polosa, 1967).

SYNAPTIC CONNECTIONS

The presynaptic fibres of the neuropil are probably all un-myelinated and approach the intermediolateral nucleus in small bundles mainly from its lateral side with a few fibres converging from the medial region of the gray matter. These fibres make re-peated contacts with dendrites and the cell bodies of preganglionic neurones (Rethelyi, 1972). Axon terminals may be classified into three groups (1) those containing clear spherical vesicles exclu-sively; (2) those containing dense cored vesicles which may well indicate they are monoaminergic and thus probably correspond to the terminals of the bulbospinal monoaminergic axons described by Carlsson, Falck, Fuxe and Hillarp (1964) and Dahlstrom and Fuxe (1965); (3) those containing flattened vesicles which might suggest they have an inhibitory action (Tibes et al., 1977). None of these terminals disappear following section of the dorsal roots indicating that there is little likelihood of monosynaptic connections at least to the neurones of the intermediolateral cell column (Petras & Cum-mings, 1972; Sato, 1971; Szentágothai, 1964).

INPUT TO THE SYMPATHETIC MOTOR NUCLEI

The inputs to the sympathetic preganglionic neurone can be divided into two main categories, peripheral and central.

Peripheral Inputs (Figure 1)

By peripheral I mean the afferent fibres which are the axons of some of the dorsal root ganglion cells. Not all primary afferent fibres influence sympathetic neurones and not all sympathetic neurones can be made to discharge by stimulation of the primary afferent fibres (Coote & Westbury, 1977; Janig & Schmidt, 1970; Sato, 1972b; Seller, 1973). The type of primary afferent fibre which may influence preganglionic cells is now well established and the extensive literature has been comprehensively reviewed (Koizumi & Brooks, 1972; Sato & Schmidt, 1973; Schmidt, 1974). All authors are agreed that the relevant afferent fibres are to be found amongst those myelinated fibres conducting below 40 m/sec and the unmyelinated fibres, i.e., the Aβ, δ and C fibres of cutaneous nerves and the Group II, III and IV of muscle nerves (Coote & Perez-Gonzalez, 1970; Henry & Calaresu, 1974b; Koizumi et al., 1970; Sato et al., 1969; Sato & Schmidt, 1966; Schmidt & Schonfuss, 1970; Schmidt & Weller, 1970) and the small myelinated and unmyelinated afferent fibres of visceral nerves (Coote, 1964; Franz et al., 1966; Sato et al., 1969).

On entering the dorsal horn the small somatic and visceral afferent fibres may synapse directly with neurones in the marginal zone, the tract of Lissauer (Earle, 1952; Kumazawa & Perl, 1976; Ramson, 1913; Schmidt, 1939; Szentágothai, 1964), the fibres of which run for 1 to 2 segments before entering the subjacent gray matter. The afferent fibres also synapse with cells in the substantia gelatinosa (Kumazawa & Perl, 1976) which may send fibres back into the tract of Lissauer where they run longitudinally making synaptic contacts for up to 6 segments (Szentágothai, 1964). This is one route enabling the afferent volley to reach up to 6 segments on either side of the segmental input, a feature of somato-sympathetic and viscerosympathetic reflexes (Coote et al., 1969; Franz et al., 1966; Koizumi et al., 1971; Sato et al., 1967; Sato & Schmidt, 1971; Sato et al., 1965). The afferent volley may also enter another propriospinal system through synapses on cells in laminae IV and V of the dorsal horn, which contribute fibres to a dorsolateral system ascending and descending via short relays of some 2 segments (Kerr, 1975). Axons of cells in these laminae may also connect to sympathetic preganglionic neurones in the same segment but as yet there is no information on how they do this. However, their general anatomical and physiological properties make it likely that they are interneurones in the somato-sympathetic reflex pathway. Lamina V cells are particularly interesting because they receive inputs from both small somatic and small visceral afferent fibres (Fields et al., 1970; Foreman et al., 1977; Pomeranz et al., 1968; Selzer & Spencer, 1969), the only cells of the dorsal horn to do so, and it is these afferents which are largely involved in sympathetic reflex activation. Many cells of these laminae have radially oriented dendrites confined to the transverse plane (Schiebel & Schiebel, 1968; Szentágothai & Rethelyi, 1973) and there is a similar arrangement of the presynaptic axons enabling the interneurones to "collect" the activity of a large number of incoming fibres (Rethelyi, 1974) hence they have large receptive fields. Other cells have more restricted receptive fields (Brown, 1976). We thus have the basis for discrete and nonspecific reflexes both of which occur in the sympathetic system.

In addition to their segmental contribution cells of laminae IV and V contribute axons to ascending tracts in the ventral funiculus and anteriolateral fasciculus (Fields et al., 1970a, 1970b; Fields & Winter, 1970) and to the dorsolateral funiculus (Brown, 1976; Bryan et al., 1973; Hongo et al., 1968). This latter region is very important from the point of view of the somato-sympathetic reflexes, since the main ascending afferent pathway for sympathetic reflexes mediated via medullary or supramedullary regions, is located there (Chung et al., 1975; Chung & Wurster, 1975, 1976; Coote & Downman, 1966; Johnson, 1962; Ranson & Billingsley, 1916).

The afferent fibres also synapse with a group of cells located just ventral and lateral to the central canal designated as the intermediomedial cell column which are thought to have an autonomic function (Bok, 1928). The axons of these cells project laterally and divide close to the lateral column nuclei to send branches cranially and caudally. It is suggested that these afferent fibres make synaptic connections with the sympathetic preganglionic neurones although undisputable evidence is lacking (Bok, 1928; Petras & Cummings, 1972; Poljack, 1924). If this suggestion is confirmed this will be the first anatomical description of a complete sympathetic reflex pathway. Petras and Cummings (1972) speculated that the intermediomedial cells act principally in spinal segmental sympathetic reflexes whereas the cells of laminae IV, V and VI in the dorsal horn probably relay afferent activity to supraspinal regions.

Central Inputs (Figure 2)

These are those which originate within the brain. Both sympathoexcitatory and sympathoinhibitory pathways descend from the brainstem, but unfortunately the origin of these fibres is not established. The stimulation and recording electrophysiological studies of Gebber, Taylor and Weaver (1973) and Henry and Calaresu (1974a, 1974b, 1974c, 1974d) are somewhat equivocal on this point but support the notion that the origin of medullary sympathoexcitatory pathways is in the lateral portion of the medullary reticular formation. Some fibres originate in the hypothalamus and traverse the medulla on its most ventral border (Loewy et al., 1973; Senapati, 1966) and join the other descending sympathoexcitatory pathways in the lateral funiculus of the spinal cord (Coote & Macleod, 1972, 1974; Foreman & Wurster, 1973, 1975; Illert & Gabriel, 1972; Kell & Hoff, 1952; Kerr, 1975). Sympathoinhibitory pathways probably originate in the ventromedial reticular formation, in the caudal raphe nuclei of the lower brainstem and in the ventrolateral portion of the medulla as well as from the hypothalamus (Alexander, 1946; Chen et al., 1939; Coote & Downman, 1969; Coote et al., 1969; Coote & Macleod, 1972, 1974, 1975; Gootman & Cohen, 1971; Kahn & Mills, 1967; Kirchner et al., 1971; Neumayr et al., 1974; Prout et al., 1964; Schiebel & Schiebel, 1968; Wang & Brown, 1956b; Wang et al., 1956; Wang & Ranson, 1939). The sympathoinhibitory pathways descend in two main regions of the spinal cord, one localised to the dorsal part of the lateral funiculus (Coote & Macleod, 1974, 1975; Henry & Calaresu, 1974c; Illert & Gabriel, 1972; Lipski & Trzebski, 1975), and the other just ventral and lateral to the ventral horn (Coote & Macleod, 1974, 1975; Dorokhova et al., 1974; Eh & Huan-Ji, 1964; Henry & Calaresu, 1974c; Illert & Gabriel, 1972; Illert & Seller, 1969). Whether these pathways terminate directly on sympathetic preganglionic neurones is unclear. On the one hand a number of studies suggest that descending fibres do not

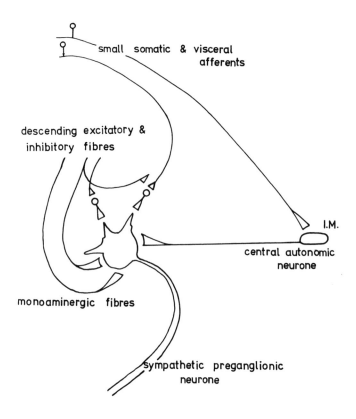

small somatic & visceral
afferents

descending excitatory &
inhibitory fibres

I.M.

central autonomic
neurone

monoaminergic fibres

sympathetic preganglionic
neurone

Figure 2. Diagram based on anatomical and neurophysiological evidence illustrating the connections of peripheral and central inputs to a sympathetic preganglionic neurone in the intermediolateral cell column. IM = intermediomedial nucleus.

terminate on sympathetic preganglionic cells but on interneurones lying close to the intermediolateral cell column although there is still the possibility that synaptic connections are made with dendrites of sympathetic preganglionic cells lying outside the sympathetic nucleus (Kirchner et al., 1971, 1975; Neumayr et al., 1974; Nyberg-Hansen, 1965; Perez-Gonzalez & Coote, 1972; Petras & Cummings, 1972; Rethelyi, 1974; Riedel et al., 1972; Wang & Ranson, 1939; Wurster, 1977). On the other hand, Carlsson et al. (1964), Dahlstrom and Fuxe (1965), and Konishi (1968) using the formaldehyde fluorescent technique for demonstration of monoamines identified abundant terminals of bulbospinal monoaminergic neurones ending close to preganglionic cell bodies and dendrites. The fluorescence disappeared after damaging the descending pathways (Coote & Macleod,

1977; Dahlstrom & Fuxe, 1965). The difference between the two sets
of results is somewhat puzzling although until further evidence is
available a convenient explanation is that the monoamine transmitter
may disappear quite rapidly but degeneration of the small unmyelinated fibres may require a much longer period of time (Riedel et
al., 1972.

   In summary it is evident that both inhibitory and excitatory
pathways from the brainstem converge onto sympathetic preganglionic
neurones. Whether these pathways are multisynaptic in their course
down the spinal cord and whether they terminate directly on the
sympathetic cells or influence them via interneurones located in
closely associated regions of the gray matter are still questions
which need further investigations (Gebber & McCall, 1976; Kirchner
et al., 1975).

   The anatomical features described are illustrated diagrammati-
cally in Figure 1 which has been modified from Petras and Cummings
(1972).

REFLEX PATHWAYS

   Stimulation of spinal afferent nerves conducting below 40 m/sec
causes a change in the activity of sympathetic neurones, mediated
over several central pathways. These are illustrated diagrammati-
cally in Figures 3 and 4.

Excitatory Effects

   Following single shock stimulation of Aβ, Aδ and C fibres of
cutaneous nerves or group II, III and IV fibres of muscle nerves,
at least four reflex waves of excitation in pre- and postganglionic
sympathetic nerves have been described. (1) Early reflex with a
central delay of 6 to 15 msec (Beacham & Perl, 1964; Coote & Downman, 1966; Coote et al., 1969); (2) intermediate reflex with a
central delay of 20 to 30 msec (Foreman, 1975); (3) late reflex
with a central delay of 40 to 50 msec (Coote & Downman, 1966);
(4) very late reflex with a central delay of 300 msec or more
(Coote & Perez-Gonzalez, 1970; Koizumi et al., 1970; Sato, 1972a,
1973; Sato et al., 1969).

   The early reflex persists with unchanged central delay after
cervical spinal cord section indicating that it is a spinal reflex
(Coote & Downman, 1965, 1966; Coote et al., 1969; Sato et al., 1967;
Sato & Terui, 1976). This reflex has been divided into three com-
ponents associated with different types of preganglionic neurone
(Lebedev et al., 1976a, 1976b). According to Lebedev et al. (1976a,

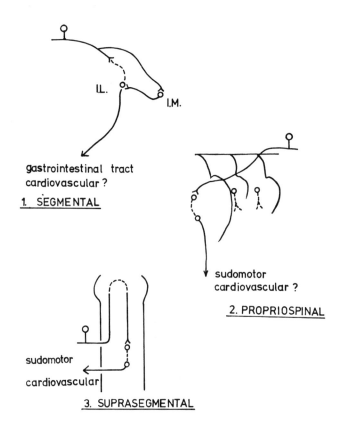

Figure 3.   Diagrams to show the three pathways which can be involved in somatosympathetic reflexes.

1976b), the earliest of these components represents activity which is evoked monosynaptically in sympathetic preganglionic neurones with axons conducting above 10 m/sec which are located in the white matter lateral to the intermediolateral cell column.   Previous esti-mates of central delay, which were too long for monosynaptic excita-tion, were determined from measurements of the conduction time in the sympathetic efferent pathway in ventral roots and white rami which was assured to be the same in the spinal cord (Beacham & Perl, 1964; Coote & Downman, 1965, 1966; Coote et al., 1969).   However, a calculation of the efferent conduction time based on a decreased intraspinal conduction velocity of the preganglionic axon suggested to the Russian workers that monosynaptic excitation was feasible for a small group of preganglionic neurones.   As emphasized earlier, there is as yet no anatomical evidence to support this (Petras & Cummings, 1972; Rethelyi, 1972, 1974; Szentágothai, 1948).

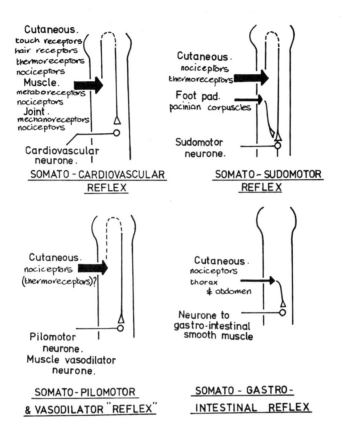

Figure 4. Diagram illustrating the central pathways by which different sympathetic preganglionic neurones are influenced by inputs
from different types of receptor. Thick arrow indicates that the
afferent input may be from anywhere on the body; thin arrow indicates that the input is localised to a specific region of the body.

    The intermediate reflex may also be spinally mediated and in
view of the latency must be dependent on quite long propriospinàl
pathways (Foreman, 1975).

    The late reflex is found by most investigators to depend on a
pathway ascending to and descending from the brainstem (Coote &
Downman, 1966; Iwamura et al., 1969; Kirchner et al., 1970; Sato et
al., 1967; Sato & Schmidt, 1971; Sato et al., 1965; Sell et al.,
1958). However, there is one account in the literature (Khayutin &
Lukoshkova, 1970) which concludes this late reflex is spinally
mediated since it was found to be still present, although somewhat

reduced, following anaemic decerebration. The case is well argued by Khayutin and Lukoshkova (1970) but evidence from such a technique of spinalisation is equivocal and will need better verification before it is acceptable.

The very late reflex in the anaesthetized animal is elicited by the unmyelinated afferent fibres (Coote & Perez-Gonzalez, 1968, 1970; Fussey et al., 1969; Koizumi et al., 1970; Sato et al., 1969). This reflex is mediated supraspinally since it disappears following acute spinal cord section (Coote, 1964; Coote & Downman, 1966; Sato, 1973). Long latency reflexes evoked by unmyelinated afferents do reappear in the spinal animal, but not until some 8 to 12 weeks after spinal cord section in the cat (Sato, 1973) which suggests some growth of synapses is necessary for the mediation of this response after the ascending and descending limbs of the reflex have been removed.

There is also another very late reflex response obtainable on stimulation of the small myelinated fibres which is present only under light chloralose anaesthesia and which is mediated via suprapontine structures (Sato, 1972a).

Apart from some small differences sympathetic preganglionic neurones show similar responses to electrical stimulation of the small myelinated and unmyelinated afferent fibres of both cutaneous and muscle nerves (Koizumi & Brooks, 1972; Sato & Schmidt, 1973).

Visceral afferent fibres may also elicit spinal and supraspinal sympathetic reflexes, and these again are only those fibres conducting below 40 m/sec (Coote, 1964; Franz et al., 1966; Khayutin & Lukoshkova, 1970; Koizumi & Suda, 1963; Kuru, 1965; Sato et al., 1969). Interestingly the central delay of the spinal viscero-visceral reflexes is longer than that of the somatovisceral reflexes (Coote et al., 1969; Franz et al., 1966). Recently EPSPs were recorded in sympathetic preganglionic neurones of the third thoracic segment following electrical stimulation of the visceral afferent fibres in T_3 white ramus (Coote & Westbury, 1977). The shortest latency EPSP observed was 7.0 msec which was some 2 to 3 msec longer than for a somatic afferent input and does not favour masosynaptic connections between visceral afferents and sympathetic preganglionic neurones, at least at this level of the spinal cord.

Participation of Various Sympathetic Preganglionic Neurones
in These Reflexes

It is quite evident from the work of Coote & Downman (1965, 1966) that not all sympathetic neurones are excited via each of the reflex pathways. For example, early or spinal reflexes are only

rarely seen in cardiac and renal sympathetic nerves (Coote & Downman, 1966; Coote & Sato, 1975, 1977), whereas they are commonly
observed in cervical sympathetic nerves (Schmidt & Schönfuss, 1970),
in mesenteric nerves (Khayutin & Lukoshkova, 1970; Koizumi & Suda,
1963) and in all of the white rami (Coote et al, 1969; Sato &
Schmidt, 1973; Sato et al., 1965).

     In a study of the characteristics of individual units in the
cervical sympathetic trunk it was found that out of 534 units only
about 30% responded to somatic afferent nerve stimulation (Janig &
Schmidt, 1970). Fernandez de Molena, Kuno and Perl (1965) and
De Groat and Ryall (1967) were unable to excite by stimulation of
somatic afferent nerves any of the preganglionic neurones from
which they recorded. Hongo and Ryall (1966) found a minority of
preganglionic neurones in T_3 and T_4 segments could be reflexly
activated and recently Coote and Westbury (1977) found that out of
a total of 79 sympathetic preganglionic neurones tested in the
third thoracic segment only 22 neurones could be caused to discharge by supramaximal stimulation of the third intercostal nerve.
Commonly neurones that were reflexly activated were spontaneously
active (Coote & Westbury, 1977; Janig & Schmidt, 1970) but the
reverse was not true. The afferent input may nonetheless converge
onto the sympathetic cells since EPSPs related to the input can be
recorded in them (Coote & Westbury, 1977). Occasionally there may
be sufficient summation of the EPSPs to fire the cell. This suggests that the reflex firing of a sympathetic preganglionic neurone
is dependent on the synchronicity of its excitatory inputs, i.e.,
the afferent volley would have to arrive at the neurone at a time
when it could summate with other excitatory inputs. These features
of sympathetic preganglionic neurones are important since they show
that the central synapses in the somato-sympathetic reflex pathways
differ in their potency, and that for the majority of cells the
major importance of the somatic afferent input is to provide a
background level of excitation to them.

     For those sympathetic neurones that could be reflexly activated
in the anaesthetized cat, Sato (1972b) and Kaufman and Koizumi (1971)
determined to what extent they served as a final common path for the
four different somato-sympathetic reflexes. Only 8% showed all four
reflexes, 18% responded only with an early reflex, 34% showed early
and late reflexes and 48% showed only late or very late reflexes.

     As a result of recent work some light can be thrown on the
question to what extent this great variety of reflex response pattern of preganglionic neurones reflects their different functional
roles and their destination to different effector organs. For example, the fact that reflex discharge into cardiac and renal sympathetic nerves is of the long latency variety involving suprasegmental pathways may be indicative that cardiovascular neurones

cannot normally be excited over a spinal segmental pathway (Kerr, 1975; Koizumi & Sato, 1972). In this connection it is interesting that such pathways do exist onto these neurones since spinal reflexes can be evoked in cardiac and renal nerves after complete cord section (Coote & Downman, 1966). This suggests that the spinal segmental pathway is inhibited in the animal with intact neuraxis. This inhibition can be removed by sectioning a descending sympathoinhibitory pathway in the ventral quadrant of the spinal cord (Coote & Sato, 1975, 1977). It looks, therefore, as though the somatic reflex pathway onto functionally different sympathetic preganglionic neurones is differentially affected by this descending inhibition. This suggests that different interneurones are involved in the spinal mediation of the somatic afferent influence on functionally different sympathetic preganglionic neurones.

Sudomotor reflexes have many features similar to the cardiovascular reflexes and it is likely that electrical stimulation of somatic afferent nerves excites sudomotor neurones also only via a suprasegmental pathway (Wang, 1964; Wang & Brown, 1956a; Wang et al., 1956). However, Janig and Rath (1977) have now shown that spinal sudomotor reflexes can be evoked by natural stimulation of receptors in the same limb (pacinian corpuscles of the pads) in cats with intact neuraxis. This opens up the possibility that there may well be other sympathetic reflexes with local sign that up to now have been obscured by electrical stimulation of bundles of afferent nerve fibres.

Spinal sympathetic reflexes are best represented in the sympathetic outflow to the gastrointestinal tract where they are easily elicited by stretch of the viscera or stimulation of mesenteric nerves in the animal with intact neuraxis (Johansson et al., 1968; Johansson & Langston, 1964) or by pinching of the skin over the abdomen (Sato et al., 1975; Sato & Terui, 1976).

Two types of sympathetic neurone, the pilomotor and the vasodilator neurones to skeletal muscle, cannot be reflexly excited by somatic afferent fibres in the anaesthetized cat (Abrahams et al., 1962; Grosse & Janig, 1976), although in the unanaesthetized hypothalamic cat both piloerection and vasodilatation in skeletal muscle occur as part of a defence reaction in response to touching or pinching the skin (Abrahams et al., 1964). It is likely that a suprasegmental pathway mediates this response in these neurones.

These different features of the somatic afferent pathways onto functionally different preganglionic sympathetic neurones suggest a high degree of organisation of the somato-sympathetic reflexes in the spinal cord.

Facilitation in the Somato-Sympathetic Reflex Pathway

Quite marked facilitation of somato-sympathetic reflexes can
be produced in the cat with intact neuraxis, but this is confined
to the late and very late reflexes. Repetitive stimulation of the
small myelinated afferent fibres at 100 Hz to 300 Hz can augment
the reflex discharge recorded from either pre- or postganglionic
sympathetic nerve bundles, by 200 to 300% (Coote & Perez-Gonzalez,
1970; Sato & Schmidt, 1971; Schmidt & Schönfuss, 1970). Such
stimulation not only increases the number of neurones firing but
also their firing rate (Sato, (1972b). The unmyelinated afferent
fibres are much more powerful at producing temporal facilitation.
The very late group IV or C fibre sympathetic reflexes can best be
elicited by the application of stimuli to afferent nerves at intervals of less than 8 sec down to 1 sec (Fedina et al., 1966;
Sato & Schmidt, 1966). Under these conditions each consecutive
unmyelinated afferent volley recruits greater numbers of sympathetic units until after about 10 to 20 stimuli a new stable level
is obtained. Such recruitment and facilitation has been demonstrated in renal nerves (Coote & Perez-Gonzalez, 1970; Fedina et
al., 1966; Koizumi et al., 1970) in lumbar white rami (Sato, 1973),
in the cervical and lumbar sympathetic trunk (Schmidt & Weller,
1970) and in sympathetic postganglionic units in muscle and
cutaneous nerves (Janig et al., 1972; Koizumi & Sato, 1972).

Facilitation seems to be absent or very weak in the spinal
animal (Beacham & Perl, 1964; Coote et al., 1969; Sato, 1972c).
This led Beacham and Perl (1964) to suggest that in the spinal cat
the afferent volley excited all the neurones in the sympathetic
pool with little subliminal fringe. There was some evidence for
this since following a conditioning volley there was 90 to 100%
occlusion of a second test somato-sympathetic reflex. However, we
now know that in the acute spinal animal there are many sympathetic
preganglionic neurones that cannot be caused to discharge by the
segmental afferent volley. Therefore, the interpretation of this
observation of Beacham and Perl (1964) must be limited to a specific group of sympathetic preganglionic neurones, and implies
that for those neurones which are especially affected by the spinal
segmental pathway the synaptic connections have a high potency.

Inhibitory Effects

Stimulation of somatic afferent fibres can inhibit sympathetic
activity via spinal and supraspinal pathways. The majority of
afferent fibres which may produce sympathetic inhibition are the
small myelinated group II and III or Aβ fibres mostly with conduction velocities above 20 m/sec. Numerous experiments have attempted to distinguish these fibres from those eliciting excitatory

effects and have encountered difficulties because when stimulating
with electrical shocks the threshold of the two sorts of afferent
fibres overlaps considerably. What has usually been described,
therefore, is a sympathetic reflex followed by a silent period
most of which results from inhibition (Schmidt & Schönfuss, 1970).
However, inhibition without prior excitation has been reported in
renal sympathetic nerves (Coote & Perez-Gonzalez, 1970), in sympathetic preganglionic neurones of the third thoracic segment of the
spinal cord (Wyszogrodski & Polosa, 1973) and of postganglionic
sympathetic units in muscle nerves (Koizumi & Sato, 1972). Some
unmyelinated afferent fibres can inhibit sympathetic neurones but
they are very selective. Thus Janig, Sato and Schmidt (1972) reported that group IV muscle afferent and cutaneous C fibres could
inhibit a high proportion of postganglionic sympathetic units to
the skin but not those to muscle. Other evidence for a selective
effect of inhibitory afferents comes from the experiments of Sato
(1972c) in which he showed that early spinal reflexes in lumbar
white rami were not so profoundly depressed by these afferent fibres
as the late medullary reflexes. Much of this reflex inhibition of
sympathetic preganglionic neurones is dependent on a pathway ascending to and descending from the brainstem since its duration
and potency are greatly reduced in acute and chronic spinal animals (Beacham & Perl, 1964; Coote et al., 1969; Coote & Perez-
Gonzalez, 1970; Kirchner et al., 1971, 1975; Sato, 1972c; Sato et
al., 1969; Wyszogrodski & Polosa, 1973). Its main effect is
probably occurring at the spinal level, at best on a select population of preganglionic neurones, because both the late medullary
reflex and the early spinal reflex which has occasionally been
recorded in cardiac and renal sympathetic nerves are inhibited by
it (Coote & Sato, 1977).

In the spinal animal the remaining inhibitory effects seem to
be organised in such a fashion that they are most pronounced at the
level of the somatic afferent input (Beacham & Perl, 1964; Coote et
al., 1969; Sato, 1972c). However, there are accessible propriospinal
pathways (Kirchner et al., 1975), since some inhibition of sympathetic activity in the spinal cat can be produced by stimulation of
limb nerves with inputs remote from the sympathetic outflow (Kaufman
et al., 1977; Koizumi & Sato, 1972; Sato, 1972c).

RELATION BETWEEN THE AFFERENT INPUT AND AUTONOMIC EFFECTORS

The question of whether somatic afferent fibres located in
particular dermatomes may evoke specific autonomic reflexes is an
important one, to which we are just beginning to find some answers.
The recent neurophysiological investigations certainly suggest that
such a capability of the afferent fibres should exist. Firstly,
experiments in visceral afferents support this notion. Stimulation

of receptors in the kidney has been shown to cause a decrease in renal blood flow via renal sympathetic nerve activation in the spinal cat (Astrom & Crafoord, 1968; Beacham & Kunze, 1969). Stimulation of some cardiac receptors can cause increases in heart rate and cardiac contractility, and of other receptors, the opposite effects, in spinal animals (Brown & Malliani, 1971; Malliani et al., 1969, 1970, 1971, 1972; Pagani et al., 1974). In these cases the afferent fibres which were stimulated enter the spinal cord in segments closely related to the sympathetic outflow to the organ concerned. Unfortunately, we do not know if these reflex responses were localised only to the organ under study. Studies in man show receptors from sensory fields remote from the effector may evoke specific cardiovascular responses. Thus deep inspiration elicits a vasoconstriction localised to the fingers in normal and spinal man (Gilliat et al., 1947). Afferent fibres in muscle excited by muscle spasm can evoke blood pressure and heart rate increases in spinal man (Corbett et al., 1971).

Somatic afferent inputs to the spinal cord at segments which are remote from the level of sympathetic outflow may also produce quite specific and differentiated sympathetic reflex responses. Thus non-noxious stimulation of the skin anywhere on the body produces an increase in the firing of sympathetic postganglionic units to cutaneous vascular bed but a decrease in the firing of sympathetic postganglionic units to muscle vascular bed. In contrast, noxious stimulation of the skin produces the opposite effect in the two sympathetic efferents (Horeyseck & Janig, 1974a, 1974b). These differential effects of the cutaneous receptors are seen only in animals with brain intact. Another pattern of response is seen in the majority of sympathetic postganglionic vasoconstrictor units to the tail skin. These respond with an increase in activity to both non-noxious and noxious cutaneous stimulation (Grosse & Janig, 1976).

However, a really important finding by Janig and his collaborators has been the identification of reflexes with local sign. Horeyseck and Janig (1974b) showed that noxious mechanical stimulation of toes of the ipsilateral hindfoot suppressed the activity only in sympathetic postganglionic vasoconstrictor units to the skin of the same limb, whereas similar stimulation of contralateral hindfoot or the forefeet had little effect. Similarly, Grosse and Janig (1976) showed that the majority of vasoconstrictor neurones to the tail skin were inhibited by noxious stimulation of the tail skin whereas they were excited by similar stimulation of the skin in other areas of the body. More recently Janig and Rath (1977) have shown that sympathoexcitatory responses in sudomotor neurones also exhibit "local sign". Evidence for this was obtained by recording the electrodermal reflexes from the pads of the feet in cats. These reflexes could be elicited by non-noxious stimulation

of receptors in the pads of each of the hindlimbs but not from any
other area of the body. This specific somato-sympathetic reflex is
localised to one dermatome, but the afferent input from the foot
pads is into segment L7 of the spinal cord whereas the sympathetic
preganglionic neurones supplying the sweat glands of the pads of
the hindlimb in the cat are located in segments T_{12} to L_4 (Langley,
1891, 1894-5; Patton, 1948). Therefore, strong functional connections exist between quite remote spinal cord segments. These experiments establish amongst other things two important principles:
(1) Some somato-sympathetic reflexes display a strong spatial organisation, and (2) a consequence of these powerful synaptic contacts onto sympathetic neurones can occur with somatic afferents
which enter the spinal cord in segments quite different from those
where the relevant sympathetic preganglionic neurones are located.
Both these points were recognised by Beacham and Perl (1964) who
found that a sympathetic unit in T1 white ramus could be inhibited
by squeezing the forelimb whilst another unit did not so respond.
In contrast, the latter unit could be activated by squeezing one
hind paw but this stimulus had no effect on the first unit. They
also showed that there were preganglionic units in one segment
which could be excited at a shorter latency by an afferent input
from an adjacent segment, than by the afferent input of the same
segment.

PHYSIOLOGICAL SIGNIFICANCE OF THE SOMATIC AFFERENT INPUT

     Experiments using electrical stimulation of large numbers of
afferent fibres in peripheral nerves have provided us with valuable
information but this technique is very artificial and may even give
misleading results. More meaningful information is now forthcoming
from studies of the response of effector organs or identified sympathetic postganglionic fibres following natural stimulation of
receptors. Good examples of this approach which has been exploited
for visceral afferent fibres are the studies on the heart by
Malliani and his collaborators (Brown & Malliani, 1971; Malliani et
al., 1969, 1970, 1972; Pagani et al., 1974) and on the kidney by
Beacham and Kunze (1969) and Astrom and Crafoord (1968). However,
it then becomes difficult to determine the pathways of these reflexes in the central nervous system. This has to some extent been
overcome in a recent series of studies on cutaneous inputs by Sato
and his collaborators (Kaufman et al., 1977; Sato, 1975; Sato et
al., 1967, 1975, 1976; Sato & Terui, 1976; Scherrer, 1966) and by
Janig and collaborators (Grosse & Janig, 1976; Horeyseck & Janig,
1974a, 1974b; Janig, 1975; Janig & Rath, 1977).

Cutaneous Afferent Fibres and Their Sympathetic Reflex Effects

The influence of a number of cutaneous receptors has been studied but so far the significance of their reflex effects has to be somewhat speculative.

(1) Nociceptors. In the normal anaesthetized animal with brain intact, mechanical or thermal nociceptive stimulation of the skin excites the sympathetic outflow to the heart (Kaufman et al., 1977) and the vasoconstrictor fibres to muscle and tail skin and the sympathetic fibres to sweat glands of the feet (Grosse & Janig, 1976; Horeyseck & Janig, 1974a, 1974b; Janig & Rath, 1977), and the sympathetic outflow to the gastrointestinal tract (Sato et al., 1975; Sato & Terui, 1976). In contrast, they depress the activity in vasoconstrictor fibres to the skin at least of the hindlimb (Horeyseck & Janig, 1974a, 1974b). The combination of excitation of vasoconstrictor fibres to skeletal muscle and inhibition of those to the skin following cutaneous nociceptive stimulation must be a consequence of the anaesthetic preventing the natural reflex. In the conscious or hypothalamic cat cutaneous nociceptive stimulation produces a defence reaction which includes excitation of the vasoconstrictor to skin and mainly an inhibition of those to muscle (Horeyseck et al., 1976) which is the opposite of that described in the anaesthetized animal.

(2) Cold and Warm Receptors. There is no doubt that stimulation of cutaneous warm and cold receptors in various regions of the body can induce changes in sympathetic outflow consistent with thermoregulation (Hensel, 1973). Stimulation of warm receptors (mainly C fibres) leads to a decrease in sympathetic vasoconstrictor activity to skin and an increase in this activity to the gastrointestinal tract and in the sympathetic supply to sweat glands (Riedel et al., 1972).

Stimulation of cold receptors (mainly Aγ fibres) leads to the opposite effects. The sympathetic outflow to the heart is excited by both types of receptor (Kaufman et al., 1977).

(3) Mechanoreceptors. Stimulation of hair follicle receptors (Aβ and C fibres) produces a decrease in the activity of sympathetic postganglionic vasoconstrictor fibres to muscle but an increase in the vasoconstrictor fibre activity to the skin of the limbs and tail (Grosse & Janig, 1976; Horeyseck & Janig, 1974a, 1974b). They have no effect on sudomotor neurones (Janig & Rath, 1977). Stimulation of Pacinian corpuscles (Aβ fibres) in the foot pads by vibration elicits a very specific sudomotor reflex in the foot pad. Janig and Rath (1977) suggest that such electrodermal reflexes may keep the hairless skin surfaces moist during movements.

Muscle and Joint Afferent Fibres and Their Reflex Effects

Our knowledge of the small myelinated and unmyelinated afferent
fibres in muscle is still rather fragmentary. This group of fibres
comprises some 48 to 75% of the total afferent component of muscle
nerves, yet they have received little attention. Some fibres are
considered to signal nociceptive information since they can be made
to fire following close arterial injections of pain-producing substances (Fock & Mense, 1976; Franz & Mense, 1975; Hiss & Mense, 1976;
Kniffki et al., 1976; Kumazawa & Mizumura, 1976; Mense & Schmidt,
1974).

However, a proportion of these small fibres can be activated
during "nonpainful" contractions of muscles and this effect can be
potentiated by prior occlusion of the blood supply to the muscles
(Coote & Thamer, unpublished observations; Tibes & Groth, 1977),
effects which characterise "exercise" type receptors (Perez-
Gonzalez & Coote, 1972) and not the muscle nociceptors (Kniffki et
al., 1976). It has been suggested that these afferent fibres are
responsible for the cardiovascular and respiratory adjustments seen
at the beginning of muscle contraction or exercise (Asmussen et al.,
1965; Coote et al., 1969, 1971; Fisher & Nutter, 1974; Hnik et al.,
1969; Kao & Ray, 1954; McCloskey & Mitchell, 1972; Mitchell et al.,
1968; Senapati, 1966; Tibes & Groth, 1977; Tibes & Hemmer, 1974;
Tibes et al., 1977). It is thought that the free nerve endings of
some of these afferent fibres, many of which lie close to arterioles
and capillaries (Stacey, 1969), may be metabolic receptors responding to metabolites released into the interstitium by the working
muscles (Coote, 1975; Coote et al., 1971; Hnik et al., 1969; Miza-
mura & Kumazawa, 1976; Perez-Gonzalez & Coote, 1972; Ramsay, 1955,
1959; Stegemann & Kenner, 1971; Tibes & Groth, 1977; Wildenthal et
al., 1968). However, more evidence is required before we can substantiate this hypothesis (Figure 5).

Natural stimulation confined to joint receptors has been shown
to elicit reflex cardiovascular and respiratory adjustments similar
but smaller than those elicited by muscle contraction (Barron &
Coote, 1973; Bilge et al., 1963; Comroe & Schmidt, 1943; Flandrois
et al., 1966, 1967). The articular receptors which are most likely
to be responsible were identified as the small myelinated and unmyelinated endings of the group III (conduction velocity 24-4 m/sec)
and IV (conduction velocity < 2.0 m/sec) nerve fibres (Barron &
Coote, 1973) which belong to the type IV receptors described by
Freeman and Wyke (1967). Many of these small fibres are associated
with ligaments and tendons of the joint although they are particularly dense in the intra- and extra-articular fat pad and fibrous
capsule (Figure 6). They comprise a high proportion of the afferent
fibre population of articular nerve yet we know little of their
properties. Nonetheless, it is likely that some of the small nerve
endings are mechanoreceptors stimulated by joint movement.

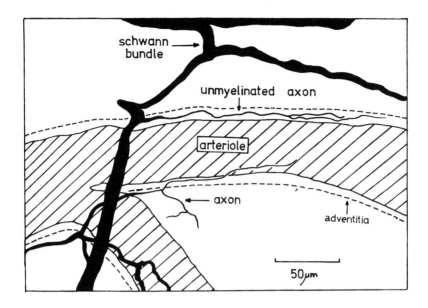

Figure 5.   Drawing slightly modified from a photomicrograph (Figure 20, Stacey, 1969) showing free nerve endings lying close to an
arteriole in a de-efferented and sympathectomised skeletal muscle.

SUMMARY AND CONCLUSIONS

Recent work on the location and synaptic connections of sympathetic preganglionic neurones has gone some way to identify clearly
the neuronal elements that form part of the sympathetic reflex arc.
Both segmental and intersegmental polysynaptic connections can be
described but we are still not able to identify with certainty the
interneurones by which somatic afferent fibres synapsing in the
dorsal horn make connections with the sympathetic preganglionic
neurone, although cells of lamina V or cells in the intermediomedial
nucleus are strong candidates.   Electrophysiological experiments
show that onto some sympathetic neurones, shorter and more powerful
pathways converge from adjacent or even more remote segments than do
from the same segment.   These pathways provide the basic circuit for
strong functional connections between specific receptors and functionally discrete preganglionic neurones.

As well as these spinal reflex pathways, sympathetic neurones
may be reflexly influenced by afferent pathways ascending to and

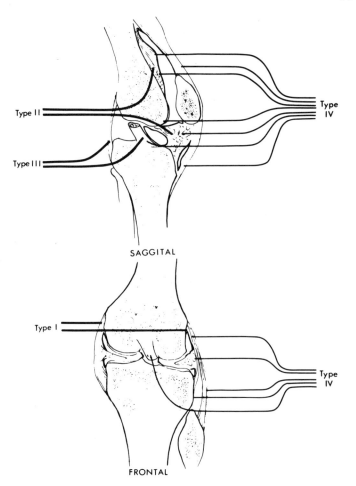

Figure 6.   Diagram illustrating the innervation of the knee joint.
The small myelinated and unmyelinated afferent fibres from the
population of type IV receptors which lie in similar regions of the
joint to the well established mechanoreceptors of type I, II and III.

descending from the brainstem.   The afferent limb of such suprasegmental somato-sympathetic reflexes ascends in the dorsal part
of the lateral funiculus.   This is a region containing axons from
cells in Lamina IV and V of the dorsal horn destined for the
brainstem and thalamus.

     Descending inhibitory and excitatory pathways from various
regions of the brainstem converge onto sympathetic preganglionic

neurones or nearby interneurones and may profoundly influence the excitability of the somato-sympathetic reflex pathways.

Not all sympathetic preganglionic neurones are similarly influenced by stimulation of somatic afferent nerves or by natural stimulation of specific receptors. Many cells do not discharge in response to a synaptic input because there is insufficient summation, illustrating there is different synaptic potency amongst the cell population. Some cells may be excited whilst others are inhibited. For example, vasoconstrictor neurones supplying muscle were excited whereas vasoconstrictor neurones to skin were inhibited following stimulation of hair follicle receptors.

Sympathetic preganglionic neurones can be inhibited or excited over both spinal and supraspinal pathways. The extent to which one is favoured may be determined by the dominance of supraspinal excitatory or inhibitory influence. It is also partly dependent on the function of the neurone and partly on the stimulus. Thus for those neurones supplying the smooth muscle of the gastrointestinal tract the segmental pathway is the more powerful, whereas for cardiovascular and sudomotor neurones often the suprasegmental pathway is preferred. Even so, specific spinal reflexes can be elicited in these neurones by stimulation of particular receptors. An example is the sudomotor reflex elicited by stimulation of pacinian corpuscles of the foot pads. Also occasionally spinal somato-cardiovascular reflexes can be evoked probably because of a decreased effect of a descending inhibitory system which normally prevents the spinal reflex. One can conclude that where somato-sympathetic reflexes are very specific then they are mediated over spinal reflex pathways, but if the stimulus is indicative of a more widespread disturbance, then the supraspinal pathway is favoured; then the afferent volley which is long circuited to medullary or supramedullary regions enables the elaboration of a pattern of sympathetic and somatic response appropriate to the locus and intensity of the stimulus. In this case the response of some sympathetic neurones to the afferent input may be the opposite to that elicited through the spinal reflex pathway. There is, therefore, a very specific organisation of the sympathetic nervous system at different levels of the neuraxis. Changes in the influence of these different levels on the sympathetic preganglionic neurone could well lead to altered autonomic motor responses.

REFERENCES

ABRAHAMS, V. C., S. M. HILTON, and J. L. MALCOLM. Sensory connections to the hypothalamus and midbrain and their role in the reflex activation of the defence reaction. *J. Physiol.* 164: 1-16, 1962.

ABRAHAMS, V. C., S. M. HILTON, and A. W. ZBROŻYNA. The role of active muscle vasodilatation in the alerting stage of the defence reaction. *J. Physiol., London* 171:189-202, 1964.

ALEXANDER, R. S. Tonic and reflex function of medullary sympathetic cardiovascular centers. *J. Neurophysiol.* 9:205-217, 1946.

ASMUSSEN, E., S. JOHANSEN, M. JORGENSEN, and M. NIELSON. On the nervous factors controlling respiration and circulation during exercise. Curarization experiments. *Acta Physiol. Scand.* 63:343-350, 1965.

ASTROM, A., and J. CRAFOORD. Afferent and efferent activity in renal nerves in cats. *Acta Physiol. Scand.* 74:69-78, 1968.

BARRON, W., and J. H. COOTE. The contribution of articular receptors to cardiovascular reflexes elicited by passive limb movement. *J. Physiol., London* 235:423-436, 1973.

BEACHAM, W. S., and D. L. KUNZE. Renal receptors evoking a spinal vasomotor reflex. *J. Physiol.* 201:73-85, 1969.

BEACHAM, W. S., and E. R. PERL. Background and reflex discharge of sympathetic preganglionic neurones in the spinal cat. *J. Physiol.* 172:400-416, 1964.

BEACHAM, W. S., and E. R. PERL. Characteristics of a spinal sympathetic reflex. *J. Physiol.* 173:431-448, 1964.

BILGE, M., T. VELIDEDEOGLU, and M. TERZIOGLU. Variations in respiration induced by passive movements of the hind limbs of the anaesthetized cat. *New. Instambal. Contr. Clin. Sci.* 6:3-19, 1963.

BOK, S. T. Das Rückenmark. In: *Handbuch der mikroscopischen Anatomie des Menschen*, edited by W. von Mollendorf. Berlin: Springer, 1928, 4:478-578.

BROWN, A. G. The spinocervical tract: Organisation and neuronal morphology. In: *Int. Symp. Sensory functions of the skin in primates*, edited by Y. Zotterman. Oxford: Pergamon, 1976, p. 91-103.

BROWN, A. M., and A. MALLIANI. Spinal sympathetic reflexes initiated by coronary receptors. *J. Physiol., London* 212:685-706, 1971.

BRYAN, R. N., D. L. TREVINO, J. D. COULTER, and W. D. WILLIS. Location and somatotopic organization of the cells of origin of the spinocervical tract. *Exptl. Brain Res.* 17:177-189, 1973.

CARLSSON, A., B. FALCK, K. FUXE, and N. A. HILLARP. Cellular locali-
    zation of monoamines in the spinal cord. *Acta Physiol. Scand.*
    60:112-119, 1964.

CHEN, M. P., R.K.S. LIM, S. C. WANG, and C. L. YI. On the question
    of a myelincephalic sympathetic centre. IV. Experimental
    localization of its descending pathway. *Chinese J. Physiol.*
    11:385-408, 1939.

CHUNG, J. M., K. CHUNG, and R. D. WURSTER. Sympathetic preganglionic
    neurons of the cat spinal cord: horseradish peroxidase study.
    Brain Res. 91:126-131, 1975.

CHUNG, J. M., and R. D. WURSTER. Localization of ascending de-
    pressor pathways in the cat spinal cord. *Federation Proc.*
    34:407, 1975.

CHUNG, J. M., and R. D. WURSTER. Ascending pressor and depressor
    pathways in the cat spinal cord. *Clin. J. Physiol.* 231:786-
    792, 1976.

COMROE, J. H., and C. F. SCHMIDT. Reflexes from the limbs as a
    factor in the hyperpnoea of muscular exercise. *Am. J. Physiol.*
    138:536-547, 1943.

COOTE, J. H. Properties of spinal autonomic reflex arcs and their
    comparison with somatic arcs. Ph.D. Thesis. Royal Free Hos-
    pital School of Medicine, London, 1964.

COOTE, J. H. Physiological significance of somatic afferent path-
    ways from skeletal muscle and joints with reflex effects on the
    heart and circulation. *Brain Res.* 87:139-144, 1975.

COOTE, J. H., and C.B.B. DOWNMAN. Comparison of reflex volleys in
    white ramus and postganglionic pathways. *J. Physiol.* 181:
    37-38P, 1965.

COOTE, J. H., and C.B.B. DOWNMAN. Central pathways of some auto-
    nomic reflex discharges. *J. Physiol.* 183:714-729, 1966.

COOTE, J. H., and C.B.B. DOWNMAN. Supraspinal control of reflex
    activity in renal nerves. *J. Physiol., London* 202:147-160,
    1969.

COOTE, J. H., C.B.B. DOWNMAN, and W. V. WEBER. Reflex discharges
    into thoracic white rami elicited by somatic and visceral af-
    ferent excitation. *J. Physiol., London* 202:147-160, 1969.

COOTE, J. H., S. M. HILTON, and J. F. PEREZ-GONZALEZ. Muscle affer-
    ents responsible for the pressor response to exercise. *J.
    Physiol.* 201:34-35P, 1969.

COOTE, J. H., S. M. HILTON, and J. F. PEREZ-GONZALEZ. The reflex
    nature of the pressor response to muscular exercise. *J.
    Physiol., London* 215:789-804, 1971.

COOTE, J. H., and V. H. MACLEOD. The possibility that noradrenaline
    is a sympathoinhibitory transmitter in the spinal cord. *J.
    Physiol., London* 225:44-46P, 1972.

COOTE, J. H., and V. H. MACLEOD. The influence of bulbospinal
    monoaminergic pathways on sympathetic nerve activity. *J.
    Physiol., London* 241:453-475, 1974.

COOTE, J. H., and V. H. MACLEOD. The spinal route of sympatho-
    inhibitory pathways descending from the medulla oblongata.
    Pflügers Arch. 359:335-347, 1975.

COOTE, J. H., and V. H. MACLEOD. The effect of intraspinal micro-
    injections of 6 hydroxydopamine on the inhibitory influence
    exerted on spinal sympathetic activity by the baroreceptors.
    Pflügers Arch. 1977. In press.

COOTE, J. H., and J. F. PEREZ-GONZALEZ. The response of some sym-
    pathetic neurones to volleys in various afferent nerves. *J.
    Physiol., London* 197:25-26P, 1968.

COOTE, J. H., and J. F. PEREZ-GONZALEZ. The response of some sym-
    pathetic neurones to volleys in various afferent nerves. *J.
    Physiol., London* 208:261-278, 1970.

COOTE, J. H., and A. SATO. A role for a descending sympatho-
    inhibitory pathway in the ventral part of the spinal cord. *J.
    Physiol.* 252:21-22P, 1975.

COOTE, J. H., and A. SATO. Supraspinal regulation of spinal reflex
    discharge into cardiac sympathetic nerves. *Brain Res.* 1977.
    In press.

COOTE, J. H., and D. R. WESTBURY. Properties of sympathetic pre-
    ganglionic neurones located in the third thoracic segment of
    the spinal cord. *J. Physiol.* 1977. In press.

CORBETT, J. L., H. L. FRANKEL, and P. J. HARRIS. Cardiovascular
    changes associated with skeletal muscle spasm in tetraplegic
    man. *J. Physiol.* 215:381-393, 1971.

DAHLSTROM, A., and K. FUXE. Evidence for the existence of mono-
    amine neurones in the central nervous system. II. Experi-
    mentally induced changes in intraneuronal amine levels of
    bulbospinal neuron systems. *Acta Physiol. Scand.* 62. Suppl.
    247:5-36, 1965.

DeGROAT, W. C., and R. W. RYALL.   An excitatory action of 5 hydroxy-
    tryptamine on sympathetic preganglionic neurones. *Exp. Brain
    Res.* 3:299-305, 1967.

DOROKHOVA, M. I., O. S. MEDVEDEV, Y. A. REZNIKOVA, and V. A. TSYRLIN.
    Some data on the presence of inhibitory vasomotor control at
    the spinal level. *Biull. Eksp. Biol. Med.* 77:3-6, 1974.

EARLE, K. M.   The tract of Lissauer and its possible relation to the
    pain pathway. *J. Comp. Neurol.* 96:93-111, 1952.

EH, S., and D. HUAN-JI.   The descending pathways of the bulbar
    cardiovascular centre. *Acta Physiol. Sinica.* 27:108-114, 1964.

FEDINA, L., A. Y. KATUNSKII, V. M. KHAYUTIN, and A. MITSANYI.   Re-
    sponse of renal sympathetic nerves to stimulation of afferent
    A and C fibres of tibial and mesenterial nerves. *Acta Physiol.
    Acad. Sci. Hung.* 29:157-176, 1966.

FERNANDEZ DE MOLENA, A., M. KUNO, and E. R. PERL.   Antidromically
    evoked responses from sympathetic preganglionic neurones. *J.
    Physiol., London* 180:321-335, 1965.

FIELDS, H. L., G. A. MEYER, and L. D. PARTRIDGE, SR.   Convergence
    of visceral and somatic input onto spinal neurons. *Expt.
    Neurol.* 26:36-52, 1970.

FIELDS, H. L., L. D. PARTRIDGE, JR., and D. L. WURSTER.   Somatic
    and visceral receptive field properties of fibres in ventral
    quadrant white matter of the cat spinal cord. *J. Neurophysiol.*
    33:827-837, 1970.

FIELDS, H. L., and D. L. WINTER.   Somato visceral pathway: Rapidly
    conducting fibers in the spinal cord. *Science* 167:1729-1730,
    1970.

FISHER, M. L., and D. O. NUTTER.   Cardiovascular reflex adjustments
    to static muscular contractions in the canine hind limb. *Am.
    J. Physiol.* 226:648-655, 1974.

FLANDROIS, R., J. R. LACOUR, J. ISLAS-MAROQUIN, and J. CHARLOT.
    Essai de mise en evidence d'un stimulus neurogenique articulaire
    de la ventilation lors de l'exercise musculaire chez le chien.
    J. Physiol,, Paris 58:222-223, 1966.

FLANDROIS, R., J. R. LACOUR, J. ISLAS-MAROQUIN, and J. CHARLOT.
    Limb mechanoreceptors inducing the reflex hyperpnoea of exer-
    cise. *Resp. Physiol.* 2:335-343, 1967.

FOCK, S., and S. MENSE. Excitatory effects of 5 hydroxytryptamine histamine and potassium ions on muscular group IV afferent units: a comparison with bradykinin. *Brain Res.* 105:459–469, 1976.

FOREMAN, R. D. Conduction in descending spinal pathways initiated by somato-sympathetic reflexes. *Clin. J. Physiol.* 228:905–908, 1975.

FOREMAN, R. D., R. F. SCHMIDT, and W. D. WILLIS. Convergence of muscle and cutaneous input onto primate spinothalamic tract neurons. *Brain Res.* 124:555–560, 1977.

FOREMAN, R. D., and R. D. WURSTER. Localization and functional characteristics of descending sympathetic spinal pathways. *Clin. J. Physiol.* 225:212–217, 1973.

FOREMAN, R. D., and R. D. WURSTER. Conduction in descending spinal pathways initiated by somato-sympathetic reflexes. *Am. J. Physiol.* 228:905–908, 1975.

FRANZ, D. N., M. H. EVANS, and E. R. PERL. Characteristics of viscero-sympathetic reflexes in the spinal cat. *Am. J. Physiol.* 211:1292–1298, 1966.

FRANZ, M., and S. MENSE. Muscle receptors with group IV afferent fibres responding to application of bradykinin. *Brain Res.* 92:369–383, 1975.

FREEMAN, M.A.R., and B. WYKE. The innervation of the knee joint. An anatomical and histological study in the cat. *J. Anat., London* 101:505–532, 1967.

FUSSEY, I., C. KIDD, and J. G. WHITWAM. Evoked activity in efferent sympathetic nerves in response to peripheral nerve stimulation in the dog. *J. Physiol., London* 200:77–78P, 1969.

GAGEL, O. Zur Histologie und Topographie der vegetativen Zentren im Rüchenmark. *Z. f. Anat. u Entwicklungsgesch.* 85:213–250, 1932.

GEBBER, G. L., and R. B. McCALL. Identification and discharge patterns of spinal sympathetic interneurons. *Am. J. Physiol.* 231:722–733, 1976.

GEBBER, G. L., D. G. TAYLOR, and L. C. WEAVER. Electrophysiological studies on organization of central vasopressor pathways. *Am. J. Physiol.* 224:470–481, 1973.

GILLIAT, R. W., L. GUTTMAN, and D. WHITTERIDGE. Inspiratory vasoconstriction in patients after spinal injuries. *J. Physiol.*
107:67-75, 1947.

GOOTMAN, P. M., and M. I. COHEN. Evoked splanchnic potentials produced by electrical stimulation of medullary vasomotor regions.
Exp. Brain Res. 13:1-14, 1971.

GROSSE, M., and W. JANIG. Vasoconstrictor and pilomotor fibres in
skin nerves to the cat's tail. *Pflügers Arch.* 361:221-229,
1976.

HENRY, J. L., and F. R. CALARESU. Topography and numerical distribution of neurons of the thoraco-lumbar intermediolateral
muscles in the cat. *J. Comp. Neurol.* 144:205-214, 1972.

HENRY, J. L., and F. R. CALARESU. Responses of single units in the
intermediolateral nucleus to stimulation of cardioregulatory
medullary nuclei in the cat. *Brain Res.* 77:314-319, 1974a.

HENRY, J. L., and F. R. CALARESU. Excitatory and inhibitory inputs
from medullary nuclei projecting to spinal cardioacceleratory
neurons in the cat. *Exp. Brain Res.* 20:485-504, 1974b.

HENRY, J. L., and F. R. CALARESU. Pathways from medullary nuclei
to spinal cardioacceleratory neurons in the cat. *Exp. Brain
Res.* 20, 505-514, 1974c.

HENRY, J. L., and F. R. CALARESU. Origin and course of crossed
medullary pathways to spinal sympathetic neurons in the cat.
Exp. Brain Res. 20:515-526, 1974d.

HENSEL, H. Neural processes in thermoregulation. *Physiol. Rev.*
53:948-1017, 1973.

HISS, E., and S. MENSE. Evidence for the existence of different
receptor sites for algesic agents at the endings of muscular
group IV afferent units. *Pflügers Arch.* 362:141-146, 1976.

HNIK, P., O. HUDLICKA, J. KUCERA, and R. PAYNE. Activation of
muscle afferents by nonproprioceptive stimuli. *Am. J. Physiol.*
217:1451-1457, 1969.

HOREYSECK, G., and W. JANIG. Reflexes within postganglionic fibres
within skin and muscle nerves after mechanical non-noxious
stimulation of skin. *Exp. Brain Res.* 20:115-123, 1974a.

HOREYSECK, G., and W. JANIG. Reflexes in postganglionic fibres
within skin and muscle nerves after noxious stimulation of skin.
Exp. Brain Res. 20:125-134, 1974b.

HOREYSECK, G., W. JANIG, F. KIRCHNER, and V. THAMER. Activation and inhibition of muscle and cutaneous postganglionic neurones to hindlimb during hypothalamically induced vasoconstriction and atropine sensitive vasodilation. *Pflügers Arch.* 361: 231-240, 1976.

HONGO, T., E. JANKOWSKA, and A. LUNDBERG. Postsynaptic excitation and inhibition from primary afferents in neurones in the spinocervical tract. *J. Physiol., London* 199:569-592, 1968.

HONGO, T., and R. W. HYALL. Electrophysiological and microelectrophoretic studies on sympathetic preganglionic neurones in the spinal cord. *Acta Physiol. Scand.* 68:96-104, 1966.

ILLERT, M., and M. GABRIEL. Descending pathways in the cervical cord of cats affecting blood pressure and sympathetic acitivity. *Pflügers Arch.* 335:109-124, 1972.

ILLERT, M., and H. SELLER. A descending sympatho-inhibitory tract in the ventrolateral column of the cat. *Pflügers Arch.* 313: 343-360, 1969.

IWAMURA, Y., Y. UCHINO, S. OZAWA, and N. KUDO. Excitatory and inhibitory components of somato-sympathetic reflex. *Brain Res.* 16:351-358, 1969.

JANIG, W. Central organization of somato-sympathetic reflexes in vasoconstrictor neurones. *Brain Res.* 87:305-312, 1975.

JANIG, W., and B. RATH. Electrodermal reflexes in the cat's paws elicited by natural stimulation of skin. *Pflügers Arch.* 369: 27-32, 1977.

JANIG, W., A. SATO, and R. F. SCHMIDT. Reflexes in postganglionic cutaneous fibres by stimulation of group I to group IV somatic afferents. *Pflügers Arch.* 331:244-256, 1972.

JANIG, W., and R. F. SCHMIDT. Single unit responses in the cervical sympathetic trunk upon somatic nerve stimulation. *Arch. Ges. Physiol.* 314:199-216, 1970.

JOHANSSON, B. Circulatory responses to stimulation of somatic afferents. *Acta Physiol. Scand.* 57. Suppl. 198:1-92, 1962.

JOHANSSON, B., O. JOHSSON, and B. LYUNG. Tonic supraspinal mechanisms influencing the intestino-intestinal inhibitory reflex. *Acta Physiol. Scand.* 72:200-204, 1968.

JOHANSSON, B., and J. B. LANGSTON. Reflex influence of mesenteric afferents in renal, intestinal and muscle blood flow and on intestinal motility. *Acta Physiol. Scand.* 61:400-412, 1964.

KAHN, N., and E. MILLS. Centrally evoked sympathetic discharge: a functional study of medullary vasomotor areas. *J. Physiol., London* 191:339-352, 1967.

KAO, F. F., and L. H. RAY. Respiratory and circulatory responses of anaesthetized dogs to increased muscular work. *Am. J. Physiol.* 179:249-255, 1954.

KAUFMAN, A., and K. KOIZUMI. Spontaneous and reflex activity of single units in lumbar white rami. In: *Research in Physiology. A Liber Memorialis in honor of Professor C. M. Brooks,* edited by F. F. Kao, M. Vassalle, and K. Koizumi. Bologna: Aulo Gaggi, 1971, p. 469-481.

KAUFMAN, A., A. SATO, Y. SATO, and H. SUGIMOTO. Reflex changes in heart rate after mechanical and thermal stimulation of the skin at various segmental levels in cats. *Neuroscience* 2: 103-109, 1977.

KELL, J. F., and E. C. HOFF. Descending spinal pathways mediating pressor responses of cerebral origin. *J. Neurophysiol.* 15: 229-311, 1952.

KERR, F.W.L. Neuroanatomical substrates of nociception in the spinal cord. *Pain* 1:325-356, 1975.

KERR, F.W.L., and S. ALEXANDER. Descending autonomic pathways in the spinal cord. *Arch. Neurol. Psychiat., Chicago* 10:249-261, 1964.

KHAYUTIN, V. M., and E. V. LUKOSHKOVA. Spinal mediation of vasomotor reflexes in animals with intact brain studied by electrophysiological methods. *Pflügers Arch.* 321:197-222, 1970.

KIRCHNER, F., A. SATO, and H. WEIDINGER. Central pathways of reflex discharges in the cervical sympathetic trunk. *Pflügers Arch.* 319:1-11, 1970.

KIRCHNER, F., A. SATO., and H. WEIDINGER. Bulbar inhibition of spinal and supraspinal sympathetic reflex discharges. *Pflügers Arch.* 326:324-333, 1971.

KIRCHNER, F., I. WYSZOGRODSKI, and C. POLOSA. Some properties of sympathetic neuron inhibition by depressor area and intraspinal stimulation. *Pflügers Arch.* 357:349-360, 1975.

KNIFFKI, K. D., S. MENSE, and R. F. SCHMIDT. Mechanisms of muscle pain: a comparison with cutaneous nociception. In: *Sensory Functions of the Skin,* edited by Y. Zotterman. Oxford: Pergamon, 1976, 27:463–473.

KOIZUMI, K., and C. M. BROOKS. The integration of autonomic system reactions: A discussion of autonomic reflexes, their control and their association with somatic reaction. *Ergeb der Physiol.* 67:1–68, 1972.

KOIZUMI, K., R. KOLLIN, A. KAUFMAN, and C. M. BROOKS. Contribution of unmyelinated afferent excitation to sympathetic reflexes. *Brain Res.* 20:99–106, 1970.

KOIZUMI, K., and A. SATO. Reflex activity of single sympathetic fibres to skeletal muscle produced by electrical stimulation of somatic and vagodepressor afferent nerves. *Pflügers Arch.* 332:283–301, 1972.

KOIZUMI, K., H. SELLER, A. KAUFMAN, and C. M. BROOKS. Pattern of sympathetic discharges and their relation to baroreceptor and respiratory activities. *Brain Res.* 27:281–294, 1971.

KOIZUMI, K., and I. SUDA. Induced modulations in autonomic efferent neuron activity. *Am. J. Physiol.* 205:738–744, 1963.

KONISHI, M. Fluorescence microscopy of the spinal cord of the dog with special reference to the autonomic lateral horn cells. *Arch. Histol. Jap.* 30:33–44, 1968.

KUMAZAWA, T., and K. MIZUMURA. The polymodal C-fibre receptor in the muscle of the dog. *Brain Res.* 101:589–593, 1976.

KUMAZAWA, T., and E. R. PERL. Differential excitation of dorsal horn and substantia gelatinosa marginal neurons by primary afferent units with fine (Aδ and C) fibers. In Int. Symp.: *Sensory Functions of the Skin in Primates,* edited by Y. Zotterman. Oxford: Pergamon, 1976, p. 67–87.

KURU, M. Nervous control of micturition. *Physiol. Rev.* 45:425–494, 1965.

LANGLEY, J. N. On the course and connections of the secretory fibers supplying the sweat glands of the feet of the cat. *J. Physiol., London* 12:347–374, 1891.

LANGLEY, J. N. Further observations on the secretory and vasomotor fibers of the foot of the cat. *J. Physiol., London* 17:296–314, 1894-5.

LARUELLE, L.   Contribution a l'étude du nevrexe vegetatif. *Comp. Rend. Assoc. Anat.* 31:210-229, 1936.

LEBEDEV, V. P., V. I. PETROV, and V. A. SKOBELEV. Antidromic discharges of sympathetic preganglionic neurons located outside of the spinal cord lateral horns. *Neuroscience Letters* 2: 325-329, 1976a.

LEBEDEV, V. P., N. N. ROSANOV, V. A. SKOBELEV, and K. A. SMIRNOV. Study of the early somato-sympathetic reflex response. *Neuroscience Letters* 2:319-323, 1976b.

LIPSKI, J., and A. TRZEBSKI. Bulbospinal neurones activated by baroreceptor afferents and their possible role in inhibition of preganglionic sympathetic neurons. *Pflügers Arch.* 356: 181-192, 1975.

LOEWY, A. D., J. C. ARAUJO, and F.W.L. KERR. Pupillodilator pathway in the brainstem of the cat: Anatomical and electrophysiological identification of a central autonomic pathway. *Brain Res.* 60:65-91, 1973.

MALLIANI, A., M. PAGANI, G. RECORDATI, and P. J. SCHWARTZ. Evidence for spinal sympathetic regulation of cardiovascular functions. *Experientia* 26:965-966, 1970.

MALLIANI, A., M. PAGANI, G. RECORDATI, and P. J. SCHWARTZ. Spinal sympathetic reflexes elicited by increases in arterial blood pressure. *Am. J. Physiol.* 220:128-134, 1971.

MALLIANI, A., D. F. PETERSON, V. S. BISHOP, and A. M. BROWN. Spinal sympathetic cardiocardiac reflexes. *Circ. Res.* 30: 158-166, 1972.

MALLIANI, A., P. J. SCHWARTZ, and A. ZANCHETTI. A sympathetic reflex elicited by experimental coronary occlusion. *Am. J. Physiol.* 217:703-709, 1969.

MANNARD, A., P. RAJCHGOT, and C. POLOSA. Effect of post impulse depression on background firing of sympathetic preganglionic neurons. *Brain Res.* 126:243-262, 1977.

McCLOSKEY, D. I., and J. H. MITCHELL. Reflex carciovascular and respiratory responses originating on exercising muscle. *J. Physiol., London* 224:173-186, 1972.

MENSE, S., and R. F. SCHMIDT. Activation of group IV afferent units from muscle by algesic agents. *Brain Res.* 72:305-310, 1974.

MITCHELL, J. H., D. S. MIERZWIAK, K. WILDENTHAL, W. D. WILLIS, and
    A. M. SMITH. Effect on left ventricular performance of stimu-
    lation of an afferent nerve from muscle. *Circ. Res.* 32:507-
    516, 1968.

MIZUMURA, K., and T. KUMAZAWA. Reflex respiratory response induced
    by chemical stimulation of muscle afferents. *Brain Res.* 109:
    402-406, 1976.

NEUMAYR, R. J., B. D. HARE, and D. N. FRANZ. Evidence for bulbo-
    spinal control of sympathetic preganglionic neurons by mono-
    aminergic pathways. *Life Sci.* 14:793-806, 1974.

NYBERG-HANSEN, R. J. Sites and mode of termination of reticulo-
    spinal fibers in the cat. *J. Comp. Neurol.* 124:71-99, 1965.

PAGANI, M., P. J. SCHWARTZ, R. BANKS, F. LOMBARDI, and A. MALLIANI.
    Reflex responses of sympathetic preganglionic neurones
    initiated by different cardiovascular receptors in spinal
    animals. *Brain Res.* 68:215-225, 1974.

PATTON, H. D. Secretory innervation of the cat's foot pad. *J.
    Neurophysiol.* 11:211-227, 1948.

PEREZ-GONZALEZ, J. F., and J. H. COOTE. Activity of muscle affer-
    ents and reflex circulatory responses to exercise. *Am. J.
    Physiol.* 223:138-143, 1972.

PETRAS, J. M., and J. F. CUMMINGS. Autonomic neurons in the spinal
    cord of the rhesus monkey: A correlation of the findings of
    cytoarchitectonics and sympathectomy with fiber degeneration
    following dorsal rhizotomy. *J. Comp. Neurol.* 146:189-218,
    1972.

PICK, J. *The Autonomic Nervous System.* Philadelphia: Lippincott,
    1970.

POLJACK, S. Die Struktureigentümlichkeiten des Ruckermarkes beiden
    Chiropteren. Zugleich ein Beitrag zu der Frage uber die
    spinalen Zentren des Sympatheticus. *Z. f. Anat. U. Entwick-
    lungsgesch.* 74:509-576, 1924.

POLOSA, C. Silent period of sympathetic preganglionic neurons.
    Can. J. Physiol. Pharmacol. 45:1033-1045, 1967.

POMERANZ, B., P. D. WALL, and W. V. WEBER. Cord cells responding
    to fine myelinated afferents from viscera, muscle and skin.
    J. Physiol., London 199:511-532, 1968.

PROUT, B. J., J. H. COOTE, and C.B.B. DOWNMAN. Supraspinal inhibi-
    tion of a cutaneous vascular reflex in the cat. *Am. J. Physiol.*
    207:303-307, 1964.

RAMSAY, A. G. Muscle metabolism and the regulation of breathing.
    J. Physiol., London 127, 30P, 1955.

RAMSAY, A. G. Effect of metabolism and anaesthesia on pulmonary
    ventilation. *J. Appl. Physiol.* 14:102-104, 1959.

RANSON, S. W. The course within the spinal cord of the non-
    medullated fibers of the spinal dorsal roots: a study of
    Lissauer's tract in the cat. *J. Comp. Neurol.* 23:259-274,
    1913.

RANSON, S. W., and P. R. BILLINGSLEY. Afferent spinal paths and
    the vasomotor reflexes. Studies in vasomotor reflex arcs VI.
    Am. J. Physiol. 42:16-35, 1916.

RETHELYI, M. Cell and neuropil architecture of the intermedio-
    lateral (sympathetic) nucleus of cat spinal cord. *Brain Res.*
    46:203-213, 1972.

RETHELYI, M. Spinal transmission of autonomic processes. *J.
    Neural Trans.* Suppl. XI:195-212, 1974.

RIEDEL, W., M. IRIKI, and E. SIMON. Regional differentiation of
    sympathetic activity during peripheral heating and cooling in
    anaesthetized rabbits. *Pflügers Arch.* 332:239-247, 1972.

SATO, A. The spinal and supraspinal somato-sympathetic reflexes.
    In: *Research in Physiology*. A Liber Memorialis in honor of
    Professor Chandler McC. Brooks, edited by F. F. Kao, K.
    Koizumi, and M. Vasalle. Bologna: Aulo Gaggi, 1971, p.
    507-516.

SATO, A. Somato-sympathetic reflex discharges evoked through
    supramedullary pathways. *Pflügers Arch.* 332:117-126, 1972a.

SATO, A. The relative involvement of different reflex pathways in
    somato-sympathetic reflexes, analyzed in spontaneously active
    single preganglionic sympathetic units. *Pflügers Arch.* 333:
    70-81, 1972b.

SATO, A. Spinal and supraspinal inhibition of somato-sympathetic
    reflexes by conditioning afferent volleys. *Pflügers Arch.*
    336:121-133, 1972c.

SATO, A. Spinal and medullary reflex components of the somato-
    sympathetic reflex discharges evoked by stimulation of group IV
    somatic afferents. *Brain Res.* 51:307-318, 1973.

SATO, A. Somato-sympathetic reflexes: Their physiological and
    clinical significance. In: *The Research Status of Spinal
    Manipulative Therapy*, edited by M. Goldstein. NINCDS Mono-
    graph 15:163-172, 1975.

SATO, A., A. KAUFMAN, K. KOIZUMI, and C. M. BROOKS. Afferent nerve
    groups and sympathetic reflex pathways. *Brain Res.* 14:575-
    587, 1969.

SATO, A., N. SATO, I. OZAWA, and B. FUJIMORI. Further observation
    of the reflex potential in the lumbar sympathetic trunk. *Jap.
    J. Physiol.* 17:294-307, 1967.

SATO, A., Y. SATO, F. SHIMADA, and Y. TORIGATA. Changes in gastric
    motility produced by nociceptive stimulation of the skin in
    rats. *Brain Res.* 94:465-474, 1975.

SATO, A., Y. SATO, F. SHIMADA, and Y. TORIGATA. Varying changes in
    heart rate produced by nociceptive stimulation of the skin of
    rats at different temperatures. *Brain Res.* 110:301-311, 1976.

SATO, A., Y. SATO, H. SUGIMOTO, and N. TERUI. Reflex changes in
    the urinary bladder after mechanical and thermal stimulation
    of the skin at various segmental levels in cats. *Neuroscience*
    2:111-117, 1977.

SATO, A., and R. F. SCHMIDT. Muscle and cutaneous afferents evoking
    sympathetic reflexes. *Brain Res.* 2:399-401, 1966.

SATO., and R. F. SCHMIDT. Spinal and supraspinal components of the
    reflex discharges into lumbar and thoracic white rami. *J.
    Physiol., London* 212:839-850, 1971.

SATO, A., and R. F. SCHMIDT. Somato-sympathetic reflexes: Afferent
    fibres, central pathways, discharge characteristics. *Physiol.
    Rev.* 53:916-947, 1973.

SATO, Y., and N. TERUI. Changes in duodenal motility produced by
    noxious mechanical stimulation of the skin in rats. *Neuro-
    science Letters* 2:189-193, 1976.

SATO, A., N. TSUSHIMA, and B. FUJIMORI. Reflex potentials of lumbar
    sympathetic trunk with sciatic nerve stimulation in cats. *Jap.
    J. Physiol.* 15:532-539, 1965.

SCHERRER, H.   Inhibition of sympathetic discharge by stimulation
    of the medulla oblongata in the rat. *Acta Neuroveg., Wien*
    29:56-74, 1966.

SCHIEBEL, M. E., and A. B. SCHIEBEL.   Terminal axonal patterns in
    cat spinal cord. II. The dorsal horn. *Brain Res.* 9:32-58,
    1968.

SCHIMERT, J.   Das Verhalten des Huiterwurzelkol lateraless im
    Rückenmark. *Z. Anat. Entwickl-Gesch* 109:665-687, 1939.

SCHMIDT, R. F.   Pre- and postganglionic neurones as final common
    path of somato-sympathetic reflexes. In: *Central Rhythmic
    Regulation,* edited by W. Umbach, and H. P. Koepchen. Stuttgart:
    Hippokrates-Verlag, 1974, p. 178-190.

SCHMIDT, R. F., and K. SCHÖNFUSS.   An analysis of the reflex activity
    in the cervical sympathetic trunk induced by myelinated somatic
    afferents. *Pflügers Arch.* 314:175-198, 1970.

SCHMIDT, R. F., and E. WELLER.   Reflex activity in the cervical and
    lumbar sympathetic trunk induced by unmyelinated afferents.
    Brain Res. 24:207-218, 1970.

SELL, R., A. ERDELYI, and H. SCHAEFER.   Untersuchungen über den
    Eifluss peripherer Nerven reizung auf die sympathische
    Activitat. *Pflügers Arch.* 267:566-581, 1958.

SELLER, H.   The discharge pattern of single units in thoracic and
    lumbar white rami in relation to cardiovascular events.
    Pflügers Arch. 343:317-330, 1973.

SELZER, M., and W. A. SPENCER.   Interactions between visceral and
    cutaneous afferents in the spinal cord: reciprocal primary
    afferent fiber depolarization. *Brain Res.* 14:349-366, 1969.

SENAPATI, J. M.   Effect of stimulation of muscle afferent on venti-
    lation in dogs. *J. Appl. Physiol.* 21:242-246, 1966.

SMITH, O. A.   Anatomy of central neural pathways mediating cardio-
    vascular functions. In: *Nervous Control of the Heart,* edited
    by W. C. Randall. Baltimore: Williams & Wilkins, 1965, p.
    34-53.

STACEY, M. J.   Free nerve endings in skeletal muscle of the cat.
    J. Anat., London 105:231-254, 1969.

STEGEMANN, J., and TH. KENNER.   A theory of heart rate control by
    muscle metabolic receptors. *Arch. Kreisl. Forsch.* 64:185-
    214, 1971.

SZENTÁGOTHAI, J. Anatomical considerations of monosynaptic reflex arcs. *J. Neurophysiol.* 11:445-454, 1948.

SZENTÁGOTHAI, J. Neuronal and synaptic arrangements in the substantia gelatinosa Rolandi. *J. Comp. Neurol.* 122:219-240, 1964.

SZENTÁGOTHAI, J., and M. RETHELYI. Cyto- and neuropil architecture of the spinal cord. In: *New Developments in Electromyography and Clinical Neurophysiology*, edited by J. E. Desmedt. Basel: Karger, Vol. 3, 1973, p. 20-37.

TIBES, U., and H. H. GROTH. Effect of K^+, osmolality (OSM) orthophosphate (Pi), lactic acid (Lac) and adrenaline on C-fiber receptors in skeletal muscle. *Proc. IUPS, Paris* XIII, 2241, 1977.

TIBES, U., and B. HEMMER. Peripheral drive on circulatory and ventilatory centers from muscle metabolic receptors. *Pflügers Arch.* 347:R47, 1974.

TIBES, U., B. HEMMER, and D. BÖNING. Heart rate and ventilation in relation to venous (K^+), osmolality, pA, PCO_2, PO_2 (orthophosphate), and lactate at transition from rest to exercise in athletes and non-athletes. *Europ. J. Appl. Physiol.* 36:127-140, 1977.

UCHIZANO, K. *Excitation and Inhibition. Synaptic Morphology.* Tokyo: Igaku Shoin, 1975.

WANG, G. H. *The Neural Control of Sweating.* Madison: University of Wisconsin Press, 1964.

WANG, G. H., and V. W. BROWN. Changes in galvanic skin reflex after acute spinal transection in normal and decerebrate cats. *J. Neurophysiol.* 19:446-451, 1956a.

WANG, G. H., and V. W. BROWN. Suprasegmental inhibition of an autonomic reflex. *J. Neurophysiol.* 19:564-572, 1956b.

WANG, G. H., P. STEIN, and V. W. BROWN. Effects of transections of central neuraxis on galvanic skin reflex in anaesthetized cats. *J. Neurophysiol.* 19:340-349, 1956.

WANG, S. C., and S. W. RANSON. Descending pathways from the hypothalamus to the medulla and spinal cord. Observations on blood pressure and bladder responses. *J. Comp. Neurol.* 71: 457-472, 1939.

WILDENTHAL, K., D. S. MIERZWIAK, N. SHELDON-SKINNER, and J. H. MITCHELL. Potassium induced cardiovascular and ventilatory reflexes from the dog hind limb. *Am. J. Physiol.* 215:542-548, 1968.

WURSTER, R. D. Spinal sympathetic control of the heart. In: *Neural Regulation of the Heart,* edited by W. C. Randall. Oxford: Oxford University Press, 1977, p. 213-246.

WYSZOGRODSKI, I., and C. POLOSA. The inhibition of sympathetic preganglionic neurons by somatic afferents. *Can. J. Physiol. Pharmacol.* 51:29-38, 1973.

DISCUSSION

DR. HORACE W. MAGOUN: If Charles Sherrington had started out
in Birmingham instead of Liverpool, my feeling is we would know a
lot more about the spinal organization of visceral reflex activity
than we do.   Obviously Dr. Coote and his associates are rapidly
filling this gap.   Who wants to open discussion?

DR. IRVIN M. KORR: John, you made two points in your paper
with which I find myself very sympathetic.   First, you made an
important distinction, I think, between what you call natural
stimuli and the artificial ones used in the laboratory.   The
natural ones are the physicochemical, environmental stimuli encountered in daily life and acting through the receptors.   The
others are based on the application of electrodes to whole nerve
trunks in which fibers of different kinds fire synchronously.   The
implication seems to be that the artificial stimulus may obscure
some important functional significance in the patterned firing of
the various receptors.

The other point that you made is that a given afferent may
have access to the same sympathetic pathway, that is, the same
group of preganglionic neurons, through segmental, propriospinal
and supraspinal pathways, and that the response to the same afferent stimulation may be quite different according to the pathway.
This it seems to me may have important clinical significance.

I have a third point, if I may.   There is, certainly in osteopathic circles, a great deal of emphasis on what are referred to
as segmental relationships.   Thus, a given segment of the body, a
dermatome or myotome, through reflex pathways, specifically reflects
disturbances in the corresponding vicerotome.   Would you, on the
basis of your experimental observations, care to elaborate on any
of those points?

DR. JOHN COOTE: One of the points brought out by Dr. Korr is
the idea that the response you get as a consequence of activating
the sympathetic system at the spinal level may be different from

129

that you get if the afferent ascends to the brain stem and evokes an output from the brain stem. The evidence for this is from work, again with natural stimulation, which I think is the really important point about this. As stated in my review, artificial electrical stimulation shows us some things but, of course, it forces all sorts of pathways to give responses which may not normally be given.

If you apply non-noxious stimulation to the skin, you activate hair receptors. The reflex response is vasoconstriction in the skin blood vessels and dilatation of the muscle blood vessels. You can show this sort of response also by recording efferent impulse activity.

If you do that in the spinal animal, following a transsection, what you get as a consequence of that input is vasoconstriction in both regions or in an increase of activity in the sympathetic outflow to those regions. That is one example of the sort of thing you are talking about--that the state of the central nervous system is very important for determining the pattern of responses.

DR. SCOTT HALDEMAN: Dr. Coote, the theories that we are trying to investigate here suggest that there is a chronic input from a musculoskeletal lesion or other somatic lesion. In your investigations or in your reading, what is the degree of habituation of the somatovisceral reflexes? Do they habituate over time, do they remain constant or do they sensitize, perhaps?

DR. COOTE: They may habituate or they may sensitize. Of course, most of the experiments I am quoting here are acute experiments but other investigators have looked at the pattern of response in the defense reaction, both the vasodilation in skeletal muscle, as well as increase in heart rate, increase in cardiac output and so on. The interesting thing is that the vasodilator component in the skeletal muscle of the cat, which has a cholinergic component, habituates very early with repeated stimulation. By "very early" I mean over a period of two or three presentations in the same number of days, whereas other responses take longer. You can get habituation of most of them so you would expect not to see any response to a given stimulus after something like, shall we say, a week.

It is interesting that there are certain animals that are very resistant to this, and they are like humans. I think there is some work being done on the renal vascular response. In those there are a few animals in which it can be shown that the vasoconstriction of the renal vascular bed is maintained very powerfully throughout the whole conditioning procedure.

DR. MICHAEL M. PATTERSON: To follow this habituation-sensitization theme: With the spread within the sympathetic system, do you ever see evidence of a habituation at the fringe of the pattern spread, followed by a sensitization within the main projection area? In response to the previous question, you mentioned habituation but do these reflexes also actively sensitize? If so, for long periods of time?

DR. COOTE: Yes. I should have completed my answer. In the chronic experiments you can also show some sensitization. Again, this occurs in only a few animals, and it is very difficult to predict which ones.

At the neuronal level, if you want me to answer from that point of view, there is very little information on how a response may be facilitated by "natural" inputs, apart from the fact that you can stimulate electrically in the CNS and you can make lesions in the CNS and show that the response pattern changes. There is no information, really, on increases in number of neurons responding on the periphery of a receptor area. One cannot answer your question really.

DR. HARRY GRUNDFEST: Do you have any information as to whether the ventral root afferents are involved in the autonomic system?

DR. COOTE: I have some information, yes. Ventral root afferents don't seem to be involved in the cat. Some years ago I published some experiments on what we call the isometric exercise response. In those experiments we tried to use the cat as a model of the response you get to isometric contractions of muscles on stimulating the ventral roots. We found that the response is dependent on an input in the dorsal roots of those segments. You cannot get a pressor effect by stimulating the ventral roots on their own.

If you stimulate the ventral roots intact and stop muscle contraction, the response is abolished, so it is dependent upon muscle contraction and intact dorsal roots. I think that there is very little effect of ventral root afferents.

DR. THOMAS ADAMS: I would like to make a comment about the segmental expression of autonomic reflexes which Dr. Coote described, and also about their chronicity. I find it particularly interesting that Pacinian corpuscles are facilitatory to atrichial sweat glands ipsilaterally in the same footpad, if I understand your comment correctly.

DR. COOTE: Yes.

DR. ADAMS: I think it might be a surprise for people who have not worked with furred animals, specifically the cat, to learn that these animals have sweat glands on their foot and toe pads. They are quite densely distributed in these areas, but probably don't serve a thermoregulatory function. The animal is most often standing on its foot and toe pads and these skin surfaces which are wetted by atrichial sweat-gland activity are not available as a site for evaporation. Also, the pads represent such a small percentage (less than 2%) of the total body surface area, that sweat-gland activity there is not going to be able to cool the body effectively. The sweat glands play a different role, I think. They are involved in altering the mechanical and thermal properties of the skin and serve to modify neurophysiological input transduction for the cat and probably for humans also.

We have demonstrated that as sweat approaches the skin surface in the distal portion of the duct, which is helical and provides a large surface area for water diffusion, the sweat distributes itself in the stratum corneum and the epidermis along both hydration and osmolar gradients. This changes the water and salt densities in the upper skin layers. We have demonstrated that for the cat's footpads, this changes not only a coefficient of friction at the skin surface, but also the pliability of the skin and its heat transfer properties. The sweat gland at the tactile surface does not provide a thermoregulatory function but, by putting water into the skin, changes its mechanical and thermal transduction characteristics.

In view of the chronicity of these reflexes, not only in the cat but also in the human, can it be presumed that eccrine or atrichial sweat-gland activity plays a role in influencing what the osteopathic physician sees in terms of skin texture, skin temperature and "drag"? These characteristics may be a function of chronic, low-level eccrine sweat-gland activity segmentally related to maintained autonomic reflexes. On the basis of our data we would predict the changes in friction at the skin surface and those in skin texture and skin temperature which the physician detects to be related to regional sweat-gland activity. We have measured that the thermal conductivity of the outer skin increases substantially when it is hydrated compared to when it is dry, and consequently transcutaneous temperature gradients change. I wonder if these data might not provide a physiological basis for some of the observations that the osteopathic physician makes about skin characteristics.

DR. MAGOUN: Before I ask for responses specifically to your question, there was an earlier physiologist named Carl Sandburg, who made the observation that the fog comes in on little cats' feet. Someone respond more directly to this query.

DR. HALDEMAN: For many years, practicioners in manipulation have made the suggestion that they could, in fact, notice changes in temperature, texture and resistance of the skin, and have developed instruments that are probably banned which measure skin temperature and skin impedance. There are techniques for rolling the skin under the fingers. Many of the textbooks describe and many of us believe that we can feel a segmental change in the area of the "lesion" or whatever it is that is causing the problem.

Because it is no more than observation and has not been investigated, it has been difficult to present data on this. It is an observation that is made continually, however; different groups- chiropractors, osteopaths, medical physicians, without contact with each other, make the same observations.

DR. ADAMS: There are associated data which I think are useful and interesting. Even though atrichial sweat glands on the cat's footpad are secreting at very low rates, about one-tenth of their potential, this changes hydration densities in the skin and changes also its osmolar and temperature gradients, but does not bring water in a liquid phase to the skin surface. My suggestion is that the sweat gland is effective in altering skin properties by its secretion well below the limit at which water is ever brought to the skin surface. Is it your experience that the skin is, in fact, wet, or is the water subcutaneous or subcorneal?

DR. HALDEMAN: Probably subcorneal because what is described as change in texture, one feels as a change in the way subcutaneous tissues role or move rather than an actual feeling of sweat. As I said, many instruments have been developed to measure temperature and skin resistance changes in these same segments.

DR. FRED E. SAMSON: To pursue that further, have there been any objective experiments in which you lay out a whole pattern, in a blind fashion, and see whether or not you can, by those measures, correlate them with palpatory findings?

DR. HALDEMAN: That's easy to answer . . . no.

DR. MAGOUN: Are there any other questions?

DR. OTTO APPENZELLER: I would like to return to Dr. Coote's paper for a moment. There is some evidence, in man at least, that the intermediolateral cell column looked at longitudinally is not uniform, but bead-like. In other words, the distribution of cells among the segments is not equal. There are segments which have large numbers of cells and others which have fewer. I wondered whether the spread of impulses that you discussed in the cat, two or three segments up or down, is, in fact, equal at all the levels or whether it refers just to some levels that you have tested. In

other words, is there some evidence, with the spread of impulses,
that in the cat there might also be a bead-like intermediolateral
cell column?

DR. COOTE: Yes, there is a bead-like intermediolateral cell
column. There have been a number of papers on this, some reporting
on cell counts. It seems there are more sympathetic neurons at one
level than another and even differences between left and right
sides. T-2 seems to have the highest number, in the cat anyway,
of all the levels of the cord.

So, the point is taken that it spreads into other segments
and may well be recruiting or affecting more neurons as a consequence. Of course, there are no studies in which one has been able
to record from the cells themselves at different levels and to see
how you get recruitment in this fashion, but one infers that it
does go on at the segmental levels.

DR. MAGOUN: I was intrigued by the broad distribution of
descending inhibitory fibers for this system as contrasted with a
rather compact excitatory column. Do you have any conception of
what is doing this or where the sources of these are and how the
excitatory and inhibitory differentiate in sites of origin?

DR. COOTE: Yes, we do. There is a lot of information on
this, provided by our own work and the work of Sesser and co-
workers in Germany. There are at least three descending inhibitory
systems. There are two inhibitory systems in the dorsolateral region, one of which seems to be coming from the raphe nuclei in the
lower brainstem, and the transmitter is probably 5HT. There is
another inhibitory system which emerges from a group of neurons
that lie close to the lateral reticular nucleus of the brainstem.
We have a lot of evidence suggesting that these are noradrenergic
in transmission. Then there is that ventral pathway which emerges
from the ventromedial reticular formation, from the region that,
in the cat anyway, is designated as the area containing the large
cells, the nucleus reticularis type. Whether there are other descending pathways from higher up, the hypothalamus perhaps, running
down with that pathway, we don't know.

As for excitatory systems, there are certainly two because
there is anatomical work describing a pathway directly down from
the hypothalamus. One can show degeneration occurring around the
intermediolateral cell column as a consequence of destruction of
regions of the hypothalamus. There are also fibers descending from
the lower brainstem.

What neurons are involved in the lower brainstem, we don't
know, outside of some equivocal evidence. The system is much more

complicated than the old textbook story of just a vasomotor center
or a sympathetic excitatory center in the brainstem. The very fact
that there is this high degree of incoming central inputs to the
sympathetic preganglionic neurons is very suggestive of an integrative role for the neurons. We can show that the output from
those cells can be altered by changing the activity in the central
inputs.

DR. RONALD GITELMAN: Dr. Coote, what are the pathways that
spread the effect to the opposite side of the cord?

DR. COOTE: It is very difficult to be absolutely certain of
any pathway but it would be fair to generalize and say there is
little spread to the opposite side. Most of the pathways are already designated to go to the side at which they pass down the
cord. There is little crossover at the spinal level.

DR. P. W. NATHAN: Two questions: One regarding the descending serotonergic pathway. The present story is that the raphe
spinal pathway comes down and inhibits the neurons of lamina 5 on
which the input arises. Therefore, you don't get any reflexes.
Are you saying, in addition to that, it does come down to the
sympathetic neuron itself?

DR. COOTE: No. I am saying that if you look at the reflex
as a consequence of stimulating a visceral or somatic afferent
nerve, you can inhibit that reflex by stimulation of raphe. You
can show that it is a consequence of 5HT transmission.

DR. NATHAN: The other question, regarding man: We have a lot
of material on cordotomies, about 120. We have 90 post-mortems.
In these, a unilateral cordotomy at the thoracic level has no obvious effect on the sympathetic. That is to say, with testing you
might find some effect but nothing functionally very obvious. But
a bilateral cordotomy somewhere in the anterolateral white matter
stops all sympathetic activity. So, the descending tract in man,
we think, lies nearer the intermediolateral column of the grey
matter and is bilateral; one side refers to both sides. We will
publish that.

DR. COOTE: That is important additional information that one
would be very pleased to see.

TRAUMATIZED NERVES, ROOTS AND GANGLIA: MUSCULOSKELETAL FACTORS AND NEUROPATHOLOGICAL CONSEQUENCES

Sydney Sunderland

Department of Experimental Neurology

University of Melbourned, Australia

The disabilities which are a central feature of this workshop have their roots in musculoskeletal systems and take the form of complaints which are a reflection of nerve and nerve root involvement. Generalising, these complaints fall into two major categories:

(1)   those indicative of nerve irritation such as paraesthesiae, pain, tenderness and muscle spasm, and

(2)   those indicative of failing nerve conduction.

In these matters it should be noted that damage to sensory nerve fibers is not necessarily painful.

Normally movements can be freely carried out over a wide range, both actively and passively. During these movements it is clear that nerves are subjected to stresses and strains which are tolerated without pain or any disturbance of neurological function. This is because of protective mechanisms which should be identified and understood for they are fundamental to any consideration of the neuropathological consequences of deranged musculoskeletal systems.

FEATURES OF NERVE TRUNKS WHICH PROTECT THEM FROM PHYSICAL DEFORMATION

1. The Course of the Nerve in Relation to Joints

With two notable exceptions, nerves cross the flexor aspect of joints. Because extension is more limited in range than flexion

this means that the nerves are subjected to less tension during
limb movements.

The significance of a routing across the flexor aspect of
joints and the tension developed in a nerve during limb extension
are illustrated when, for example, the median nerve is severed in
the mid-upper arm. There is no separation of the nerve ends when
the forearm is fully flexed but when it is extended the nerve ends
are drawn apart. The two notable exceptions are the ulnar nerve
which crosses the extensor aspect of the elbow joint and the
sciatic nerve where it crosses the extensor aspect of the hip
joint. As a result these two nerves are repeatedly subjected to
undue tension during full flexion at the elbow and hip respectively.

2. The Slackness of the Nerve Trunk and Nerve Fibers

The nerve trunk runs an undulating course in its bed, the
funiculi run an undulating course in the epineurium and the nerve
fibers run an undulating course inside the funiculi (Figure 1).
This means that the length of nerve fibers between any two fixed
points on the limb is considerably greater than the distance
between those points.

The initial effect of stretching the nerve is to take out the
undulations in the nerve trunk. With continued stretching this is
followed by the elimination of the undulations in the funiculi and
finally the undulations in the nerve fibers. It is only at this
last point that the nerve fibers are subjected to tension. With
further stretching, conduction in the nerve fibers is next impaired, then fails, until, finally, the nerve fibers fracture
inside funiculi. The perineurium is the last component to fail
structurally.

These structural features of nerve trunks mean that during
limb movements the delicate conducting elements of the nerve are
adequately protected against traction deformation.

3. The Elasticity of Nerve Trunks

When a nerve is subjected to a gradually increasing tensile
load, once the undulations in the funiculi have been removed and
the funiculi begin to take load, there is a linear relationship
between load and elongation until a certain point is reached beyond
which the nerve ceases to behave as an elastic structure. The
principal component imparting elasticity to the nerve trunk and
giving it tensile strength is the perineurium. The percentage
elongation has been recorded for a number of nerves at the elastic

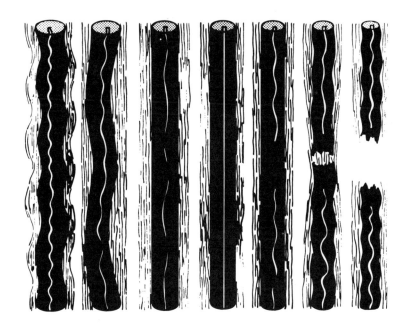

Figure 1.   Behaviour of the funiculi and contained nerve fibers of a nerve trunk stretched to the point of mechanical failure.

limit, beyond which stress is no longer proportional to strain, and at the point of mechanical failure.   Data from tensile tests on nerves followed through to their destruction are shown in Table 1.

4.   The Cushioning Effect of the Epineurium

A special feature of peripheral nerves is the large amount of epineurial connective tissue that separates the funiculi and holds them together.

(i)   The epineurium varies in amount along the nerve, at corresponding levels on the two sides of the body, and from nerve to nerve and individual to individual.   Despite these variations, individual nerves (e.g., radial, median, ulnar) present regional differences and peculiarities as regards the proportion of the cross-sectional area devoted to this tissue.   These details are not relevant to the present discussion.   In general, values for the

Table 1.   Percentage elongation of human nerve trunks under tensile
loading.   Rate of elongation 7.5 cm/min .

NERVE	AT THE ELASTIC LIMIT		AT MECHANICAL FAILURE	
	Range	Mean	Range	Mean
Ulnar	8 to 21	15	9 to 26	18
Median	6 to 22	14	7 to 30	19
Medial popliteal	7 to 21	17	8 to 32	23
Lateral popliteal	9 to 22	15	10 to 32	20
Anterior spinal roots	9 to 15	11	9 to 21	15
Posterior spinal roots	8 to 16	12	8 to 28	19

epineurial tissue range from 30 to 75 per cent of the cross-
sectional area of the nerve. An exception is the sciatic nerve in
the gluteal region, where this tissue usually occupies 70 to 80 per
cent of the cross-sectional area of the nerve.

(ii) The epineurium, by providing a loose matrix for the
contained funiculi, cushions them against deforming forces.

(iii) Nerve fibers are more susceptible to compression where
the nerve trunk is composed of large and closely packed funiculi
with little supporting epineurial tissue. Where, on the other
hand, peripheral nerves are composed of a large number of small
bundles that are widely separated by a relatively greater amount
of epineurium they are more favourably constituted to withstand
compression. With the former arrangement forces fall maximally on
the main content of the nerve trunk which is funicular tissue and,
therefore, nerve fibers. In the latter, the effects of compression
are minimised, the damaging forces being dispersed and cushioned by
the epineurial packing, while the funiculi, being more loosely
arranged, are more easily displaced within the nerve which reduces
the effects of the deforming force (Figure 2).

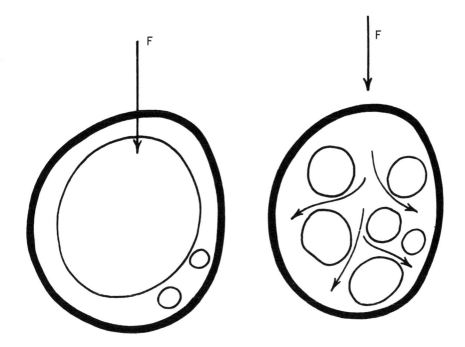

Figure 2

It is of interest that where nerves cross joints they are
composed of many small funiculi separated by large amounts of epineurial tissue. This is particularly so in the case of the sciatic
nerve where it crosses the extensor aspect of the hip joint. This
is probably a special protective feature for we spend much of our
time sitting on the sciatic nerves with the thighs flexed.

PROTECTIVE MECHANISMS AND THE VULNERABILITY OF
NERVE ROOTS TO PHYSICAL DEFORMATION

Nerve roots differ from peripheral nerves in several respects
but importantly the nerve fibers of the former are arranged in
parallel bundles and are loosely supported by endoneurial tissue
alone. In the absence of perineurial tissue they lack the tensile
strength of peripheral nerves and so are more vulnerable to stretch.
Lacking any protective epineurial packing they are also more
susceptible to compression.

In addition it has been known for a very long time that forces
generated by traction on a peripheral nerve are transmitted to the

corresponding nerve roots. Thus fully flexing the hip and extend-
ing the knee puts tension on the lumbosacral nerve roots in the
spinal canal. Finally, the intervertebral foramen remains as a
region of potential danger to the contained neural elements.

Despite these vulnerable features, the nerve roots are not left
without any form of protection.

There are three anatomical arrangements which prevent nerve
roots from being overstretched. One concerns the arrangement of
the dura at the intervertebral foramen, another the attachment of
certain spinal nerves to the vertebral transverse process and the
third is the elastic properties of the nerve roots.

NEURAL RELATIONS AT THE INTERVERTEBRAL FORAMEN

Opposite the foramen each pair of anterior and posterior nerve
roots invaginates the dura and arachnoid to form a funnel-shaped
depression at the bottom of which each perforates the meninges
independently carrying with it, as it does so, an individual and
separate bilaminar sleeve of dura and arachnoid (Figure 3). The
arrangement is such that the subarachnoid space is continued along
the nerve roots usually as far as the ganglion, occasionally to involve its inner pole but never to envelop it completely. Laterally
the dural layer of the sleeve blends with the anterior root and the
ganglion to form an outer fibrous sheath for these structures. This
sheath is continued outwards to become the strong perineurial sheath
of the single bundle of nerve fibers of the spinal nerve formed by
the fusion of the two roots. The epidural tissue on the surface of

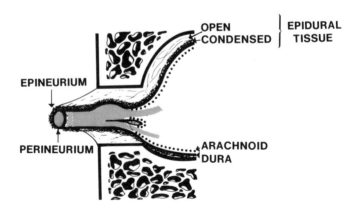

Figure 3. The relationship of the nerve root – spinal nerve
complex to the meninges in the intervertebral foramen.

the dura is continuous with the epineurium of the spinal nerve. The
formation of this perineurial-epineurial connective tissue sheath
adds to the thickness of the spinal nerve so that its cross-
sectional area exceeds the combined cross-sectional areas of the
nerve roots from which it is formed.

The two roots of each spinal nerve remain separate as far as
the ganglion and so may be selectively involved in pathological
processes central to this level. Immediately distal to the ganglion,
the nerve fibers are contained in a single funiculus in which the
motor fibers are concentrated antero-inferiorly (Figure 4). The
eighth cervical to the second lumbar nerve roots and those of the
second, third and fourth sacral nerves, contain sympathetic (C8-L2)
and parasympathetic (S2,3,4) elements. Within a few millimeters
the single funiculus of nerve fibers divides into several bundles
which engage in plexus formations. This effects the first mixing
of sensory and motor fibers.

The nerve root - spinal nerve complex with its connective tissue
sheath occupies 35 to 50 per cent of the cross-sectional area of the

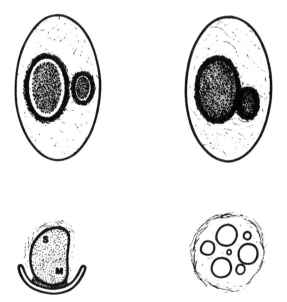

Figure 4. Transverse sections at and just distal to the intervertebral foramen illustrating the transition from nerve roots to spinal
nerve, the localisation of sensory and motor nerve fibers and the
attachment of a lower cervical spinal nerve to the vertebral
transverse process.

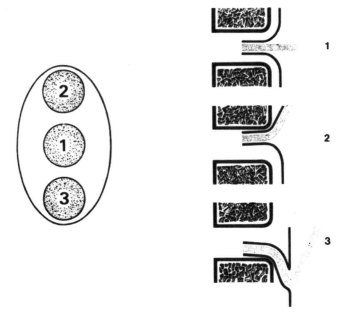

Figure 5. Variations in the position occupied by the nerve complex in the intervertebral foramen. For simplification the complex has been represented as a single bundle.

foramen so that normally there is ample space for the complex. The latter is enveloped by loose areolar connective and adipose tissue containing the spinal artery, and its anterior and posterior branches, with numerous veins which often surround the complex, lymphatics and the recurrent meningeal nerve. Particular attention is directed to the size and number of the veins surrounding the nerve complex.

The position of the neural complex in the intervertebral foramen is subject to some variation. The first cervical root is aligned horizontally while the remaining roots are directed downwards with gradually increasing obliquity until the lumbar and sacral roots descend vertically to reach their respective foramina.

The usual arrangement is for the nerve roots to pass through the dura, ensheathed in their meningeal sleeves, opposite the corresponding foramen so that the neural complex occupies a central position in the foramen (Figure 5). Variations in the level at which this occurs may bring the nerve roots closer to the upper or the lower margin of the foramen; in the case of the obliquely and vertically aligned roots an increasingly superior position on entry is favoured. However, it is common in the lower cervical and upper thoracic regions, for the nerve roots to descend intradurally by as much as 8 millimeters below the foramen which they are to enter before perforating the dura in the usual way. They must then ascend acutely, enclosed in their dural sleeves, in order to reach the foramen over the lower margin of which they are again angulated as they pass outwards.

THE MOBILITY OF THE NERVE COMPLEX
IN THE INTERVERTEBRAL FORAMEN

The arrangement of structures in the foramen is such that the nerve complex is permitted to move freely within and through the foramen. There is abundant evidence, dating from Dana's observations in 1882 down to the present time, that traction on peripheral nerves during limb movements tenses nerve roots. The position of the complex in the foramen also changes with movements of the head and neck. With ventroflexion the nerve roots are tensed and the complex is drawn inwards and upwards toward the upper margin of the foramen; in dorsal extension the complex is relaxed and returns to its original position. The nerve roots maximally involved in this way are the eighth cervical to the fifth thoracic, but ventroflexion of the cervical spine also tenses the lumbar and sacral nerve roots.

All this means that the forces generated during limb, trunk and neck movements are responsible for the repeated "piston-like" movement of the nerve complex in the intervertebral foramen.

Overstretching of nerve roots by transmitted forces generated in the manner indicated is normally prevented by the following mechanisms:

(1) Because the dura becomes adherent to and part of the nerve complex laterally, traction on the spinal nerve pulls the entire system outwards so that the dural funnel is drawn laterally into the foramen and, being cone-shaped, plugs the foramen in such a way as to resist further displacement of the nerve (Figure 6). Thus the integrity of the system is due, not to any strong meningeal attachment at the foramen, but to the continuity of the nerve sheath with the dura.

(2) During the wide range of movements occurring at the cervical spine, shoulder girdle, and shoulder joint, additional strains are generated which fall maximally on those spinal nerves forming the brachial plexus which, if transmitted directly to the corresponding short cervical nerve roots, would expose them to traction injury. In order to protect the roots against such injuries, the fourth, fifth, sixth, and seventh cervical nerves are securely attached to the vertebral column. Each, on leaving the foramen, is

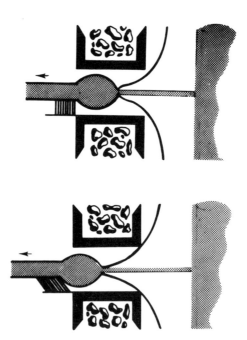

Figure 6. Displacement of the nerve complex laterally through the
foramen is resisted by the attachment of the spinal nerve to the
cervical transverse process and subsequently, and where there are
no such attachments, by the plugging action of the dural funnel
which is drawn into the foramen.

immediately lodged in the gutter of the transverse process to which
it is securely bound by its sheath, by reflections of the prevertE-
bral fascia and by slips from the musculo-tendinous attachments to
the transverse processes. The significance of this attachment
emerges when the relative susceptibility to avulsion injury of the
several nerve roots contributing to the brachial plexus is examined.
Traction injuries, which do not avulse nerve roots, more commonly
involve the upper spinal nerves of the plexus whereas the incidence
of avulsion injuries is much higher in the case of the lower nerve
roots, which anatomically are at greater risk. Such protective
attachments are not needed for the other spinal nerves.

     (3) The elastic properties of the nerve roots allow them to
accommodate to the tension generated during limb, neck and trunk
movements though there are limits to their elasticity. In this
respect it has already been noted that the roots lack the tensile
strength of peripheral nerves and that they fail under increasing
tension before peripheral nerves. The greater vulnerability of
nerve roots to traction deformation is due to structural differences.

NEUROLOGICAL COMPLICATIONS OF MUSCULOSKELETAL PATHOLOGY

Relevant generalisations are:

1. Adhesions which fix a nerve trunk in its bed or reduce its mobility, and changes in the connective tissue of a nerve which reduce its elasticity, prejudice nerve fibers by lowering the threshold at which stretching begins to produce structural and physiological effects.

2. Whereas normal nerve fibers show a remarkable tolerance to mechanical deformation, damaged nerve fibers are particularly susceptible to physical deformation and ischaemia.

3. Pathology rendering nerve fibers more vulnerable to involvement in musculoskeletal disorders includes:

(i) The neuropathies of toxic or metabolic origin. Subclinical neuropathies may remain latent until precipitated by some traumatic or ischaemic incident.

(ii) Intercurrent infection. Some febrile condition of viral or other origin may combine with an existing musculoskeletal lesion to implicate nerve fibers with the appearance of neurological disturbances.

COMMON SITES OF NERVE INVOLVEMENT

Three potential sites of nerve involvement immediately suggest themselves.

1. The peripheral tissues.

2. Where a nerve pierces fascia or runs in a confined space with rigid walls. This is the entrapment lesion.

3. At the vertebral column.

The Peripheral Tissues and Fine Sensory Terminals

The lid of this Pandora's box will not be disturbed other than to comment that the biochemical milieu of fine sensory filaments may be altered in a manner and to a degree which leads to spontaneous discharges and/or renders them unduly sensitive to stretch and compression. The outcome is spontaneous pain or pain precipitated by even the slightest movement or pressure.

The Nerve Trunk and the Chronic Entrapment Lesion

This is a convenient time to discuss the genesis of the chronic entrapment lesion.

Musculoskeletal sites of nerve entrapment are legion but, to generalise, nerves are at risk where (1) they run in confined spaces with unyielding walls, e.g., the median nerve in the carpal tunnel, the facial nerve in the facial canal, and the neural contents of an intervertebral foramen though the last named will be considered separately later; and (2) they traverse muscle, fascia or ligamentous tissue, e.g., the greater occipital nerve (occipital neuralgia) and the lateral cutaneous nerve of the thigh (meralgia paraesthetica).

Here the entrapped nerve becomes involved as the result of local pathology which brings about its harmful effects on the nerve by (1) chronic compression and/or (2) the formation of restrictive and constrictive adhesions.

THE NERVE LESION DUE TO CHRONIC COMPRESSION

Any nerve, which in its course passes through an opening or tunnel with unyielding walls, may be selected as a model to illustrate the manner in which a vascular mechanism produces the initial lesion when the nerve is subjected to slowly increasing pressure. Essential features to keep in mind in the following discussion are:

1. For simplification one funiculus in the nerve has been isolated for consideration (Figure 7).

2. The only vessels found inside funiculi are capillaries. These are fed by arterioles and drain to venules and veins all of which are located in the epineurium; venous vessels outnumber arterial. The nutrient vessels take an oblique course through the perineurial sheath which leads to their closure where there is any swelling of the bundle.

3. The tensile strength and diffusion barrier properties of the perineurium are well documented.

4. There is a normal intrafunicular pressure which is maintained by the perineurium.

5. Veins succumb to pressure before arteries.

6. There are at least five interrelated pressure systems in the tunnel (Figure 7): (i) the pressure in the nutrient arteries

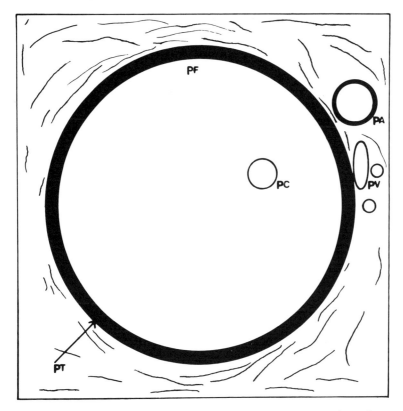

Figure 7. A single funiculus, with its related vessels, from a multifuniculated nerve in an entrapment situation.

in the epineurium P^A; (ii) the capillary pressure inside the funiculus P^C; (iii) the intrafunicular pressure P^F; (iv) the pressure in the veins in the epineurium draining the funiculi P^V; the pressure within the tunnel P^T.

In order to maintain an adequate circulation through the funiculus for the nutrition of the nerve fibers, the pressure gradient across this system must be:

$$P^A > P^C > P^F > P^V > P^T.$$

These various pressure systems are in delicate balance in a confined space which offers little margin for safety in the event of an increase in pressure in the compartment.

With any pathology leading to a gradual increase in the pressure in the tunnel, such as occurs when the lumen is reduced or the

contents slowly enlarge or become swollen, the first constituents
in the compartment to succumb are the venules in the epineurium.
Obstruction to the venous return from the nerve originating in this
way leads, both directly and indirectly, to pathological changes,
the most damaging of which take place inside the funiculus. These
pathological changes pass through the following stages each of which
represents a lesion of increasing severity.

Stage 1. Obstruction to the venous outflow from a funiculus
leads to a slowing of the intrafunicular capillary circulation,
capillary congestion, an increase in the intrafunicular capillary
pressure, and then, because of the tensile properties of the perineurium, to an increase in the intrafunicular pressure. This still
further embarrasses the intrafunicular circulation and in this way
a vicious circle is introduced. As the capillary circulation slows
and the intrafunicular pressure rises, the incarcerated nerve fibers
are compressed and their nutrition impaired by hypoxia to a point
when they become hyperexcitable and commence to discharge spontaneously. In this respect the large myelinated fibers are known to be
more susceptible and to suffer earlier than the thin finely myelinated or nonmyelinated fibers. This is the painful lesion.

At this stage in the development of the lesion, not all funiculi
or all fibers would be affected to the same degree while whatever
minor structural changes have occurred are fully and rapidly corrected by any change or procedure which relieves the pressure on
the nerve and thereby improves the circulation through it.

Stage 2. The capillary circulation finally slows to a point
where the resulting anoxia damages the capillary endothelium which
leads to the leakage of protein into the tissues which become
oedematous. As protein steadily leaks through the capillary wall
it accumulates in the endoneurial spaces because it cannot escape
across the perineurial diffusion barrier. As the endoneurial tissue becomes increasingly oedematous there is a further increase in
the intrafunicular pressure. This and the related anoxia combine
to threaten the survival of nerve fibers by (1) interfering with
their nutrition and metabolism, (2) deforming them, and (3) promoting the proliferation and increased activity of fibroblasts with
the formation of constrictive endoneurial connective tissue.

Inside the funiculus thinned nerve fibers become thinner and
undergo segmental demyelination. Finally some axons are interrupted within their endoneurial sheaths and these nerve fibers then
degenerate. At this point the lesion is of a mixed variety. More
resistant fibers may still be conducting normally but in most of
the surviving thinned fibers conduction velocity is reduced, a third
group has sustained a first degree or conduction block injury, and
for still a fourth group the deformation will have injured fibers

to a degree which will be followed by Wallerian degeneration. A
further development is the formation of ephaptic synapses which
could provide the basis for abnormal activity in sensory nerve
fibers.

With advanced structural changes the sensory and motor deficit
deepens as more and more fibers are affected. At this stage, providing whatever is responsible for the compression subsides or the
nerve is decompressed, the circulation through the compressed segment is restored, the oedema is gradually resolved and the pressure
inside the funiculi falls. Motor and sensory recovery is delayed
depending on whether individual nerve fibers have sustained first
or second degree damage and the extent to which irreversible
changes may have developed.

Stage 3. If long-standing pressure on the nerve is allowed to
continue, the lesion takes on a more permanent state, a stage being
reached when the arterial supply to the nerve is affected in addition to its venous return. Fibroblasts proliferate in the intrafunicular protein exudate and promote the development of an irreversible fibrosis which results in the constriction of increasing
numbers of nerve fibers. The final stage is reached when nutrient
vessels are obliterated and the affected segment of the nerve becomes converted into a fibrous cord in which only a few fine nerve
fibers survive inside fibrosed funiculi which are encased in a now
dense relatively avascular epineurium.

THE NERVE LESION ASSOCIATED WITH THE PASSAGE
OF THE NERVE THROUGH OTHER TISSUES

Pain in the distribution of the affected nerve is the presenting symptom in these cases and the site where the nerve passes
through muscle, fascia or ligamentous tissue is the site of maximal
tenderness.

Details of the local pathology, both somatic and neural, in
these cases is scanty. Inference leads us to believe that the
basis of the lesion is a fibrosis secondary to mechanical irritation in which the nerve is involved as the result of the formation
of restrictive and constrictive adhesions. Movement aggravates the
condition presumably because it leads to traction on the pathological segment of the nerve at the site of entrapment. The nature
of this nerve pathology is unknown. It could be that friction
fibrosis constricts and fixes the nerve, and impairs its circulation in a manner similar to that outlined in the previous section.

But all this is speculative. The biopsy specimens that I
have had the opportunity of examining histologically have shown

surprisingly little to account for the distressing pain associated
with the entrapment.

NERVE ROOT AND SPINAL NERVE INVOLVEMENT AS THE RESULT OF
PATHOLOGY IN AND ABOUT THE INTERVERTEBRAL FORAMEN

1. Anatomical Considerations

Cervical region. The first and second cervical spinal nerves
are unusual in that they leave the spinal canal behind the joint
system (Figure 8). The first occupies a groove on the upper surface of the posterior arch of the atlas where it is behind and a
little below the capsule of the atlanto-occipital joint and beneath
the vertebral artery. In this situation the nerve and the vessel
traverse an osseofibrous foramen outlined by the bony arch and the
lower border of the posterior atlanto-occipital ligament. The second cervical nerve crosses the arch of the axis immediately behind
and in contact with the capsule of the lateral atlanto-axial joint.
Here it leaves the spinal canal through a small osseo-fibrous opening formed by a deficiency in the bony attachment of the ligamentum
flavum. The arrangement in both nerves represents a potential site
for an entrapment lesion.

In the case of the third to the seventh spinal nerves, the
nerve is lodged in the gutter formed by the articular pillar posteriorly, the pedicle of the subjacent vertebra and the extension
upwards of the crested lateral lip (processus uncinatus) of the
vertebral body anteriorly (Figures 9a, b and c). The foramen is
completed superiorly by the pedicle of the vertebra above. The
eighth cervical nerve emerges from the foramen between the last
cervical and first thoracic vertebrae and then descends to unite
with the first thoracic nerve anterior to the neck of the first rib.

The loose joint capsule of the articular pillar is located
postero-superiorly with, further medially, the lateral margin of
the ligamentum flavum (Figure 9c). The intervertebral disc and the
neuro-central joint space, if such exists, form the antero-superior
boundary of the foramen.

Thoracic region. The level of the apophyseal joint with reference to the nerve varies. In the upper thoracic region the joint
is situated postero-superiorly as in the cervical region. It then
gradually moves down the posterior wall of the foramen until it is
finally located postero-inferiorly as in the lumbar region. The
intervertebral disc forms the antero-inferior margin of the foramen
(Figure 10).

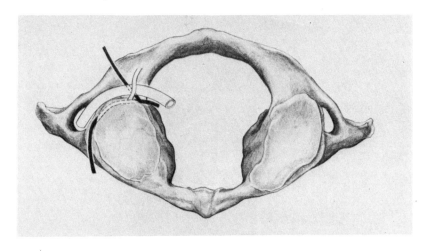

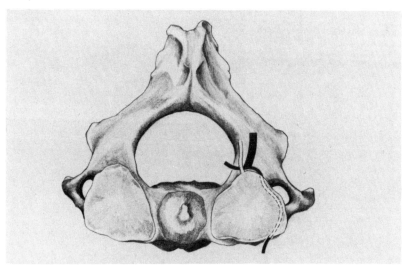

Figure 8. The first and second cervical vertebrae and the course taken by the first and second cervical spinal nerves.

Lumbar region. As they descend in the spinal canal, the lumbar nerve roots cross the disc immediately above the foramen through which they are to leave the spinal canal (Figure 11). They then enter the foramen beneath the pedicle forming its upper margin with the ligamentum flavum posterior and the body of the vertebra anterior (Figure 12). As the nerve inclines downwards, outwards, and forwards, it crosses the anterior aspect of the joint, but, by the time

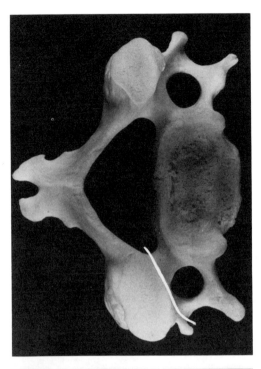

Fig. 9b

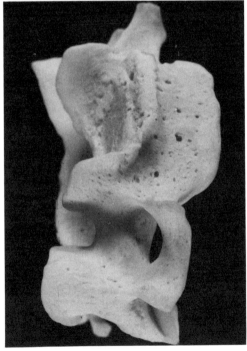

Fig. 9a

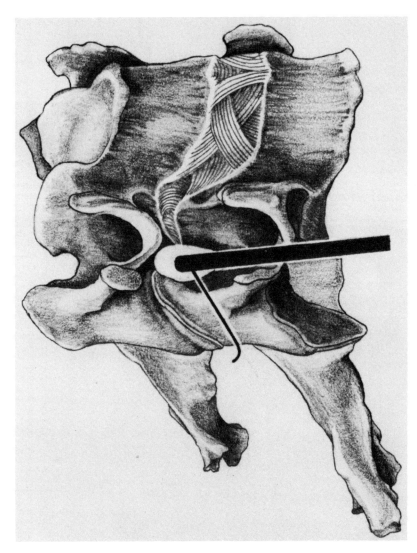

Fig. 9c

Figures 9a, b, c. The relations of a typical lower cervical spinal nerve to the vertebra, intervertebral disc and apophyseal joint.

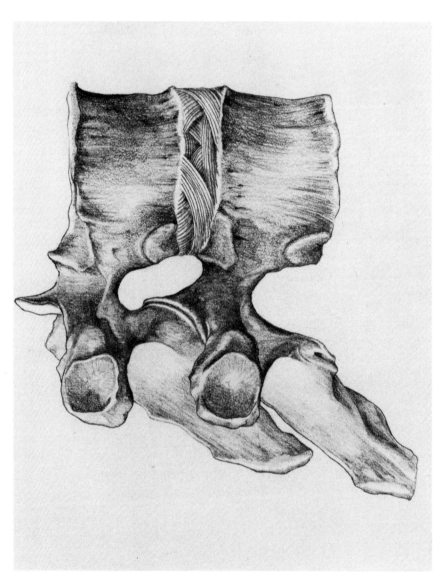

Figure 10. Diagram of a typical thoracic intervertebral foramen. The apophyseal joint, shown behind the nerve complex, occupies a superior position in the upper thoracic region, a mid-position in the mid-thoracic region and an inferior position in the lower thoracic region.

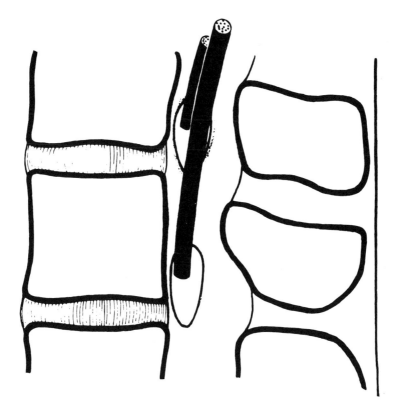

Figure 11. The relationship of nerve roots to the intervertebral discs as they descend in the spinal canal to reach their respective foramina. The nerve roots leave the foramen proximal to the disc forming its lower anterior boundary but they are directly related to the disc above.

it is at the level of the disc, it has emerged from the foramen to pass, with the exception of the fifth, between the slips of origin of the psoas to enter the substance of that muscle.

Summary. The apophyseal joint is behind and above the nerve complex in the cervical region, directly behind it in the mid-thoracic region and behind and below it in the lumbar region. The sensory fibers of the spinal nerve are intimately related to the joint.

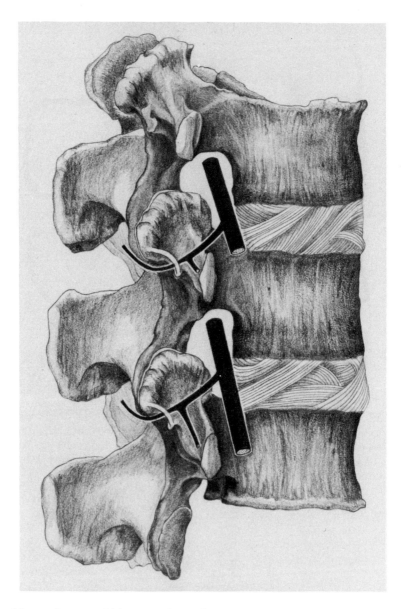

Figure 12. Diagram illustrating the passage of the lumbar nerve
through the upper part of the intervertebral foramen where it is
behind the vertebral body and immediately below its pedicle. The
course of the dorsal ramus across the lateral surface of the articular process is also shown along with the passage of the medial
branch of the ramus through a tunnel beneath the ligamentous tissue
joining the mammillary and accessory processes - only the lateral
fibers of this ligamentous arch are shown.

2. Pathological Considerations

While pathology in and about the foramen may reduce its dimensions and lead to nerve compression, more likely causes of nerve involvement at this site are friction over osseo-fibrous irregularities or traction on a nerve or nerve roots fixed in the foramen by adhesions.

SPINAL NERVE - NERVE ROOT LESIONS DUE TO COMPRESSION

Two relevant generalisations are:

(i) Though the neural structures are at risk as they pass through the foramen they normally have ample room in this situation and are also well cushioned by fat-containing connective tissue. In addition, the narrowing of the foramen, which occurs with extension of the vertebral column, does not embarrass its contents.

(ii) Nerves will tolerate remarkable degrees of deformation, providing this occurs sufficiently slowly and does not impair their blood supply.

Pathology which may reduce the dimensions of the foramen and cause nerve compression involves (1) the intervertebral disc, (2) the apophyseal joint, and (3) the ligamentum flavum.

Tuberculous lesions and benign and metastatic tumours of the vertebral column will not be considered.

1. Intervertebral disc pathology includes:

(i) Atrophy and narrowing of the disc. Because of the position of the vertebral apophyseal joint, any reduction in the thickness of the disc in the cervical region has little, if any, effect on the vertical diameter of the foramen. In the thoracic region, narrowing of the disc results in slight subluxation of the apophyseal joint and some reduction in the vertical diameter but this is not usually sufficient to embarrass the neural contents of the foramen. However, in the lumbar region narrowing of the intervertebral disc leads to subluxation of the apophyseal joint so that the inferior articular process of the vertebra above moves downwards toward the pedicle of the vertebra below, the overall effect being to significantly reduce the dimensions of the intervertebral foramen and its cross-sectional area. The veins are the first to suffer and venous congestion impairing the return of venous blood from the nerve is probably the basis of the early neurological signs and symptoms.

(ii)   A herniated disc and osteophyte formation involving the rim of the vertebral body may encroach on the foramen anteriorly.

2.   Apophyseal joint pathology includes:

(i)   Inflammatory swelling of the joint. Magnuson (1944) has shown that injecting saline into the joint narrows the foramen by 2 mm.

(ii)   Osteophyte formation.

3.   The ligamentum flavum. With hypertrophy, this tissue may encroach on the foramen posteriorly.

SPINAL NERVE - NERVE ROOT LESIONS DUE TO CHRONIC IRRITATION

Osteoarthritic changes may destroy the smooth contour of the foramen replacing it with irregularities which irritate and traumatize the nerve as it is continuously drawn in and out of the foramen during movements of the limbs, neck and trunk. The damaging effects are increased when nerve roots, on entering the foramen, are angulated across its upper or lower margin. Chronic irritation and trauma originating in this way involve the nerve in a friction fibrosis which imperils nerve fibers by (1) constricting them, (2) interfering with their blood supply, and (3) forming adhesions which fix the nerve in the foramen so that traction on the nerve aggravates the deformation of nerve fibers.

INVOLVEMENT OF THE DORSAL RAMI OF THE SPINAL NERVES

On its way to the posterior compartment of the back each dorsal ramus is accompanied by an artery and its associated vein to form a neuro-vascular bundle. This bundle and the medial and lateral branches into which it divides establish important relations with the apophyseal joints. The cervical dorsal rami diminish rapidly in size from above downwards (Figure 13). The dorsal ramus of the first nerve has no cutaneous distribution but provides a sensory innervation to the atlanto-occipital joint, the ligaments of the region and the suboccipital muscles for which it also provides a motor supply. The dorsal ramus of the second nerve is the largest of the spinal series. It carries some motor but mostly sensory fibers and divides into a small lateral and large medial branch. The latter, after a circuitous course as the greater occipital nerve, pierces the semispinalis and then the trapezius muscle at its attachment to the skull where it traverses a tendinous tunnel or passes under a tendinous arcade to become cutaneous. Those of the third

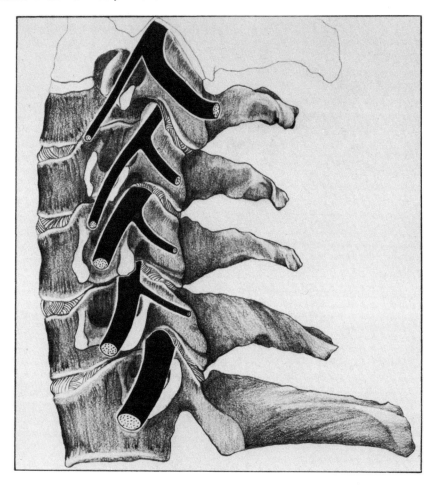

Figure 13. Diagram illustrating the course of the cervical dorsal rami in relation to the articular pillars. The rami diminish in size from above downwards.

to the seventh cervical nerves cross the lateral surface of the articular pillar which is grooved to carry the nerve, the groove being converted into an osseo-fibrous tunnel by the posterior inter-transverse ligament and muscle. On emerging from the tunnel the ramus gives branches to the vertebral joint above and below. On its way posteriorly the eighth ramus crosses and grooves the upper surface of the first rib. It then establishes a relation with the vertebral joint which is essentially the same as that to be described for the thoracic nerves. Each ramus terminates behind the articular pillar by dividing into a larger medial and smaller lateral division. Both send branches to ligaments and muscles. In

addition, the medial provides further twigs to the joint before becoming cutaneous just lateral to the midline to innervate the skin.
Cutaneous fibers may be absent from the lower cervical rami.

Each thoracic dorsal ramus passes backwards across the apophyseal joint to enter a roomy osseo-fibrous opening formed medially
by the apophysis, superiorly by the transverse process, inferiorly by
the neck of the rib and the upper border of the subjacent transverse
process, and laterally by the superior costo-transverse and inter-
transverse ligaments and the intertransverse muscle. In its course
the nerve is in contact with the joint capsule to which it sends
branches. Posteriorly the nerve curves medially for a short distance before dividing into medial and lateral branches. The medial
continues inwards and downwards to give articular, muscular, ligamentous and, in the case of the upper thoracic nerves, cutaneous
branches. The lateral branch runs outwards between the layers of
the superior costo-transverse ligament to reach and innervate the
deep muscles of the back; those of the lower thoracic nerves also
have a cutaneous distribution.

The dorsal ramus of each lumbar nerve runs downwards and backwards across the lateral surface of the adjacent superior articular
process from a point immediately above and anterior to the vertebral
joint, to which it gives twigs, to reach and cross the upper surface
of the base of the transverse process, where the ramus divides into
medial and lateral divisions as do the accompanying vessels (Figures 12, 14a, b). The site of this branching is readily located on
the transverse process at the bottom of a connective tissue plane
between the multifidus muscle medially and the longissimus group
laterally (Figure 15).

The finer medial branch, somewhat less than 1 mm in diameter,
continues freely before entering the groove between the accessory
and mammillary processes beyond which it curves medially following
the lower border of the joint (Figures 12, 14a, b). In the groove
and over this infra-articular section the neurovascular bundle is
covered and tightly bound to bone by exceedingly dense tissue formed
by fibrous extensions from the capsule of the joint, the inter-
transverse ligament and the tendinous attachments of the longissimus
thoracis, multifidus, rotatores, and medial intertransverse muscles.
After a course of about 1 cm in this tunnel, the nerve emerges to
pass on to the lamina. It sends branches upwards before turning
downwards to descend for some distance, branching as it does so, to
combine with corresponding branches of neighbouring rami to form an
openly arranged plexus. The medial branch innervates ligaments and
muscles medial to the line of the vertebral joints, while the joint
itself is richly supplied by multiple articular twigs from both the
parent ramus and its medial branch. In the curved transverse section of its course the medial branch also sends twigs downwards to
the capsule of the joint below.

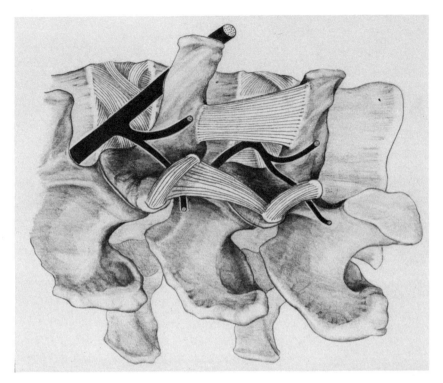

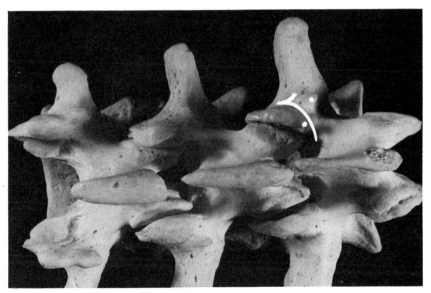

Figures 14a, b. The course of the lumbar dorsal rami. The medial branch passes through an osseo-fibrous tunnel outlined by the ligamentous and musculo-tendinous tissue arching between the mammillary and accessory processes.

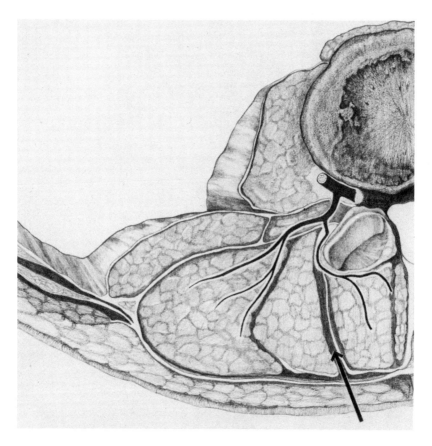

Figure 15. Diagram illustrating the site of branching of a lumbar
dorsal ramus on the transverse process at the bottom of a tissue
plane between the multifidus muscle medially and the longissimus
muscle laterally. The course of the medial branch is also shown
in relation to the vertebral joint.

The passage of the medial branch of the lumbar dorsal ramus
and its accompanying vessels through an osseo-fibrous tunnel and
the intimate relationship of this neurovascular bundle to the capsule of the apophyseal joint represents a potential site of fixation
and entrapment following pathological changes involving the joint.

Particular attention is directed to this feature for it is
relevant to the symptomatology in disc pathology.

Narrowing of the lumbar intervertebral space, whatever the
cause, results in the subluxation of the apophyseal joints in which

the facet of the vertebra above is displaced inferiorly across the
surface of the vertebra below. As a result of this displacement
the medial branch of the lumbar dorsal ramus, which is fixed in
this region (see above), is involved in two ways: (1) inflammatory
swelling of the joint reduces the lumen of the tunnel containing the
neurovascular bundle, and (2) the superior articular pedicle comes
to press directly on the nerve.

The larger lateral branch of the dorsal ramus passes outwards
and downwards to innervate muscles and ligaments lateral to the
line of the vertebral joints. In the case of the twelfth thoracic
and upper three lumbar nerves the lateral branch descends through
muscle to pierce the lumbo-dorsal fascia just above the iliac crest
before descending vertically across the crest to innervate the skin
of the buttock as far down as the greater trochanter.

The fifth lumbar ramus crosses the sacrum immediately lateral
to the lumbosacral joint where it divides into medial and lateral
branches. The former turns inwards below the joint to supply it
before continuing on to terminate in the multifidus. The lateral
is lost in the sacroiliac ligament.

On emerging from the posterior sacral foramina each dorsal
ramus divides into a finer medial and a larger lateral branch.
These are in turn linked by a complicated system of overlapping
branchings and anastomotic loopings to form a plexus which is
deeply situated on bone and ligamentous tissue beneath the multifidus and sacrospinalis muscles with extensions between the deep
and superficial parts of the posterior sacroiliac ligament. The
plexus is joined by the descending medial divisions of the fourth
and fifth lumbar rami which reach as far distally as at least the
second sacral segment. Terminal medial branches of the system
innervate muscles while the lateral are distributed to muscles
along with the sacroiliac, sacrotuberous, sacrospinous and ilio-
lumbar ligaments; in addition, those branches derived from the
first three sacral nerves send cutaneous branches through the
gluteus maximus muscles to the skin.

The passage of the cutaneous branches through the muscles and
fascia of the back should not be overlooked as potential sites of
entrapment. This applies particularly to the greater occipital
nerve and the cutaneous branches of the dorsal rami of the upper
three lumbar nerves.

When investigating the problem of low back pain, one cautions
against concentrating exclusively on the intervertebral disc as the
site of the offending lesion lest this obscure the significance of
aetiological factors originating elsewhere in the vicinity. In
this respect the passage of the medial branch of the lumbar dorsal

ramus and its accompanying vessels through an osseo-fibrous tunnel and the intimate relationship of this neurovascular bundle to the capsule of the apophyseal joint represents a potential site of fixation and entrapment following pathological changes involving the joint.

REFERENCES

DANA, C. L.   The mechanical effect of nerve stretching upon the spinal cord. *Med. Rec.* 22:113-115, 1882.

MAGNUSON, P. B.   Differential diagnosis of causes of pain in the lower back accompanied by sciatic pain. *Ann. Surg.* 119:878-891, 1944.

SUNDERLAND, S.   Anatomical perivertebral influences on the inter-vertebral foramen. *The Research Status of Spinal Manipulative Therapy.*   NINCDS Monograph No. 15:129-140, 1975.

SUNDERLAND, S. *Nerves and Nerve Injuries* (2nd ed.).   Edinburgh: Churchill Livingstone, 1978.   In press.

ACKNOWLEDGEMENTS

The illustrations in this text are from the author's publications listed above and have been used with the permission of the publishers.

DISCUSSION OF EXCITATION AND CONDUCTION IN TRAUMATIZED NERVES

Harry Grundfest, Initiator of Discussion

Trauma affects excitation and conduction of impulses through alterations in the processes which generate these impulses. The processes involve, primarily, changes in the permeability of the cell membrane to specific ions.

The neuron is essentially an electric telegraph system in which information is received and appropriate messages are generated at one (input) end of the cell, propagated along the axon (cable) which is the characteristic feature of a neuron and, arriving at the nerve terminals (output), are passed on (transmitted) to other cells.

A telegraph system must incorporate an electrical power source, keying and modulating elements which generate impulses and encode them into a message, amplifiers that ensure against distortion of the signals, and transducer devices which decode the message. These elements of a commercial telegraph system comprise huge electrical generators, well-insulated, low-resistance metallic conductors, and intricate electrical and/or mechanical keying and transducing devices. The neuron performs the functions of a complete telegraph system within the confines of a single cell, utilizing the biological processes that are common to all living cells, and incorporating the various functional elements of a telegraph in the structure of the cell membrane, which has undergone remarkable evolutionary adaptation in the formation of neurons.

The membrane maintains an asymmetric distribution of ions between the interior of the cell and the external bathing fluid. The asymmetric distribution of K--high inside and low outside--and the reverse distribution of Na are of major importance for the axon. They give rise to an inside negative K-battery and an inside positive Na-battery approximately according to the Nernst relation:

$$E_K = 58 \text{ mV} \cdot \log \frac{K_o}{K_i}; \quad E_{Na} = 58 \text{ mV} \cdot \log \frac{Na_o}{Na_i}.$$

The cell membrane is effectively much more permeable to K than to Na. The K-battery therefore has a much lower effective resistance, and the cell interior is therefore an inside-negative potential at rest.

The axonal membrane is electrically excitable, i.e., sensitive and reactive to changes in its potential. The resting potential is a negative bias on the membrane, and a small electrical depolarization (shift to lesser negativity) increases the permeability of the membrane to Na. The resistance of the Na-battery becomes less, there is an inward flow of Na from its high external concentration and the Na-current induces further depolarization with further increase in permeability to Na and more Na-influx. This positive feedback proceeds regeneratively to a maximum inside-positivity. Thus, the electrical excitability of the axon membrane operates to cause a flow of current utilizing the ionic batteries as a source of electrical power.

The shift from the resting inside-negativity to positivity is terminated by other membrane processes which are highly regular in a well-behaved axon. The result is a transient electrical current generated as an impulse of constant amplitude and duration. This is the all-or-none spike which, once generated, propagates without decrement along the axon.

Decrementless propagation along a cable is not easy to achieve. The current that enters a telegraph line at one point not only flows along the metallic conductor but also leaks out across the insulation. The rate of decrement of the signal increases as the resistance of the conductor increases and as the resistance of the insulation decreases. After some hundreds of miles the signal may become too small and too distorted in form to remain intelligible. With the advent of electronic amplifiers long-lines transmission became practical by inserting these devices at appropriate points in the cable, so as to restore signal intelligibility.

The loss of current along the axon is much more significant because the insulation of the cell membrane is poorer by many orders (ca 6 or more) than the thick nonconductor of the cable, and the interior of the axon is a far poorer electrical conductor than is a wire. An electrical signal imposed at one end of an axon decays markedly within a few millimeters or centimeters, as contrasted with hundreds or thousands of kilometers in the cable. Amplification, by which a small amount of power can produce a larger power output, is essential and is achieved in the axon by a very different mechanism, again utilizing the electrical excitability of the membrane. Once initiated by a small input signal, the larger spike can trigger a similar spike in the adjacent, as-yet-resting membrane, and this spike in turn triggers another and identical impulse further downstream. Propagation in the axon is not a purely electrical event generated at one point as in a cable. It involves local electrically-induced changes in the properties of the cell membrane much as temperature-induced changes trigger propagation along a fuse.

Conduction of the nerve impulse becomes limited by the kinetics of the local changes in the membrane which generate the spike, and is slow relative to propagation in a cable. The conduction velocity is approximately proportional to the diameter of the axon and, particularly in invertebrates, the requirement for rapid delivery of information to mediate aggressive or defensive reactions promoted the evolution of giant axons, which can, in some animals, reach a diameter of 1 to 2 mm. Conduction velocity was increased more elegantly in the myelinated axons of vertebrates. The myelin provides very high insulation in addition to that of the relatively low-resistance membrane. Leakage of current outward is minimized and the current flowing in the axon is conserved. However, the region between adjacent Schwann cells--the node of Ranvier--lacks myelin and the current can escape at this site, triggering a nerve impulse. The impulse thus jumps from node to node, bypassing the continuous point-to-point spread in the unmyelinated axons. Conduction is as rapid in a 10 to 20 μm vertebrate axon as in an invertebrate fiber of several hundred micrometers.

Through their common dependence on the electrical excitability of the axon membrane, the processes of excitation and conduction therefore are linked events. The initiation of an impulse at the input of a neuron and its transmission at the output involve rather different phenomena which are related to their specific functional requirements. If transmission resembled conduction and were mediated by the flow of current from cell to cell there would arise the possibility of crosstalk. A nerve containing hundreds and thousands of nerve fibers could become a horizontal Tower of Babel, each fiber spewing out an electric current. The messages of the individual axons would become garbled and incomprehensible to the cells for which they were destined.

Isolation of message channels is accomplished by another physiological adaptation, incorporating into the membrane regions which are capable of electrically-inexcitable electrogenesis. As a general rule, the specialized membrane at the input of neurons and effectors is of this type. Thus, sensory receptors respond preferentially to specific stimuli rather than to electric currents -- except in the specialized electroreceptor organs, where electrical excitability is obligatory. The specificity of the sensory input membrane thus provides a means for encoding messages for different sensory modalities--chemical, mechanical, photic or thermal. Transmission to a cell that has an electrically-inexcitable input membrane must necessarily involve a chemical signal from the preceding (presynaptic) cell. Here again, the organisms have adapted a general property of cells, their capacity for secretion. The synaptic vesicles of nerve terminals are storage sites of specific chemical agents that are released into the synaptic space under the command of the electrical impulses. There is an obligatory relation between pre- and postsynaptic cells. The presynaptic neuron must be capable of manufacturing the precise transmitter agent to which the postsynaptic membrane is responsive. The latter membrane may have several regions that are sensitive to different transmitters and produce different types of synaptic electrogenesis. One innervating neuron can act on a region which produces depolarizing electrogenesis--an excitatory postsynaptic potential--which can initiate impulses in the postsynaptic cell so that the processes of excitation and transmission are renewed in this cell. Another presynaptic neuron acting at a different postsynaptic site may produce inhibitory signals which tend to suppress impulses.

In certain cases, the resistance between cells is normally low enough so that there may be electrical interaction from one cell to another. Electrical transmission is particularly useful where synchronized massive discharge of cells must be evoked rapidly. But this type of transmission lacks the subtlety and flexibility which are made possible by the interplays of excitatory and inhibitory activities in the vertebrate central nervous system.

The nature and site of trauma determine the changes produced in the various physiological components that initiate, conduct and transmit impulses. Toxic agents, ischaemia or anoxia, which may themselves be sequelae of mechanical trauma, may cause selective damage, reversible or irreversible, to specific regions of the neuron. The chemically-excitable synaptic-membrane components frequently are specifically sensitive to various agents. Manufacture and delivery of metabolic or secretory material may be slowed or disrupted. Local changes in body fluids may cause changes in the ionic environment which might alter the resting potential and increase or decrease negative bias on the electrically-excitable membrane. Metabolic changes may affect the ion pumps which normally maintain the ionic asymmetry across the membrane. These changes may alter excitability or transmission, or they can affect conduction velocity. Differential effects in different neurons may

disrupt the patterns of the normal message traffic which are
extremely important in the decoding of information.

Of particular importance in the present context is localized
trauma to the axons. If the trauma disrupts the axon, but leaves
the sheaths intact (axonotmesis), the axon may regenerate along the
original pathway and may reform its contact with the next cell.
Nerve block is then temporary and recovery of function may be very
good. When the discontinuity is complete, leading to Wallerian degeneration, recovery of normal function is almost hopeless, since
it is unlikely that the new growth will be able to discover its
normal target, without the aid of the wiring diagram for the original connections. Hopes for successful regrowth following suture of
sectioned nerves were high at one time, but have proved illusory.

The past few decades have witnessed an extraordinary development in the knowledge of the electrophysiological mechanisms of
excitation, conduction and transmission of impulses, largely because electrical methods of measurement are relatively simple and
the techniques are highly developed. However, new techniques and
insights are making possible many new types of study on the morphological and chemical activities of nerves and neurons. These
studies reveal the extraordinary complexity of chemical and structural interrelations within each cell and of the interdependence of
different kinds of cells. To a considerable degree the electrophysiology is rather simple and stereotyped compared to other
aspects of neuronal activity, which will be discussed later in
this Workshop.

DR. FRED SAMSON: Would you comment on the relative vulnerability of the synaptic zone as compared to the axon? I have a
feeling that the sort of things we are talking about here are
subtle, and that the axon behavior may not be the place to look.

DR. GRUNDFEST: Your feeling is probably correct. For example,
we were discussing pain in relation to pressure on nerves. Pain is
a peripheral and central phenomenon. It is not a phenomenon of
conduction or absence of conduction. You are perfectly right.
Dr. Sunderland emphasized that pressure blocks of various kinds
are not the cause of pain.

There is some evidence that the synapses are indeed vulnerable.
For example, you can pull away nerve terminals from a motor end
plate. This is even being used as an experimental technique these
days. The synaptic complex is also a region which is much more
accessible to chemical agents than is the nerve. By chemical agents
I mean the whole gamut of things that are going on in the body. The
vulnerability will be greater there.

DR. MICHAEL M. PATTERSON: What can you say about the susceptibility either at the terminal or along the axon, during various
types of trauma, to the possibility of ephaptic connections?

DR. GRUNDFEST: In general, the mammalian nervous system
operates via chemical transmission but there are certain kinds of
structures where the passage of an electrical current is facilitated. For example, in the septa of the crayfish or earthworm
giant axons and in the central nervous system of electric fishes
there are certain electrical connections which are made easy by a
gap-type junction. There, a current can jump from one cell to the
other. Now, how much of this occurs normally in the higher animals
and during disease states is problematical. Electrical transmission can occur, undoubtedly, but whether this is a general phenomenon, I really don't know.

DR. HORACE W. MAGOUN: Would you give us your impressions of
what is sometimes described as electrotonic transmission between
dendrites in the central nervous system in areas where neuropil
makes up much of the substance? This is said to occur in the cerebellar cortices, in the tectum of the mid-brain and in the neo-
cortex and hippocampus, where there seems to be a fairly open
opportunity for interneuronal excitation without involving the
secretion of chemical transmitters.

DR. GRUNDFEST: This is a condition of this ephaptic or
electrical transmission.

DR. MAGOUN: But it is not ephaptic in the old sense of the
word where there was a traumatized nerve. Rather, it is a normal
pattern of transmission in the functional nervous system.

DR. GRUNDFEST: Yes, these things occur, of course, but I
think that they would not be as effective as synaptic transmission.
Synaptic transmission, basically, has an amplifier effect. There
is a chemical agent which can open up a lot of channels and produce a large postsynaptic potential of some kind. In electrical
transmission the areas involved are relatively small. The amount
of current flow that can occur is relatively small.

DR. MAGOUN: You don't feel, then, that they possess much
capacity for being important functional phenomena to which attention has not previously been directed?

DR. GRUNDFEST: The central nervous system is such a complex
thing that you can have all kinds of mish mash to which attention
has not previously been directed. One of the problems with electrical transmission is that it is a nonspecific effect. Also, if
anything occurs at all, it causes a depolarization of the next cell

so that it is primarily an excitatory effect. I agree with Sherrington, that inhibition is at least as important as, and maybe
even more important than, excitation.

DR. IRVIN M. KORR: My question is related to one asked by
Dr. Patterson. The early work of Granit, Leksell and Skoglund,
which is still widely quoted, showed that in areas of injury there
was "crosstalk", as neurologists call it, between fibers. Has that
been confirmed? I know Arvanitaki and others dealt with the electrical field accompanying an impulse and that in injured areas the
thresholds of neighboring nerves have been lowered so that they
responded to those ordinarily minor voltages.

DR. GRUNDFEST: Well, you remember there are some papers by
Gardner on crosstalk of that kind. I don't think the evidence is
that good. There certainly must be some kind of crosstalk, but
under conditions which are really very special, as shown by Therman
and Renshaw around 1940. This is not a strong kind of transmission
effect. Theoretically, of course, there might be lesions which
would produce interfiber transmission but I would rather question
it as being very important.

DR. KORR: I do remember that this occurred especially where
calcium was lowered. I wonder if it can occur in areas of inflammation, for example, where connective tissue elements of nerves
were inflamed.

DR. GRUNDFEST: Well, Arvanitaki, of course, showed that if
you lowered the excitability threshold so that you got a smaller,
depolarization-produced triggering of an impulse, then the minute
current that could pass from one axon to the next would be sufficient to set up electrical transmission. She reduced the calcium
concentration to an extremely low level so that the axon was already nearly firing. Again, you would have to have special
conditions.

DR. P. W. NATHAN: Professor Wu has looked for ephaptic transmission in preparations of the rat, cutting the rat's sciatic nerve
and then getting a neuroma. He has never found it. He thinks the
original Skoglund and Granit experiments were badly done and that
they let the nerve dry out.

DR. SIDNEY OCHS: You might, while you are at it, lay to rest
another old problem, the repetitive discharge in injured areas.
That has been mentioned on and off for many years.

DR. GRUNDFEST: I really don't feel capable of talking about
repetitive discharge. Repetitive discharge normally occurs in certain kinds of cells and neurons where the accommodation process,

the sodium inactivation is low or potassium activation is short
under normal conditions, sensory nerves tend to fire repetitively
in many cases, while motor axons do not.

There is another possibility for repetitive activity. In recent years, most people have come to realize that not just sodium
and potassium are involved in forming the ionic batteries but that
one may have a calcium battery and, perhaps, other kinds. The calcium battery has the possibility that once you start the current
going it doesn't end quickly as it does with the sodium current.
It can keep on going so that the calcium spikes in certain cells
are of long duration. Certain kinds of heart muscle exemplify
this. It is possible that persistent calcium activation may produce a battery which can fire the cell repetitively.

On the other hand, there is also the possibility that you increase the potassium concentration locally, which is what happens
when you cause cell damage and potassium leaks from the cell. By
the way, I should also mention that in some cases entrapment may
very well involve accumulation of potassium, say, in local regions
of the extra-axonal spaces. You now have a depolarizing agent
which is producing repetitive stimulation.

You can do that very nicely experimentally. We know that
accumulation of potassium in extra-axonal spaces may be quite
marked. Hence, this kind of repetitive excitation might occur
in damaged regions.

DR. JOHAN SJÖSTRAND: I think there is a clinical situation
in which the electrical crosstalk between axons may be relevant.
You sometimes see patients in whom trigeminal neuralgia is combined with hemifacial spasm. The electrical coupling there has
been much discussed because you can't find any pathways between
the nuclei. Often you find a tumor pressing near the foramen, near
the base of the skull. I wonder if that is an indication of electrical crosstalk in compressed nerves.

I would also like to address a question to Dr. Sunderland.
You said that after the traction forces had been taken up by the
dural sac, the nerve root became the susceptible area. Could it
be that the attachment site for the dural fibers, where they mix
with the perineurium, is the site of lower resistance? You could
have shear forces in just that area when you have traction of the
nerve. You could have a site with breakdown of the barrier at that
site.

DR. SUNDERLAND: At that transition zone which we mentioned in
the intervertebral foramen? I think there could be effects there
but, of course, what happens in these cases is that you avulse the

nerve root at the site of its attachment to the spinal cord. But
before you do that you could get an effect short of actual rupture
of the fibers or you may get the rupture of some fibers but not a
total rupture of the nerve root. You never see a rupture of the
nerve root at the intervertebral foramen. It is always torn from
the surface of the cord.

DR. SJÖSTRAND: But my question was that before you have a
rupture you have a constant and repetitive traction at that site
that will damage the perineurial barrier, not making an avulsion
of the nerve, but a site of constant irritation.

DR. SUNDERLAND: Oh, certainly, I would agree with that, yes.

DR. GRUNDFEST: Before I close I would like to add a comment
to your question. In a Louisiana shrimp, there is one case of a
very small axon, something of the order of 10 μm, which is situated in a very heavy sheath. It sends branches out through this
sheath. The conduction velocity of this 10 μm axon is something
like 200 m/sec, which is ridiculous from other physiological data.
The interpretation probably is that the current which is confined
in the thick sheath now can come out through the region and this
acts as a node, essentially, so that you have saltatory conduction
over long distances. That will now give high conduction velocity.

In the case that you mention where there are two axons in
nerves going through a constriction, it is possible to find interfiber transmission, particularly if, as you suggested, the nerve
might be drying out.

DR. A. J. McCOMAS: A comment and a question: There is one
situation where it has clearly been shown now that you may have
ephaptic transmission. This is in the ventral root fibers of
dystrophic mice. These mice are born with amyelination of their
ventral root fibers. Admittedly, the axons which are of quite
large diameter are closely apposed to each other. It has been
shown not only that you may have transmission from one axon to
another, but that the amyelinated segments may actually act as
generators of spontaneous activity.

The question is for Sir Sydney Sunderland. You mentioned that
it was possible to elongate a peripheral nerve, chronically, to
something like three times its resting length. In those situations,
do you get new nodes formed or does the myelin sheath disappear?

DR. SUNDERLAND: I think that is a very interesting question.
We see this where nerves are slowly deformed over an enlarging
tumor. A classical example is the facial nerve over an acoustic
neuroma. Again, we have seen examples of an adenoma of the

pituitary escaping from the sella turcica and passing out just under the third nerve, gradually elevating it and distorting it to such a degree that, in fact, you cannot identify either the facial nerve or the third nerve over the tumor surface. When you examine it histologically, the only things that are really surviving are the axons.

This has interested us in another context, and that is what is the relationship between fiber structure and fiber function under those circumstances? This is rather tricky. I mentioned those two instances because we have had personal experience in both of them and found no disturbance of function at the periphery--nothing referable to the ocular motor field, nothing referable to the facial nerve field. What can often happen under these circumstances, of course, is that even when the surgeon exercises the greatest care in removing the neuroma, there is clearly sufficient trauma to a now-structurally-modified nerve that he precipitates a facial nerve palsy.

You ask me about the nodes, and we can't say because we cannot identify them. The question, of course, to the physiologist, is this relationship of structure to function. What they would say under these circumstances is that conduction is modified but there are adjustments at a central level to compensate for it so that function at the periphery is not, in fact, disturbed. I don't know whether or not that is an acceptable explanation but that is the one that has been advanced. Once again, you can certainly deform nerves and modify their original structure. I don't know about disturbing conduction but you certainly do not disturb function.

We carried out some experiments in the early days in which we were testing the effect of suture materials on peripheral nerves in order to discover the most favorable material for nerve sutures. We decided not to divide the nerve because it complicated the issue in that you were then examining not only the reaction to the suture material but the reaction to the transsection. So we merely transfixed nerves with the suture material. Catgut produced an amazing reaction. When you terminate the experiment--it can be at 21 days or 120 days after suturing--you get a massive round-cell reaction to the catgut, very little in the way of a fibroblastic reaction. On either side of the round-cell infiltration, you have normal nerve. When you make microscopic sections in the area where you commence to get round-cell infiltration, there you simply cannot identify nerve. You go on sectioning past the round cells, and you are back to normal nerve. Yet, all the tests we could apply showed that there was no disturbance of function at all.

In those days we just did not have the equipment or the time to test conduction. This work was repeated, subsequently, in

Germany. I forget the name of the person who confirmed these results. I have an idea that he did find a slowing of conduction
across the area of change. It is clear that you can get remarkable
changes. Clearly there is axonal continuity because there is no
disturbance of function at all at the periphery in the experimental
animal. Some curious things go on in nerves without disturbing
function.

DR. GRUNDFEST: Dr. McComas' point is a good one. If the
nerves that you were talking about before are stretched to three
times their length and no new nodes are formed, they you should
have a high conduction velocity because with the increased inter-
nodal distance you would have a high rate of saltatory conduction.

On the other hand, are there any changes in the axonal sheaths
or in the Schwann cells? The myelin, after all, is a product of
the Schwann cells.

DR. SUNDERLAND: There is great difficulty in identifying
them. They seem to be completely thinned out. They are obviously
in continuity but they are not identifiable.

SOMATOAUTONOMIC REFLEXOLOGY - NORMAL AND ABNORMAL*

Otto Appenzeller

University of New Mexico School of Medicine

Albuquerque, New Mexico

My contribution to this workshop is limited to clinical observations of somatoautonomic relationships; the neural pathways
for some remain entirely unknown and are subject for further study.

Perhaps it is appropriate to begin with a common phenomenon
which has so far not been fully investigated. Subjects who receive
a blow on the front of the chest become, for a few seconds, apneic,
though they remain fully conscious. This apnea is frightening and
gives way soon to grunting, inspiratory efforts finally with return
of normal respiration. This is commonly encountered in motor ve-
hicle accidents where the driver is thrown forward during the impact
on to the steering wheel and, though fully conscious, may be severely
incapacitated by this reflex phenomenon. One explanation for the
reflex arrest of respiration is the sudden stretch imposed upon
intercostal muscles and the diaphragm by the blow on the chest which
leads to reflex activation of stretch receptors and muscle spasm
interfering with further expiration for a few seconds. To my
knowledge, no experimental study of this common phenomenon has been
published. A similar clinical entity well known in boxers occurs
with the knockout due to a sudden blow on the epigastrium or lower
sternal region; the so-called solar plexus blow. In this condition,

*References and a review of the literature are given in *The Autono-
mous Nervous System: An Introduction to Basic and Clinical
Concepts,* 2nd edition. New York: North-Holland Publishing Company and American Elsevier Company, 1976.

179

however, no arrest of respiration is reported, but a clouding of consciousness occurs due to global cerebral ischemia. For obvious reasons no experimental studies of this reflex have been reported, but a possible explanation is a sudden increase in intravascular pressure in the low pressure intrathoracic vasculature which reflexly leads to peripheral vasodilatation (inhibition of sympathetic tone) thus causing a fall in cardiac output and decreased cerebral perfusion leading to unconsciousness. These interpretations are entirely hypothetical.

TEMPERATURE REGULATION

Vasodilatation in the hand after immersion of the opposite extremity in hot water is well known. This vasodilatation is dependent upon warm blood reaching some central structures because it can not be produced with an arrested circulation when the limb is heated. In paraplegics, heating of the lower limbs induces normal vasodilatation in the innervated upper limbs and also the administration of warm saline intravenously causes vasodilatation which is directly related to the amount of heat infused with the saline. Central structures in man concerned with temperature regulation are involved in this reflex vasodilatation which depends for its afferent limb on warm blood reaching the structures. There is another mechanism in which central heat regulating structures can be affected. This reflex seems to have its afferents in the skin. If a limb with an arrested circulation is immersed in cold water, vasoconstriction occurs within a few seconds in the other limb. This reflex was thought at first to be in part dependent upon the unpleasant sensation which accompanies cold immersion, but it is now well established that it depends on neural afferents from the stimulated area and on functioning sympathetic efferents to the blood vessels of the skin. In those with clinically complete high spinal cord lesions, reflex vasoconstriction of the hands cannot be induced after the application of a cold stimulus to the feet and this is therefore not a spinal reflex. In patients with advanced Tabes dorsalis, the application of cold to the feet also does not produce reflex vasoconstriction in the hands even though the cold stimulus is recognized as such. On the other hand, in patients with Leprous neuritis, cold stimulation to the feet without thermal sensibility (which is lost in Leprous neuritis) but with preserved joint positions and vibration sense, produces normal reflex vasoconstriction in the hands. These observations suggest that reflex vasoconstriction in response to cold stimulation is different from constriction due to non-specific psychic stimuli, but normally the two may be difficult to separate. It is likely that afferent structures subserving reflex vasoconstriction in response to cold

are closely associated with or identical with those serving
vibration and joint position sense.

Heating the skin of the chest with a heat cradle (radiant heat)
induces reflex vasodilatation in the hand. This increase in hand
blood flow occurs within 10 sec of heating and promptly subsides to
resting levels after cessation of the stimulus. The vasodilatation
is obtainable when the circulation of a heated limb is arrested and
is not due to lack of cold receptor activity but is associated with
an actual fall in central body temperature. Reflex vasodilatation
thus induced can be abolished by sympathectomy of the heated area
even though this procedure does not interfere with normal temperature sensation of the skin subjected to radiant heat. The conscious
appreciation of warmth on the other hand is also not necessary for
normal reflex vasodilatation since it can be induced by the small
amount of energy emitted from an ultraviolet light source which
does not elicit a sensation of warmth in the irradiated area.
After the application of a rubefacient cream to the skin of the
chest (which causes an intense feeling of warmth due to local
capillary vasodilatation), no increase in hand blood flow occurs.
This shows that the appreciation of warmth is not the cause of
reflex vasodilatation. However, the loss of pain and temperature
sensation due to nervous system lesions in the spinal cord or
upper brainstem abolishes reflex vasodilatation in the hand if the
skin is heated below the level of the lesion. There is evidence,
therefore, that the pathway involved in this reflex extends above
the brainstem, but no good evidence has been presented that it
reaches the hypothalamus, though it is likely that it also is
subserved by temperature-regulating neurons in this area. The
efferent path for reflex vasodilatation as well as the vasomotor
changes produced by the action of warm or cold blood on central
structures are sympathetic. The responses of hand vessels can be
abolished by cervical sympathectomy. In patients with chronic
peripheral neuropathies, vasomotor reflexes in hand vessels may
also be absent, presumably because of involvement of postganglionic
autonomic fibers.

There are therefore two factors which normally act on central
temperature-sensitive structures and effector systems in man. One
of these is activated by neural afferents from the skin and the
other is dependent upon the temperature of the blood. The relative
importance of these two mechanisms in temperature regulation, however, is still uncertain. It is probable that skin receptor activity is responsible for vasomotor adjustments induced by rapid
environmental temperature swings, whereas the effect of blood temperature is to compensate for changes in heat production and to
prevent over-compensation by skin reflexes.

EFFECTS OF RESPIRATION ON HAND BLOOD FLOW

Vasoconstriction is easily elicited in hand vessels after a gasp. This vasoconstriction is not simply a reflection of alterations in blood pressure that occurred during the respiratory effort. Similar vasoconstriction can be induced by passive chest inflation with air under positive pressure and by sudden chest compression in those with paralysis of respiratory muscles. It cannot, however, be induced by inspiratory or expiratory efforts through an obstructed airway nor after forced expiratory efforts. No definite evidence for the location of receptors which are responsible for this type of reflex vasoconstriction has been found, but it is known that the afferents enter the spinal cord in the upper thoracic region. In patients with lesions of the spinal cord above the sympathetic outflow to hand vessels, inspiratory vasoconstriction is preserved. This is an example of a purely spinal reflex complete in the thoracic cord in man. The efferent fibers to hand vessels which mediate inspiratory vasoconstriction are sympathetic and are sometimes affected in patients with peripheral neuropathy in whom this reflex may be absent.

CHANGES IN BLOOD VESSEL CALIBER AND ENVIRONMENTAL TEMPERATURE

The rate of blood flowing through and the density of blood vessels in limbs of man are largely responsible for cooling and the development of temperature gradients through the tissues on exposure. The blood vessels in the extremities are arranged to heat superficial and cool deeper structures. The arteries are deep veins and the venae comitantes which accompany arteries form a draining system like a counter-current heat exchanger which cools the inflowing arterial blood while warming the returning venous blood. The application of cold causes local vasoconstriction, but vasodilatation after strong cooling of certain body parts has been recognized. For example, when fingers are removed from ice cold water the temperature of the finger rises above the original level. When the temperature is monitored during longer periods of immersion in ice cold water, it is found that an increase in finger temperature appears within a few minutes of cooling, waxing and waning thereafter due to vasodilatation and constriction. This feature of cold vasodilatation is called Lewis' shunting reaction. The cold vasodilatation is believed to result from episodic shunting of blood through arteriovenous anastomoses. It can be obtained in sympathectomized hands and in patients with chronically denervated fingers. Because of this, it is attributed to a direct effect of the surrounding temperature on blood vessels, but other factors such as slowed nerve conduction and histamine release may play a part.

There are numerous skin areas from which cold vasodilatation
can be elicited. These include the head and neck, except the vertex
of the skull, the olecranon, the fingers and palms, the buttocks,
the patellae, the perianal region, the toes and soles of the feet.
For this reason the assumption is made that these areas are suitably
supplied with arteriovenous anastomoses to allow cold vasodilatation.
An attempt has been made to use this phenomenon to explain the origin and possible survival function of Northern Asian man's distinctive facial features. Detailed anthropometric measures taken on
subjects of Japanese and European ancestry correlated with cold-
induced vasodilatation and various facial sites. Both Europeans
and Japanese had cycles of vasodilatation and vasoconstriction of
the face. These were most prominent on the forehead and nose, and
were more frequent in Europeans, which accounted for a higher final
temperature at the end of cooling. European face shape is associated with higher surface temperature than the Oriental face, and
temperature remains lower in the presence of high cheek thickness,
protrusive malar bones and a shorter head. It has been suggested
that from an evolutionary point of view, the head has a primary
thermoregulatory function, but the findings of anthropometric
measurements are contrary to the so-called cold-engineered face
which is said to be particularly resistant to frostbite. Inhabi-
tants of cold regions seem to have acquired the art of avoiding
facial frostbite which of course reduces frostbite as a selective
force in the evolution of their facial features.

ABNORMALITIES IN BODY TEMPERATURE

A recognized hazard during cold months in temperate climates
is accidental hypothermia which affects predominantly the old and
infirm. Otherwise healthy old people may have low body temperatures in cold environments and function reasonably well. Serious
hypothermia with impaired consciousness in the aged seems to be
associated with particular social conditions, concomitant disease
and medication, but whether these are directly related to symptomatic hypothermia is not known. Exposure of old people to cold
causes a smaller increase in oxygen consumption; the fall in
rectal temperature is greater and in skin temperature less than in
young people. It remains to be determined how much of this is
directly attributable to malfunction of central thermoregulatory
structures, perhaps induced by hypothalamic blood flow changes with
age, abnormalities in efferent neural pathways or blood vessels
directly concerned with thermoregulatory mechanisms.

Temperature regulation in elderly survivors of accidental
hypothermia has also been studied. In such subjects, the resting
temperature was low; when they were again exposed to cold, the
temperature fell progressively and abnormally rapidly.   These

abnormalities were attributed to impairment in the normally occurring increase in heat production and decrease in heat loss on exposure to cold. The disturbance in temperature regulation was
present up to three years after recovery from accidental hypothermia. All cases examined showed impaired temperature regulation
and it is thought that survivors of accidental hypothermia are
liable to recurrences upon re-exposure to even moderate cold. While
the abnormalities in temperature regulation are attributed to disease of the nervous system, the patients themselves show only slight
disorders of central nervous system function and it is impossible to
assess the probable site or extent of the lesions.

Increased participation in outdoor activities has led to the
recognition that many deaths which occur outdoors and are attributed
to exposure are in fact due to hypothermia. In many cases, victims
often wear unsuitable clothing which, when wet, may provide less
insulation than clothing ordinarily worn in cities on warm sunny
days. Many outdoor accident victims are handicapped further in the
maintenance of their body temperature by self-administered or prescribed medications. Hypothermia, once it occurs, can lead to loss
of circulatory reflexes with orthostatic hypotension. This is
clearly important to rescue crews who often have to transport the
casualty victim down steep mountain slopes.

Hypothermia occurs also in patients with recognizable disease
of the central nervous system. It may be episodic or continuous.
Thermoregulatory mechanisms in such patients have been only rarely
and usually inadequately studied. In some patients, a diminished
ability to maintain body temperature on heating or cooling was found,
or normal responses to heating and pyrogen occurred and it was concluded that the hypothermia was associated with a normal temperature-
regulating mechanism functioning at a lower set level. Some central
nervous system lesions may give rise to poikilothermia with functioning peripheral thermoregulatory mechanisms, but without response to intravenous injection of pyrogen, which acts on central
structures.

A study of patients with hydrocephaly showed autonomic
failure of central origin, whereas patients with hydrocephalus
have normal thermoregulatory function. Autopsy examination of two
such patients showed marked abnormalities of hypothalamus; the rest
of the autonomic nervous system was histologically normal. In
cerebral giantism autonomic failure with persistent fever has also
been demonstrated. This was due to abnormalities in central
thermoregulatory structures subsequently confirmed histologically.

In patients with Parkinson's disease, unusual tolerance to
cold is often found, but accidental hypothermia occurs and is
associated with reversible electroencephalographic abnormalities

which mimic those seen in rapid progressive dementia with fatal
outcome. The relationship of accidental hypothermia in these
patients to the demonstrated abnormalities in autonomic ganglia
is not understood, but Lewy bodies are found not only in the substantia nigra, but also in sympathetic chain ganglia. Apart from
accidental hypothermia, Parkinsonian patients also suffer from
sialorrhea, seborrhea, excessive sweating, constipation, dysphagia,
postural hypotension, blue mottled skin and other vasomotor abnormalities, heat intolerance and impotence. Autonomic function
studies in patients with this disorder are consistent with a central
failure of autonomic control due to dysfunction of the hypothalamus
which is perhaps complicated and aggravated by peripheral degenerative changes in autonomic ganglia.

HEAT ILLNESS

Heat illness occurs in high environmental temperatures and may
be subdivided into four varieties: heat stroke in which very high
body temperatures occur in a setting of delirium, convulsions, and
impairment of consciousness; heat hyperpyrexia in which the body
temperature is higher than $41^{\circ}C$, but the subjects have none of the
other clinical features of heat stroke and which is attributed to
an abnormality in thermoregulation; anhidrotic heat exhaustion in
which subjects, because of sweat gland abnormalities, slowly cease
to sweat until the hot environment causes an abnormal temperature
rise; and an acute variety of anhydrotic heat exhaustion which occurs
in very hot and humid climates and may be associated with mild infections. The first symptom of infection may be cessation of sweating rather than the usual chill and rigor. Patients with acute anhidrotic heat exhaustion notice a sudden diminution or cessation of
sweating, particularly after exertion. They may complain of headache, anorexia and confusion, and they may be ataxic. Their skin
is hot and dry but otherwise normal, and sweating returns within
a day or two with complete recovery after the infection has been
overcome and they have been appropriately cooled.

During heat waves, the death rate from heat-related disease is
often much higher in urban areas. This results from climate modification due to urbanization and the smaller differences between day
and night temperatures in cities than in urban areas. In cities,
radiant heat load is much greater and wind speed often much lower.
During heat waves, city dwellers have to endure sustained thermal
stress both day and night, while their rural neighbors get relief
at least during sleep. The excess deaths in cities during heat
waves are attributed to the effect of urbanization on ambient
temperature.

Heat stroke is associated with high mortality. It occurs when
excessive heat storage is present, together with an inability to

dissipate the heat by radiation, convection and sweat evaporation.
Understanding of the pathogenesis of heat stroke makes it prevent-
able and might reduce the mortality rate during heat waves (4,000
per year in cities around the United States). Prevention of the
effect of heat is best achieved by education of those exposed to
heat and humidity; to recognize conditions that can cause excessive
heat load when physical work must be limited. Intake of salt and
avoidance of dehydration are also necessary. Severe hyperpyrexia
can be precipitated by exercise in patients on phenothyazine medication. High central temperatures have been recorded and death has
been reported. While in some patients hyperpyrexia occurred with
overdosage, others have had hyperpyrexia with therapeutic levels
of phenothyazines and without associated exercise. The potent
anticholinergic action of these drugs inhibits sweating and this
might be a factor in precipitating hyperpyrexia. Heat stroke can
occur during prolonged exercise, even at moderate temperatures, in
poorly trained individuals. This is not infrequent in marathon
runners, particularly when they attempt their first race with
inadequate hydration and physical training.

THE EFFECT OF COLD ON NERVES

The mechanism of cold perception is not fully understood, but
the response to cold stimulation varies in different parts of the
skin. The face is very sensitive. Sudden cooling may cause cessation of respiration, generalized vasoconstriction and momentary
cardiac arrest. Responses to cold exposure vary in different races
and individuals. When Andean natives are exposed to cold,
they maintain substantially warmer extremity temperatures than do
Caucasian subjects. There are also some sex differences. Studies
on hand temperature, blood pressure and heart rate of Highland
Quechuan Indians during cold immersion of the hand for 20 min showed
that females maintained warmer skin temperatures and had most marked
cold-induced vasodilatation and reactive hyperemia. They also had
a lesser increase in systolic cold pressor responses and heart rates
during cold water immersion. White males participating in the same
study were least tolerant to cold.

There is a decline in heat production with advancing age. The
rate of decline varies amongst species, but a fixed minimum of heat
production is usually reached near senescence and appears to be independent of species, reaching a value of about 20 calories per
kilogram per day at the age of approximately 100 years in man. It
has been suggested that survival is related to minimum heat production which is necessary for life of homeotherms.

Intensive cooling of the hand is associated with pain which
reaches its peak after about 1 min. With further cooling, the pain

gives way to deep-seated ache and paresthesia which improve with
periods of cold vasodilatation. During the first 5 min of cold immersion there is a rise in blood pressure which is related to the
intensity of the pain. When the hand is kept in cold water for
about 30 min, the elevated blood pressure is replaced by a fall in
blood pressure which can cause a faint with typical pallor, sweating
and loss of consciousness. Fibers in peripheral nerves which mediate cold pain are remarkably resistant to anoxia since the pain can
still be produced after 45 min of circulatory arrest by which time
touch and appreciation of pain from pin prick have been lost.

Nerve conduction slows with cooling but there are considerable
differences between species and in nerves of the same animal in the
temperature at which nerve conduction ceases. Cooling the skin over
nerve trunks in man causes a loss of light touch and cold sensibility after which motor power, vasoconstrictor fiber paralysis and,
lastly, pain and pressure sensation are abolished. The sequence of
sensory loss is different from that observed after local anesthetic
or compression block in which cold sensibility is not the first to
be lost.

                              SHIVERING

Shivering in man and an associated increase in metabolism occur
in response to cold. In adults the metabolic increase in response
to cooling is entirely due to shivering since it can be abolished by
muscular paralysis. When the skin is cooled there is shivering, an
increase in metabolic rate and elevation of the central temperature.
In this situation, shivering is provoked by skin receptor activity
because the rise in central temperature does not inhibit shivering.
In normal subjects shivering appears to be entirely dependent on a
reflex initiated from the skin, but in patients with spinal cord
lesions it can be shown that shivering occurs in normally innervated muscles above the site of the lesion when the central temperature falls due to cooling of the legs. In these studies, the skin
above the lesion was kept warm and no patient felt the cold. Therefore, there must exist in man central structures, capable of inducing
shivering when the temperature of the blood falls, which appear to
play no role in normal subjects, however. Such studies have also
shown that the perception of cold is predominantly dependent upon
skin receptors and not on central temperature. This has importance
in subjects who are accidentally exposed to cold in outdoor winter
accidents. If, as sometimes happens, alcohol is given to the victims, skin vessels dilate because of a direct effect of alcohol on
blood vessels, and a feeling of warmth may give an inappropriate relief from shivering. The dilated skin vessels lead to further cooling of the blood, and with increasing rate of fall in central temperature serious hypothermia may occur. In fever, shivering occurs,

but in those with paralyzed muscles, shivering can be observed only in muscles normally innervated. Therefore, this type of shivering must be initiated by the activity of pyrogens on central structures.

NON-SHIVERING THERMOGENESIS

Non-shivering thermogenesis (NST) is heat production due to the release of chemical energy which does not involve muscle contraction. Heat production in basal conditions, at rest and in the thermal neutral zone, is for the most part the so-called obligatory or basal NST, which maintains the energy demands of the homeothermic animal. Regulatory NST occurs at environmental temperatures which are below thermal neutral zone; this may include heat production by the specific dynamic action of food. NST occurs predominantly in cold-adapted animals. In those not acclimated to cold exposure, low ambient temperatures cause shivering which appears to be the only source of regulatory heat production in non-acclimated animals. In adapted animals, however, NST occurs in addition to shivering and this increases resistance to cold exposure. NST is of great importance in thermoregulation of newborn animals and man and is influenced by the relationship between skin temperature and the temperature of the anterior hypothalamus. In experimental situations it has been shown that the lower the body surface temperature, the warmer the anterior hypothalamus has to be to avoid induction of NST. On the other hand, when hypothalamic temperature is low, a small decrease of skin surface temperature is sufficient to induce NST. Like so many other thermoregulatory activities, NST regulation seems to be intimately associated with the preoptic and supraoptic areas of the hypothalamus.

The effector part of NST is the sympathetic nervous system. NST is stimulated by norepinephrine which is liberated from sympathetic nerve endings and can be blocked by the administration of β-adrenergic blockers. However, during NST there is not only sympathetic activation, but also stimulation of the parasympathetic nervous system. Many experiments suggest, but do not conclusively prove, that other hormones than norepinephrine, including thyroid hormone, ACTH, and corticosteroids, have calorigenic effects and participate in NST.

Food intake is associated with an increase in metabolism. In man this is accompanied by increased peripheral blood flow which in turn results in greater heat loss from the body. The dynamic action of food in man is usually not available for thermoregulation. Increased heat production occurs mostly in the liver during metabolism of amino acids, but it is not known whether its magnitude can be regulated. NST causes increased cardiovascular and pulmonary activity (increased heart rate, cardiac output and oxygen utilization).

Blood flow through various organs of the body is also increased, but this is most marked in brown and white adipose tissue, pancreas, heart, diaphragm, and muscles. Regulation of the metabolism of cells during NST appears to depend on the following scheme: Sympathetic stimulation leads to norepinephrine release which interacts with cell membranes (brown adipose tissue). This leads to membrane depolarization and stimulation of the Na^+-K^+ pump. By an unknown mechanism, adenylcyclase is activated, increasing the availability of cyclic AMP; this in turn leads to an increase in lipolysis and higher levels of free fatty acids and glycerol. An increased oxygen uptake occurs accompanied by greater heat production. Whether the intensity of oxidative processes stimulated by norepinephrine in other organs is similar to that found in brown adipose tissue is not known. The precise role of NST and of catecholamines in thermogenetic activity has not been fully elucidated in man and further study is necessary for an understanding of cold adaptation and perhaps for the differential susceptibility to exposure of various racial groups.

SWEAT GLAND ACTIVITY AND DISTURBANCES OF SWEATING

The term sympathetic dermatome has been used to designate the area of cutaneous distribution of sympathetic nerves in a given segment. The sympathetic dermatomes do not coincide with the corresponding sensory dermatomes and their outlines are often irregular and asymmetric. In some completely denervated areas which encircle the body, a gap of normal sympathetic activity may remain in the midline, either anteriorly or posteriorly. Cessation of thermoregulatory sweating in circumscribed areas of the skin due to lesions of the sympathetic ganglia or rami is often associated with hyperhydrosis in surrounding zones. Extensive denervation may lead to excessive sweating in normally innervated areas, perhaps because of compensatory thermoregulatory activity. Sympathectomy does not lead to obvious anatomic changes in denervated structures even if this is performed early in life. There is no atrophy of denervated smooth muscles, and sweat glands remain histologically unaffected.

Man, in common with the mole, has sweat glands which are not associated with hair follicles, called atrichial sweat glands. Sweat glands of almost all other mammals are next to hair follicles and are part of a unit. These sweat glands are termed epitrichial. Not all hair follicles have an associated sweat gland; animals with dense hair coats do not always have high densities of sweat glands. For example, the density varies from 20 to 30/cm^2 in the pig to over 2,000/cm^2 in Zebu cattle. Because of an anatomical arrangement, sweat is often mixed with sebum before it reaches the surface of the skin. This has an effect on skin texture and may contribute to some hyperhydrotic states.

Two types of sweating are generally recognized, thermoregulatory sweating which occurs over the whole body in response to changes in ambient temperature, and emotional sweating which is confined to palms, axillae soles and some areas of the face. It is still not entirely clear whether thermoregulatory sweating is due to a rise in blood temperature which activates central structures responsible for thermoregulation, or whether a peripheral heat-sensitive receptor reflexly activates central structures and induces heat loss by sweating. Under certain circumstances either of these mechanisms alone or in combination may produce sweating. Sweating can be inhibited temporarily in a hot environment by cooling a part of the body or by ingestion of ice. If the circulation to the cooled limb is arrested, the effect remains unaltered. The temporary inhibition of thermoregulatory sweating by these maneuvers is a reflex due to stimulation of cold receptors. The mechanism by which sweating is initiated in hot environments varies with the thermal adaptation of the individual. In non-adapted subjects, an abrupt rise in ambient temperature causes sweating after a delay, which correlates with a rise in rectal and tympanic membrane temperatures, but is not related to skin temperature. Adapted subjects under similar conditions show an immediate onset of sweating related to the rise in skin temperature and which increases as the rectal temperature rises. In endurance-trained subjects, sweating is also initiated by active muscles normally used in exercise, irrespective of skin or central body temperature. A second and third wave of sweating occurs after skin temperature rises and when central temperature reaches levels which activate the thermal eye in the hypothalamus.

In a warm environment, sweating occurs within 1 to 2 sec after the beginning of muscular exercise. The stimulus for this sudden appearance of sweating is neurogenic rather than thermal since it is seen when a limb is exercised with the circulation arrested. When exercises stop with continued circulatory arrest the sweat rate drops, so that it is unlikely that local heat receptors in exercised muscles or veins participate in this response. In a warm environment, therefore, sweating with exercise is, in part at least, independent of hypothalamic temperatures, but it is not clear what neural mechanisms are responsible for this phenomenon.

Postural influences on sweating, which seem to be related to pressure, have also been recognized. When a subject lies on his back in a hot environment, sweating is about equal over the body. Lying on one side, however, causes a remarkable increase in sweating on the uppermost side, and inhibition of sweat gland activity on the other side. The palm, which is not usually concerned in thermoregulatory sweating, does participate in this response. Standing after recumbency is also associated with a change in sweat secretion which increases on the upper part of the body and is inhibited in the legs. The initiation of these reflexes is by pressure applied

to the skin. These hemihydrotic reactions can be obtained most
readily by pressing the axillae or adjacent pectoral regions. Other
skin areas require much stronger pressure. These responses are
limited to either the upper or lower half of the body and are separated by an ill-defined border about the iliae crests. The reflex
increase in sweating on the trunk and decrease in sweating of legs
on standing is probably related to a similar mechanism since the
reduction in sweat-gland activity on the legs can be induced by
pressure on soles or hips. These postural sweat reflexes may influence results of experimental studies in man and it is not
understood whether they are related to observations of unilateral
hyperhidrosis in patients confined to bed with a variety of diseases which may have no relation to sweat-gland dysfunction.

Reflex sweating can be elicited locally by faradic stimulation.
This is an unusual way of causing sweat-gland activity and does not
occur physiologically in normal subjects. This activity is induced,
however, by the same peripheral mechanism as that brought about by
normal activation of sweat glands. Sweating after faradic stimulation can be inhibited by atropine and augmented by prostigmine. It
depends on a local axon reflex, mediated by post-ganglionic sympathetic fibers; many overlapping axon systems are involved in this
response.

Sweating can also be induced by the ingestion of fluids in de-
hydrated subjects regardless of the tonicity of the fluid. However,
the intensity and duration of sweating is related to the tonicity of
the fluid. This response is not gustatory sweating, since the latter
is usually confined to the face and head and depends, in normal subjects, on excitation of pain receptors within the oral cavity.

The response to ingestion of fluid in non-dehydrated subjects
is not an uncontrolled reflex, but it can be shown to be a quanti-
tatively controlled active response which consists of a thermal
component and a part which is related to the volume of the ingested
fluid. The volume component could be related to distention of the
stomach or it may be a response to deglutation as if it were a reflection of extra work and associated with a rise in metabolism.
The tonicity of the fluid has no effect on this type of sweating
response in non-dehydrated subjects, provided it is kept within the
range of from 0 to 9% of sodium chloride per liter. The ingestion
of hypertonic saline, on the other hand, is associated with a marked
depression of sweating.

Though it is generally agreed that pain is an emotional stimulus, yet even severe pain does not induce sweating under laboratory
conditions in normal subjects except for ischemic forearm exercise
which significantly increases the rate of sweating.

In patients with pheochromocytoma, sweating is often a prominent feature, but its exact cause is not fully understood. Whether this is the result of the effect of circulating norepinephrine on sweat glands or due to an activation of the nerve supply to the sweat glands has not been determined. Recent studies have suggested that in patients with pheochromocytomas, sweat glands are activated by cholinergic sudomotor nerves rather than by circulating levels of catecholamines acting directly on the glands. These studies support the view that attacks of sweating in patients with pheochromocytoma may be the result of activation of thermoregulatory structures by circulating catecholamines which then in turn activate the sweat glands through normal cholinergic sympathetic fiber activity.

The relation of sweat secretion to cutaneous blood flow is complicated and varies with skin area. In some parts of the body, vasodilatation of the skin may be dependent upon the release of vasodilator substances in the sweat and both these thermoregulatory activities occur concurrently. In the skin of the hand, however, vasodilatation in response to a rise in central temperature may be abolished in patients with the Guillain Barré syndrome, for example, and yet sweating occurs normally. Moreover, in freshly amputated limbs without circulation, sweating can be elicited for some time by direct electrical stimulation of the nerves.

ABNORMALITIES OF SWEATING RELATED TO DISEASES OF THE NERVOUS SYSTEM

Disturbances in sweating produced by lesions in the nervous system in man yield information about pathways involved in this function. Such studies have been mainly concerned with peripheral lesions in which complete sympathetic paralysis is produced and have led to the recognition of certain grouping of symptoms such as Horner's syndrome. In its full-blown form, capillary constriction, dilatation of conjunctival vessels, drooping of the eyelid, anhidrosis and vasodilatation of the vessels of the face on the ipsilateral side are seen. This complete syndrome is usually evident only after lesions interrupting the cervical sympathetic pathways. Lesions in the medulla, which involve descending autonomic pathways, rarely give rise to all the features of autonomic paralysis in the face. Unfortunately, most studies of autonomic function in man lack precision, and correlation with anatomic findings is not wholly satisfactory. Nevertheless, it is believed that fibers related to sweating vasoconstriction in response to cooling of the body, dilatation of the pupils and retraction of the upper eyelids pass through the lateral medullary area. These pathways are mostly uncrossed below the medulla, but some fibers from the opposite side contribute to innervation because the Horner syndrome is incomplete with lesions

in this site.   In degeneration of the intermedial lateral cell columns of the spinal cord, thermoregulatory sweating is impaired, but
not completely absent.   Similarly, in unilateral spinal cord lesions
and in syringomyelia, sweating may be impaired but not abolished.
Lesions above the level of the medulla rarely abolish sweating, but
are associated sometimes with hyperhidrosis.   In infarction involving the insular cortex, hyperhidrosis on the contralateral side of
the body may occur.

    Recent clinical studies of the innervation of sweat glands on
the face after section or block of the facial and trigenimal nerves
or of the perivascular nerve plexuses around the internal carotid
artery have shown that in man all sweat glands of the face are
stimulated by sympathetic and not parasympathetic fibers.   The
facial sweat glands differ from the rest of the body because of a
dual innervation, both from sympathetic fibers which join the
branches of the trigeminal nerve distal to the Gasserian ganglion
and from sympathetic fibers which accompany the external carotid
artery and its branches.   It has also been shown in man that innervation reaching sweat glands from one or other sources is interchangeable, and if there is interruption or failure of one,
compensatory re-innervation from the other pathway is possible.

    Excessive perspiration on the face is common.   Sometimes it
may be confined to one-half of the face and be associated with
tearing and nasal discharge or sweat may appear only on the cheeks.
This type of sweating is provoked by emotional or gustatory stimuli.
Exaggerated sweating of this sort seems to be mediated by accessory
sweat fibers, except sweating confined to the cheek, which occurs
sometimes after injury or surgical operations in the region of the
parotid gland and may be related to diffusion of acetyleleoline,
released by the activity of the parotid secretory nerves.   The
ordinary fibers supplying sweat glands in the face are sympathetic
so that anhidrosis is the usual result of cervical sympathectomy.
In some subjects, however, when the sympathetic supply is interrupted the accessory fibers become active and hyperhidrosis occurs.
This can be observed in about 35% of patients after sympathetic
denervation of the upper lip and it occurs after an interval of
weeks or years.

    The auriculotemporal syndrome is paradoxical reflex gustatory
sweating seen after nerve injury in the face.   Sweating and flushing
of the skin supplied by the auriculotemporal nerve occurs during
eating, particularly of spicy or sour foods.   Because the auriculotemporal nerve carries both sympathetic preganglionic fibers to
vessels and sweat glands and parasympathetic preganglionic secretomotor fibers to the parotid gland, it has been suggested that reflex
sweating during eating is due to cross-excitation between parasympathetic and sympathetic fibers.   The auriculotemporal syndrome

has been successfully treated by division of the 9th nerve, suggesting that the impulses initiating this abnormal sweating are
carried through parasympathetic fibers. The auriculotemporal syndrome has been reported in infants and in children where it is
attributed to injury to the auriculotemporal nerve during forceps
delivery. In the auriculotemporal syndrome, thermoregulatory
sweating is abolished or markedly reduced in the area of reflex
gustatory sweating. Gustatory sweating can be abolished by
anesthetizing the tongue, the otic ganglion, or auriculotemporal
nerve, but not by anesthetizing the cervical sympathetic chain.
Parenteral pilocarpine provokes sweating and this can be inhibited
by atropine, but the sweat glands responding to gustatory stimuli
are hypersensitive to intradermal injection of acetylcholine. The
electrolyte content of sweat in the auriculotemporal syndrome is no
different from sweat produced by thermal load. However, the normally observed decrease in sodium and chloride content of sweat
after administration of 9-α-fluorohydrocortisone does not occur in
sweat glands responsive to gustatory stimuli; this difference in
the control of electrolyte secretion has not been explained.

The chorda tympani syndrome is gustatory sweating in the sub-
mental region. This occurs after surgical trauma in that region
and is attributed to cross-excitation of sympathetic fibers from
parasympathetic secretory fibers to the submaxillary gland, both
of which are in close proximity in this region. This syndrome is
relieved by local anesthetic block of the lingual nerve carrying
chorda tympani fibers, but not by blocking the stellate ganglion.
It has been pointed out that paradoxical sweating is not seen after
trauma or sympathectomy in lower limbs where sympathetic and parasympathetic fibers are anatomically widely separated.

Diabetic anhidrosis is a condition in which sweating is absent
in the lower limbs and trunk of patients with diabetic neuropathy.
Patients with this disorder are intolerant to heat and may also
complain of excessive perspiration on the head, face and neck.
Such hyperhidrosis may be compensatory thermoregulatory sweating.
In diabetic neuropathy sympathetic denervation is predominantly in
the lower limbs and is evidenced by the absence of sweating and by
disturbed vasomotor control. Sweating during eating has been found
in a group of diabetic patients where it was considered a feature
of autonomic neuropathy. Profuse facial sweating at meal times
embarrassing enough to be socially unacceptable was found. The
sweating occurred up to the level of the 3rd of 4th cervical dermatome and was always confined to the territory of the superior
cervical ganglion. The intravenous administration of atropine
inhibited gustatory sweating after cheese and thus established that
cholinergic mechanisms were involved in these patients. All patients
had abnormal autonomic function tests showing that the autonomic
nervous system and autonomic supply to other organs were involved.

If, as has been postulated, gustatory sweating in diabetic neuropathies is a result of sprouting or cross-innervation of fibers,
then in this condition, in spite of the persistence of the metabolic
abnormality, regeneration of axons is possible.

During percutaneous radio-frequency lesions of the Gasserian
ganglion for trigeminal pain it was observed that the application
of the coagulation current to the tissue is accompanied by dense
erythema confined to the division of the trigeminal nerve which is
being interrupted. This blush of the face does not appear if the
lesion is applied in a situation where the sensory root, the
ganglion or the sensory division of the 5th nerve has been interrupted prior to electro-coagulation with consequent facial anesthesia. The facial blush can be used surgically to determine the
extent of subsequent analgesia and by proper technique the blush
can be confined to a single division of the trigeminal nerve. This
blush is attributed to stimulation of a vasodilator system whose
anatomical course has not yet been defined.

In children with congenital heart disease sweating is increased. The increase in sweating in such patients could predict
those who were about to go into cardiac failure. No similar increase in sweat-gland activity was found in patients with congenital
heart disease without a tendency for heart failure. The increased
sweat-gland activity in patients with congenital heart disease and
heart failure was attributed to a compensatory thermoregulatory
activity and thought to be due to the peripheral vasoconstriction
which occurs in impending and during heart failure and which
decreases heat loss by conduction, convection and radiation.

Spinal cord lesions above the sympathetic outflow abolish most
thermoregulatory activity. Patients with such lesions may retain
some ability to react to environmental temperature changes due to a
direct effect of the temperature on vessel walls. Usually, however,
as the ambient temperature rises they are unable to sweat and their
skin temperature reaches approximately the same level as the surroundings. This, in part, is probably due to the effect of the
increasing temperature accelerating tissue metabolism. Patients
with chronic lower cervical cord lesions have little control over
rectal temperature when exposed to hot and cold environments. Those
with lesions of the 4th thoracic segment are not much better off in
hot ambient temperatures, but cool less rapidly in cold surroundings.
Lesions at the level of the 8th thoracic segment or below do not interfere with normal temperature regulation even though there is no
thermoregulatory activity in the lower limbs. All this is in keeping with the suggestion that there is no thermoregulatory center in
man below the level of the 5th cervical cord segment. The study of
thermoregulatory activity in paraplegic patients is of value also to
determine the completeness of the cord lesion, because the only sign

of an incomplete transection may be a preserved sympathetic response
in one or another limb.

In spinal cord lesions usually of the traumatic variety, "border
zone sweating" is often seen. This has been attributed to the "mass
reflex". In high spinal cord lesions sweating is part of the mass
reflex and occurs over the face and upper part of the body and limbs,
whereas in lower cord lesion the excessive sweating is usually over
the lower trunk and lower limbs. At the edge of an area of skin recently deprived of normal sympathetic supply because of a cord
lesion, excessive sweating may also be seen. Hyperhidrosis in connection with cord lesions may appear in the absence of a mass reflex
and then it could represent compensatory hyperhidrosis because of the
inability to sweat in extensive areas of the body below the lesion.

Excessive sweating in patients with severe scoliosis which may
be confined to shoulder, arm or patches on the chest has also been
noted. Whether this occurs because of injury to the spinal cord or
to efferent preganglionic sympathetic fibers has not been determined,
but such patients, if socially embarrassed by their hyperhidrosis,
can be cured by sympathectomy including the ganglia supplying the
appropriate hyperhidrotic segments.

Disturbances of autonomic function have been described after
surgical lesions placed in the thalamus for the treatment of
Parkinsonism, dystonia and torticollis. These consist of ptosis,
miosis, and meianhidrosis on the side of the lesion. The difference
in the size of the pupil is very striking but ptosis is incomplete
and patients can elevate the involved lid voluntarily, but often less
well than the normal one. There is a tendency for these disturbances
to improve with time. The miotic pupil, although responsive to light
dilates slowly again after the end of the stimulus and never reaches
a normal diameter. The psychosensory reflex, which consists of
pupillary dilatation to noise, is impaired on the affected side also.
The ipsilateral loss of sweating involves the whole of the side of
the body and is far more extensive than is usually seen with peripheral sympathetic lesions. The lesions in the thalamus which are
associated with these autonomic deficits are medial and caudal to
those placed in the thalamus anteriorly and rosterally which are not
associated with sympathetic dysfunction. Most of the lesions were
ventral and caudal to the nucleus ventralis oralis posterior of the
thalamus. In a few patients the lesions were placed close to the
red nucleus and included the pre-rubral fibers of the capsule of
the red nucleus. The site of the lesions which produced autonomic
deficits suggests that descending sympathetic fibers from the hypothalamus are interrupted and that the observed autonomic deficits
are due to interruption of these descending fibers. Though there
is experimental evidence to show that autonomic fibers are located
in this area, the evidence does not specifically relate to the

deficits described. However, some clinical evidence has been obtained for the localization of autonomic fibers in the mesencephalon. In one patient, after the sudden onset of hemiballismus, a miotic pupil and ptosis were noted and at autopsy there was an infarct in the corpus Luysii and slight demyelination of the medial part of the capsule of the red nucleus on the side of the pupillary abnormality. In all these studies the eye and sweating abnormalities were the predominant interest. However, the suggestion that efferent autonomic fibers are not scattered but can be interrupted by discrete stereotactically-placed lesions in the mesencephalon might allow a new surgical approach to the treatment of intractable hypertension. The intensive study in post-thalamotomy patients of cardiovascular responses in which the autonomic nervous system is involved is, therefore, of great interest.

In untreated patients with Parkinson's disease, thermoregulatory sweating has been found abnormal with compensatory hyperhidrosis on the face and neck. Patients with Parkinson's syndrome have long been known to sweat excessively but it was not clear whether this clinical observation referred to hyperhidrosis on the face or to excessive sweating on the entire body. More recent observations suggest that excessive sweating on the face in some patients with Parkinson's syndrome, like in diabetic neuropathy, might be the result of failure of thermoregulatory sweating on other parts of the body.

Anhidrosis or hypohidrosis occurs also in patients with postural hypotension who suffer from intermedial lateral column degeneration. In such patients the anhidrosis is a part of other functional deficits involving multiple autonomic activities including sexual impotence, orthostatic hypotension, and clinical evidence of multiple neurologic system degeneration. Segmental anhidrosis may be the first manifestation of the disorder. Patients later develop generalized anhidrosis and the other signs and functional deficits of intermedial lateral column degeneration. The appearance of extensive autonomic deficits may be delayed for years and some patients with so-called "forequarter anhidrosis" may in fact later develop the full-blown syndrome.

Sweating abnormalities have been found in patients with multiple sclerosis. It has been suggested that the plaques of multiple sclerosis involve the descending sudomotor pathways of the spinal cord which appear to be widely distributed and probably are intermingled with other fiber systems. Abnormalities in sweating were related to the severity of the disease. Patients with less severe disease had normal thermoregulatory sweating. Abnormal sudomotor responses were found in severely affected patients, with total anhidrosis in a few, facial sweating only in some and no sweating below the waist in some other patients. Spinal reflex sweating induced by distention of the urinary bladder was not found in patients with sudomotor abnormalities and multiple sclerosis. This suggests that such patients had incomplete transections of the spinal cord. Because intravenously-administered pilocarpine, which acts peripherally by stimulating sympathetic cholinergic fibers, induced sweating in normal amounts, it was concluded that the abnormal thermoregulatory sudomotor activity in multiple sclerosis was due to interruption of central descending sudomotor connections and not the result of peripheral denervation or sweat-gland abnormalities.

Hyperhidrosis is sometimes seen in patients with peripheral neuropathies or in those with traumatic lesions to peripheral nerves. It is usually a sign of incomplete peripheral nerve interruption. When it is associated with causalgia it occurs most commonly in median or sciatic nerve injuries and is associated with a swollen, cyanotic, painful extremity. In such patients, sympathectomy does relieve the pain, excessive sweating and other symptoms of causalgia. In patients with other peripheral nerve lesions, hyperhidrosis usually disappears after a time, concomitant with progression of the lesion, and in advanced peripheral nerve disease there is usually anhidrosis of the distal parts of the extremities. Some patients with cervical ribs may present with hyperhidrosis of the affected limb in a segmental distribution. This usually disappears after surgical resection of the rib and must be attributed to local irritation and pressure of the rib on nerves.

Pink disease or acrodynia is associated with numerous manifestations of autonomic dysfunction, but excessive sweating also occurs. This disorder is attributed to the ingestion of mercury which has been used in "teething powders" given to infants. Ganglion blocking agents have been successful in the treatment of the hyperhidrosis, but chelating agents to remove the metal from the body are essential for eventual cure.

Hyperhidrosis is also seen in patients with tetanus. It is part of an overactivity of the sympathetic nervous system in this disorder.

Sympathectomy leads to anhidrosis in appropriate segments of the body which is usually permanent, whereas vasomotor paralysis can recover after some time. However, "escape areas" where sweating is preserved after sympathectomy are sometimes found, usually in the lower limbs, and can be attributed to intermediate ganglia in the rami communicantes.

In patients with collagen disease, particularly with rheumatoid arthritis and polyarteritis modosa, abnormalities of sweating have been described. This may be a manifestation of mononeuritis

multiplex which is often present. Anhidrosis corresponding to
cutaneous branches of peripheral nerves is a feature of some types
of leprosy also and of great diagnostic value when small anhidrotic
patches appear on the skin, occurring in areas not corresponding to
the major cutaneous distribution of peripheral nerves. This is a
clinical manifestation of involvement of cutaneous nerve twigs by
the disease.

A number of drugs used for the treatment of hypertension impair
sympathetic function and decrease sweating. Anticholinergic drugs
also block sweating. The use of such medication should be suspected
in patients with otherwise unexplained hyperthermia.

SOMATOAUTONOMIC RELATIONSHIPS AND THE CIRCULATION

In conscious subjects, stimulation of the anterior cingulate
region results not only in affective responses but also in other
physiologic changes. These changes have been observed also in anesthetized patients on stimulation of the cingulum below and in front
of the genu of the corpus callosum and from the anterior cingulate
region. Autonomic responses occur on stimulation of structures included in the Papez circuit. These responses are being used to
identify appropriate sites for interruption of the circuit,
as employed in psychosurgery for affective disorders. The close
association between emotional and autonomic pathways and their
anatomic separation from pathways related to memory make ablation
operations on the two parts possible. Anterior cingulate or posterior cingulate lesions do not affect memory, but lesions of the
Papez circuit which involve the hippocampus, fornix, mammilary
bodies and mammillo-thalmic tract impair recent and long-term
memory.

A relationship between the cortex and cardiac and vasomotor
activity in intact man is suggested by several phenomena. Some
persons are capable of voluntary cardiac acceleration and emotional
stress causes excitation of of vasodilator fibers to blood vessels
in human muscles. If normal subjects are frightened while their
forearm blood flow is measured, an eight- to tenfold increase in
blood flow can be observed. This occurs without change in arterial
blood pressure and is due to significant vasodilatation. Vasodilatation in the forearm during emotional stress is confined to
muscles but is usually associated with vasoconstriction in skin
vessels. Similar responses are obtained after mental arithmetic.
T h e   r e s u l t s   of stress vasodilatation elicited after treatment
of the forearm with atropine and bretylium tosylate suggest that
this phenomenon is mediated, at least in part, by sympathetic
vasodilator fibers.

In man, angiotensin or phenylephrine has been used to elicit short bursts of increased arterial pressure to stimulate baroreflexes. When the heart rate intervals are plotted against systolic pressure during baroreflex activity, a measure of baroreceptor activity is obtained. Baroreflex activity thus can be assessed during normal behavior and during sleep. In the majority of normal subjects, an increased baroreceptor sensitivity occurs during sleep, but the sensitivity is maximal during REM sleep. Using the same technique, it was also possible to show that the sensitivity of the baroreflexes is decreased in hypertensive patients and that this decreased sensitivity is also found with advancing years in otherwise normal subjects. Baroreflex sensitivity also decreases during exercise and more so with increased workloads. At a heart rate of 150 beats/min, no effect on baroreflexes was detectable in normal subjects in spite of an increase of 25 to 30 mm of mercury in arterial pressure. This has been interpreted to show that the hypothalamus influences baroreflexes in man. Though this interpretation is not unreasonable, some animal experiments with more elaborate instrumentation suggest that there might be species differences and do not entirely support the findings of a hypothalamic influence in man.

NEUROGENIC CONTROL OF THE CUTANEOUS CIRCULATION

Changes in hand blood flow are largely due to alterations in blood flow through the skin since this is the predominant tissue in the hand, just as the forearm blood flow reflects largely flow through muscles. No definite evidence has ever been found for active vasodilatation in skin vessels and it has been concluded that the vasomotor control of hand vessels is achieved by release of constrictor tone without the participation of vasodilator fibers.

In the forearm the increase in blood flow observed with body heating has been shown to be confined to the skin; and the forearm skin is extremely vascular. The rich blood flow in the human forearm is regulated almost exclusively by a vasodilator mechanism contrary to what is seen in the hand where regulation is achieved through the release of constrictor tone. Vasodilator nerve activity does not, however, account entirely for the very marked increase in blood flow in the forearm skin during body heating and it has been suggested that a large part of the vasodilatation is due to sweat-gland activity for it can be shown that sweat contains an enzyme forming a vasodilator polypeptide. The relationship between forearm sweating and vasodilatation is a variable one, although in general sweating is always accompanied by vasodilatation. For example, in cholinergic urticaria, in gustatory sweating and in insulin hypoglycemia, vasodilatation does accompany sweat-gland activity, but in shock and fainting profuse sweating is seen when

the skin is pale and vasocontriction is present. The relation of
sweating to vasodilatation in the forearm skin is a complicated one
and at present not fully understood, but it appears that, apart
from a vasomotor mechanism, some other factors may play a part.

CIRCULATION IN SKELETAL MUSCLES

The blood vessels in skeletal muscles are supplied by sympathetic vasoconstrictor and sympathetic vasodilator fibers. The
constrictor fibers are activated mainly through baroreceptor activity which originates in the chest. Blood vessels in skeletal
muscles do not participate in reflex vasodilatation induced by body
heating. This vasodilatation is confined to skin vessels. Vasoconstrictor fibers in muscles are not activated by emotional stimuli,
mental arithmetic, pain, a deep breath, or the application of cold,
all of which would normally produce intense vasoconstriction in
skin vessels. There are, however, a number of stimuli which alter
vasoconstrictor tone in muscle vessels. Raising the legs passively
in a recumbent subject causes reflex vasodilatation in the forearm
but not in the hand. This maneuver results in an increase in oxygen
saturation of the blood taken from the deep veins of the forearm
draining muscles but not in superficial veins draining the skin.
The vasodilatation in muscle vessels of the forearm induced by
changes in posture is due to alterations in vasoconstrictor tone,
rather than to activity of vasodilator fibers. Other stimuli which
decrease vasoconstrictor tone in muscle vessels include negative
pressure breathing, squatting, and large intrathoracic pressure
transients.

Stimuli increasing vasoconstrictor tone in muscles are tilting
from recumbent to standing position, positive pressure breathing,
Valsalva's maneuver, radial acceleration and hypercapnia. In
inactive muscles during exercise there is also an increase in vasoconstrictor tone. The main effect of vasoconstriction in resting
muscles during exercise is to prevent an increase in flow through
them, which would otherwise result from the increased blood pressure
which accompanies exercise. Vessels in active muscles dilate by
powerful local vasodilator mechanisms which overcome reflex constriction. In patients with severe mitral stenosis, unable to further increase their cardiac output with exercise, this reflex vasoconstriction in inactive muscles is very efficient and accounts for
the maintenance of blood pressure in spite of vasodilatation in active muscles. In patients with orthostatic hypotension, on the
other hand, mild exercise in the recumbent or head-down position,
where pooling of blood is unlikely to occur, is associated with a
marked drop in blood pressure. This fall in blood pressure is
attributed to failure of compensatory vasoconstriction in other
vascular beds. The afferent pathways and receptors of these reflex

responses in the vessels of skeletal muscles are not known, but it
may be that they are not initiated by arterial baroreceptors since
raising or lowering effective pressure in the carotid sinus produces the well known changes in arterial pressure and heart rate
only, but does not alter the resistance to blood flow in the forearm.

Vasodilator cholinergic fibers to muscle blood vessels are found
in animals and man. They are not involved in reflex changes in
muscle blood flow during postural changes or exercise. These vasodilator fibers are activated by emotional stress and by hypothalamic
electrical stimulation which results in a large increase in muscle
blood flow. This emotional vasodilatation in skeletal muscle vessels
is believed to be responsible for emotional fainting, because during
a faint, blood flow in the forearm increases.

REFLEX CHANGES IN VENOUS TONE

The veins are capable of constriction and dilatation. They
are low-pressure-capacity vessels and normally control the filling
pressure of the heart which in turn affects stroke output. This,
through its action on arterial baroreceptors, influences peripheral
venous tone. An acute decrease in filling pressure, stroke output
and arterial pulse pressure induced by sudden tipping from recumbency to the erect position or by Valsalva's maneuver causes reflex
constriction in veins and arteries. In young subjects there is a
direct relation between the reduction in pulse pressure and the
degree of arterial and venous constriction. The vasoconstriction
appears 5 to 7 sec after the reduction in pulse pressure and when
the filling pressure to the heart returns to normal there is a
transient overshoot in arterial pressure. This results not only
from reflex arterial constriction but also from an increase in
stroke output caused by reflex venous constriction.

The regulation of cardiac output is markedly affected by
venous reflexes. These reflexes occur after Valsalva's maneuver,
a deep breath, hyperventilation, mental arithmetic, cold, head
up-tilt and exercise. The efferent pathways depend entirely upon
stimulation of α-adrenergic receptor activity.

High-altitude pulmonary edema is likely to occur in susceptible
individuals during the first several days after exposure to altitude.
In such patients a large central but normal total blood volume is
found; therefore, a shift from capacitance vessels - the peripheral
veins - to the central circulation occurs. In normal subjects at
altitude there is significant peripheral venoconstriction and the
venomotor responses to exercise become more intense during early
exposure to altitude. In subjects with high-altitude pulmonary
edema, the venoconstriction is more intense and in such patients

and others exposed to altitudes, the urinary excretion of norepinephrine and vanilmandelic acid is increased, suggesting that these
responses are mediated by the sympathetic nervous system.   The
peripheral blood flow and venomotor tone are influenced predominantly
by hypocapnia and the venoconstriction is facilitated by hypoxia.

In anemia and beri-beri, venous constriction is marked and is
associated with arterial vasodilatation.   This venous constriction,
together with the increase in plasma volume in such disorders, accounts for the very marked increase in cardiac output.   The mechanism
of the venous constriction in anemia and in beri-beri is unknown.

CLINICAL IMPORTANCE OF AUTONOMIC DYSFUNCTION

Most drugs used in the treatment of hypertension diminish or
abolish reflex adjustments of the circulation to falls in cardiac
output such as those induced by postural changes.   If such drugs are
given to patients, whether with or without inadequate baroreceptor
function, they may induce profound falls in blood pressure.   They
should therefore be avoided in diabetics and alcoholics with peripheral neuropathy in whom baroreceptor function is often defective.
In the acute phase after a cerebrovascular accident, these drugs
should not be given either, because baroreceptor activity may be
temporarily abolished or worsened until some return of neurologic
function occurs.   In such patients early postural changes should
also be avoided.

Long-standing absence of baroreceptor function is usually not
associated with symptomatic postural hypotension, presumably because
of residual venous tone which assures an adequate return of blood to
the heart.   This abnormality can only be recognized by intro-arterial
beat-to-beat pressure measurements during and after a sudden reduction in cardiac output, which can be achieved by Valsalva's
maneuver, lower body suction or tilting to an upright position.
Such patients, if subjected to extra loads on the circulation,
may become symptomatic due to postural hypotension, though ordinarily they can maintain an adequate supply of blood to the brain.
A significant number of elderly subjects have inadequate baroreceptor function and in these, barbiturates, psychotherapeutic and
hypotensive agents, alcohol and other substances affecting baroreceptor function should be avoided since a decrease of venous tone
caused by these agents may lead to profound falls in blood pressure.

Orthostatic hypotension, with hypertension in the recumbent
position, can be a disabling symptom.   Investigation of the renin
angiotensin system to explain these paradoxical blood pressures has
shown that in some patients with orthostatic hypotension an increase
occurs in plasma renin activity upon stimulus of upright posture.

But in most with diabetic orthostatic hypotension, this normal increase in renin with the upright posture is not found. Plasma
renin levels in idiopathic orthostatic hypotension have been studied
in subjects in whom the orthostatic pressure drop is due to either
efferent or afferent baroreflex impairment. In patients with the
Holmes-Adie syndrome, in whom the baroreflex block is on the afferent side, repeated tilting to the upright position leads to a
progressive increase in plasma renin concentration. In other patients with orthostatic hypotension, in whom baroreflexes were
interrupted on the efferent side, no such increase in plasma renin
concentration in response to head up-tilt can be found. In patients
with high spinal cord transections and orthostatic hypotension, a
change of posture can induce an elevation of plasma renin concentration and these patients may have high resting renin values.
These elevated renin values may in part play a role in the adaptive
circulatory responses to the upright posture which is seen with time
after spinal injury. In chronic hemodialysis patients severe hypotension may occur and though in the past this has been attributed
to volume depletion, it is clear that the peripheral neuropathy of
chronic uremia also plays a part. Circulatory responses to
Valsalva's maneuver and the response to hypotension induced by
the inhalation of amylnitrite are defective.

Impaired reflex vasoconstriction also occurs in chronically
hypoxemic patients. There is prompt improvement in such patients,
however, when the hypoxemia is temporarily corrected. In these
patients the abnormal sympathetic function is probably of central
and/or peripheral origin and may be related to an impairment in
neural transmission rather than to permanent autonomic neuropathy.

In primary amyloidosis, hypotension in the upright posture may
be a disabling symptom. Abnormal sweating also occurs and these
reflex abnormalities are presumably the result of widespread involvement of the peripheral, autonomic and somatic nervous systems
by amyloid.

The role of systemic hypotension in the genesis of transient
focal cerebral ischemia is not clear; however, a number of mechanisms which might cause temporary falls in systemic blood pressure
and perfusion pressure are thought to be significant in transiently
reducing blood flow in a diseased part of the vasculature supplying
the brain which may lead to symptoms of focal ischemia. Impairment of baroreceptor function after the age of 40 is found in the
recumbent position and is further aggravated in upright normal
subjects. This is probably the result of pooling of the blood
below the heart in an incompletely constricted vasculature. A
possible morphologic basis for the observed deterioration in baroreflex activity with age has been found in the reduction of inter-
nodal lengths of white rami communicantes in the human paravertebral

sympathetic chain. This observation is interpreted to show that
Wallerian degeneration and segmental demyelination occur in white
rami communicantes with increasing frequency with advancing years
and regenerative processes do not keep pace with successive degenerative events. These abnormalities could result in a temporal
dispersion of impulses with impaired ability of the nerve to transmit synchronous volleys which in turn could affect baroreflex
activity.

The lack of symptomatic orthostatic hypotension under ordinary
circumstances in patients with chronic baroreflex block is poorly
understood, but it could be that compensatory cerebral vasodilatation which ordinarily assures adequate flow despite a falling perfusion pressure plays a part in this adaptive mechanism also.

Postural hypotension has been demonstrated in Wernicke's
disease. The lesion in this disorder is in the hypothalamus, but
on physiologic grounds the disturbance of autonomic function is
thought to be due to dysfunction in the efferent sympathetic fibers,
intermediolateral columns or peripheral nerves.

The occurrence of strokes in association with meals has been
anecdotally recognized, but this relationship is not fully understood. A possibility that such patients lose vasomotor control in
relationship to meals, and a change of posture then leads to significant fall in perfusion pressure of the brain, jeopardizing
blood flow in an already diseased part of the vasculature, has been
suggested. The administration of oral glucose decreases baroreflex
activity in all subjects and it may lead to complete baroreceptor
block in some in whom this baroreflex function is already impaired.
The ingestion of carbohydrates during a meal is a potent stimulus
to the release of insulin and the intravenous administration of
insulin leads to circulatory changes which are independent of the
induced hypoglycemia. The magnitude of the impaired baroreflex
activity after insulin differs in subjects with normal or impaired
baroreflex function. It is possible, therefore, that the ingestion
of glucose releases endogenous insulin and has a similar effect upon
the circulation.

A congenital condition called familial dysautonomia is characterized by many disturbances of autonomic nervous system function.
These include diminished lacrimation, hyperhidrosis, blotching of
the skin, abnormal swallowing reflexes, impaired vestibular reflexes, labile blood pressure and disturbed temperature control.
Emotional instability, severe vomiting, poor coordination and insensitivity to pain, including diminished deep tendon reflexes, are
usually found. The pathogenesis of this disorder is not fully
understood, but diminished dopamine-β-hydroxylase levels in the
plasma have been documented, though this does not distinguish

between a deficient norepinephrine synthesis and a defect in catecholamine release which is thought to be important in this disorder.
Cholinergic dysfunction in familial dysautonomia also is present.
Cholineacetyl transferase was absent or low and this may account
for some of the ocular abnormalities that occur in this disorder.

Hypothetically, nerve growth factor has been implicated in the
pathogenesis of familial dysautonomia. The suggestion has been made
that a developmental arrest of migration of neurons from the neural
crest could explain the decrease of unmyelinated fibers and absence
of large myelinated fibers, including muscle spindle afferents in
peripheral nerves. There is also a similarity in the morphologic
findings in familial dysautonomia and those experimentally induced
by nerve growth factor antiserum.

The Lesch-Nyhan syndrome is a disorder of purine metabolism
characterized by hyperuricemia and excessive production of uric
acid. These patients have self-mutilating behavior to varying
degrees. In those with severe self-mutilating activity, a unique
pattern of adrenergic dysfunction has been documented. They have
an elevated plasma dopamine-β-hydroxylase which catalyses the formation of norepinephrine from dopamine. The level of this enzyme
serves as a quantitative index of adrenergic function. Clinical
tests of adrenergic responsiveness in patients with the Lesch-Nyhan
syndrome have shown a positive cold pressor test in those without
self-mutilating behavior. The relationship of the plasma dopamine-
β-hydroxylase levels to the bizarre behavioral manifestation of
this disorder is not clear.

An experimental disorder of vasomotor function can be produced
in rabbits by the injection of human sympathetic tissue mixed with
Freund's adjuvant. Affected animals have a circulating antibody
specific to sympathetic tissue, but no pathognomonic, microscopic
or ultrastructural lesions have been found. The disease is thought
to be an experimental model for acute pandysautonomia; a self-
limiting total failure of autonomic function which occurs in a
setting of otherwise normal peripheral and central nervous system
function in man.

TROPHIC DISORDERS APPEARING AFTER BIRTH

Parietal wasting has been well described and numerous cases
are on record. This may occur after injuries to the parietal lobe,
either in the perinatal period or in childhood. Clinically, there
is wasting of muscles on the opposite side to the parietal lobe
lesion, but occasionally minor wasting may occur ipsilaterally.
Parietal atrophy may occur after vascular accidents and may develop
within a day or two, although usually taking a week or more with

slowly progressive lesions such as tumors or degeneration. Usually upper limbs are more affected than lower limbs and, rarely, half the tongue, palate or face may be wasted. A progressive decrease in tone and in tendon jerks usually accompanies wasting. Such wasting is also characterized by the presence of shiny thin skin, usually of warm hands which are slightly moist, but on occasion colder; the fingers are tapered and nails brittle and the hair on the affected side may be lost. Deformities are not common. X-rays of the bones are not often remarkable, though in long-standing cases hypoplasia or demineralization may be present. There are some cases on record where parietal wasting occurred without the presence of motor weakness and it has been recognized that unilateral wasting with astereognosis is a parietal lobe sign. This phenomenon is not understood but numerous theories have been advanced to explain it.

THE INFLUENCE OF THE NERVOUS SYSTEM IN THE TRIPLE RESPONSE OF LEWIS

The flare component of the triple response of Lewis is absent in denervated skin, but it can be elicited for a few days after section of the appropriate nerve until the nerve degenerates. Thereafter, only the wheal and central red area, without the spreading flare, are seen. Transection of the dorsal roots has no effect on the flare, but it is abolished seven or more days after dorsal root ganglionectomy in man. This gives direct evidence that the integrity of afferent fibers which arise in dorsal root ganglion cells is essential for the diffuse cutaneous vasodilatation (flare) which forms part of the normal response to injury of the skin. In subjects with intact peripheral nerves, however, the central nervous system modulates the extent of the flare and thus in turn influences the response to injury. In patients with lesions in the deep and superficial territory of the middle cerebral artery associated with impaired sensation, the flare response is enhanced on the contralateral side of the body. Lesions of the spinothalamic tract or thalamus decrease the extent of the flare on the contralateral side of the body in which also a decrease of sensibility is found. In cord lesions, a decrease of the flare in dermatomes below the lesion has also been demonstrated. The mechanism by which the central nervous system affects this peripheral axon reflex is not clear, but trophic changes and painful syndromes, occasionally seen after central lesions, may be related to the modulation of the flare by the central nervous system after injury to the skin.

INFLUENCE OF THE NERVOUS SYSTEM ON MYOEDEMA

Contractions after percussion of skeletal muscles normally give rise to small waves which leave a knot at the margin of percussion.

This wave lasts only a few seconds and electromyographic studies
have shown that action potentials which are irregular and persist
throughout the visible contraction and perhaps beyond accompany the
small waves. Two responses have been recognized; an immediate electrical response which is triggered by mechanical stimulation of the
muscle and a delayed electrical response which is a spinal reflex.
Myoedema is characterized, however, by a local contraction (mounding) in response to percussion of the muscle which is not associated
with a recordable electrical discharge. Moreover, this mounding is
fatigable.

Myoedema has been recognized in patients with wasting disorders
and at one time it was considered important in the recognition of
cavitary tuberculosis when atrophy of pectoral muscles was usually
found overlying an apical cavity. In addition to syndromes associated with malnutrition, such as sprue, the cachexia of cancer,
acute infections, gastritis and the debility of chronic alcoholism,
myoedema has also been recognized in myxedema. The exact mechanism
of the production of myoedema is not clear, but it persists after
death and it has been attributed to an abnormal but inherent muscular excitability predominantly related to the contents of the
muscle fiber rather than depolarization of the membrane. There is
no reasonable doubt now that myoedema is a physiologic phenomenon,
its duration and ease of demonstration at the bedside being largely
dependent upon skin and muscle thickness. The possibility that the
intensity of myoedema is modulated by the nervous system has been
explored. The phenomenon is always symmetric and is most commonly
found in the brachio-radialis muscle in patients with peripheral
neuropathies. Myoedema does not seem to be affected by lesions of
the cortico-spinal tract in patients with or without myxedema. But
in some patients with a pure sensory stroke and in others with involvement of the spino-thalamic pathways, myoedema was elicited
only on the uninvolved side of the body. It is clear that this
phenomenon is widespread in patients with neurologic disease and
is not confined to those with clinical evidence of malnutrition or
endocrine disturbances. It persists in the face of corticospinal
tract lesions, but seems to be suppressed by lesions in the thalamus
or spinal-thalamic tracts. It is clear, therefore, that though the
phenomenon is a manifestation of activities of muscles, this can be
influenced by lesions in the central nervous system. Whether this
is a direct effect of the central nervous system on muscle or due
to removal of trophic function by the lesion has not been established. It is yet another example of central nervous system
modulation of what appears to be a purely peripheral phenomenon.

NEUROARTHROPATHIES

Experimentally it can be shown that joint denervation in association with trauma produces the characteristic changes of neuropathy. Denervation alone, however, is not effective. It seems that continued function of a denervated joint is necessary before the characteristic clinical features of excessive mobility subluxation and finally dislocation appear. Later this is associated with heterotrophic cartilage and bone formation.

After a hemiplegic event, several ill understood but well recognized phenomena have been described which affect the paralyzed limbs and include swelling, cyanosis, excessive sweating and the shoulder-hand syndrome. Less commonly recognized is the protective effect of hemiplegia on the development of rheumatoid or osteoarthritis with Heberden's nodes. In this situation it seems that the hemiplegia has to precede the onset of arthritis and that no evidence has so far been produced to show that hemiplegia will affect an established arthritic change. In the cases reported, the interval between the clinical onset of arthritis and pre-existing hemiplegia was variable and ranged from 10 years to 8 months.

Peripheral nerve lesions preceding the onset of arthritis appear to afford some protection to the involved parts also. The mechanism of this protective effect of nervous system lesions on a generalized arthritic condition is not understood but it is clearly not related to immobilization alone because many protected joints remain quite useful. It might, however, be due to the alteration in the inflammatory response which is modulated by lesions of the nervous system or to a relative disuse since the paretic parts would naturally be used less frequently.

EFFECT OF MUSCLE HYPOACTIVITY AND HYPERACTIVITY

At some stage of neuromuscular disease, weakness of some muscles and hyperactivity of others unaffected by the process occurs. Both hypoactivity and hyperactivity of muscles lead to changes in muscle bulk. When an injured nerve is prevented from re-establishing contact with its muscle, the fiber size spectrum of the nerve remains unimodal and contains numerous small demyelinated fibers. When such a nerve is allowed to regenerate and re-innervate its muscle without interference, it regains a normal fiber size spectrum. Thus there is a demonstrated influence of neuromuscular connections on fiber size of regenerating peripheral nerves. It has also been suggested that the level of activity of muscle might influence fiber diameters in peripheral nerves. Studies on this aspect of trophic function of muscle on nerves have shown that fiber densities of nerves innervating hypoactive or hyperactive muscles change reciprocally with time. Small fibers behave differently from large fibers. Examination of cyclic AMP content of such nerves also showed a time-dependent, but reciprocal, relationship on the hypoactive and hyperactive size. This suggests that workload establishes a set-point of fiber size in peripheral nerves. Information is relayed through the axon. The time delay or inertia of the system carries it past its equilibrium point and oscillations in fiber size spectra and cyclic AMP occur. Information to and from the controller might be transmitted by axoplasmic flow or cyclic AMP from the muscle to some central site which controls fiber size spectra in peripheral nerves.

HYPERTROPHIC OSTEOARTHROPATHY

This condition is characterized by clubbing of the fingers and toes, periostitis with new bone formation, and arthritis. Most patients with this condition have disease of the lung, heart, liver, gastrointestinal tract and occasionally thyrotoxicosis. Rarely is it seen in syringomyelia. Pathologically, the lesion is an inflammatory periostitis and arthritis and involves the adjacent subcutaneous tissue. Nowadays, the commonest association of this syndrome is with carcinoma of the lung, although previously pulmonary suppurative processes were common also. There is no satisfactory explanation for this disorder, but occasionally it regresses within days after section of the vagi. It is thought that the interruption of an abnormal pulmonary vascular reflex by this procedure may account for the decrease in the peripheral circulation which accompanies the improvement of hypertrophic osteoarthropathy.

SLEEP DISORDERS

There are four clinically recognizable sleep disorders: (1) when patients complain they sleep too much (hypersomnia); (2) when sleep is disturbed (insomnia); (3) where relatives complain about their sleep being disturbed by the patients; and (4) when other illness affects sleep secondarily. The best known of sleep disturbances is narcolepsy. It has also been labelled hypersomnia, but evaluation of the duration of sleep in narcoleptics shows that sleep rarely exceeds the normal amount in a 24 h period. Narcolepsy is characterized by attacks of sleep associated with cataplexy, sleep paralysis, hypnagogic hallucinations and a general disruption of nocturnal sleep.

A sudden loss of muscle tone characterizes cataplexy. This is associated with an inability to perform any voluntary movement. The severity of the attack varies from total loss of motor function to impairment of voluntary activity of certain muscle groups only. Extraocular muscles are not involved. Most commonly, there is sagging of the jaw, a forward droop of the head, and buckling of the knees. In severe attacks, however, a sudden loss of muscle tone may lead to falls. Cataplexy usually occurs after emotional stress, fatigue and sometimes after large heavy meals.

It has been shown that the only condition in which there is a spontaneous, non-reciprocal motor inhibition in man is during REM sleep. During cataplectic attacks, the same phenomenon is observed with total simultaneous inhibition of EMG activity in different muscle groups. This, incidentally, is also associated with abolition of tendon reflexes. The sparing of motor inhibition of the extraocular muscles parallels the lack of inhibition of electromyographic activity in these muscles in normal subjects during REM periods. This sparing of extraocular muscles is of course also seen in patients with narcolepsy who may present with paralysis and areflexia during a cataplectic attack though they are able to execute voluntary movements with their eyes. This explanation of cataplexy does not account for the attacks induced by strong emotions. How emotions can inhibit tonic muscle discharges is not known.

BREATHLESSNESS

Breathlessness is a purely subjective sensation and can only be defined by those who have experienced it by referring to the circumstances in which it occurs. Normal subjects may be breathless when breathing is mechanically impaired or when the volome of breathing is increased. Increased breathing on exercise is rarely unpleasant whereas hindered breathing such as when wearing masks, tight garments, or in disease is always unpleasant. The most obvious neurologic condition in which breathlessness is a prominent feature occurs in patients with paralysis of respiratory muscles. Such patients, however, may complain of breathlessness, although they are still able to maintain adequate ventilation and they may even overbreathe. The mechanism of this phenomenon is not clear. Moreover, in some conscious subjects with central neurogenic hyperventilation, but without respiratory muscle paralysis, dyspnea may be denied even though the ventilation rate is some six times higher than normal. The breathlessness sometimes seen in behavioral disorders remains unexplained mainly because of a lack of known neurophysiologic changes in such patients. Two patterns have, however, been recognized: hyperventilation presumably due to excessive respiratory drive initiated by cortical mechanism, and variations in lung volume at which tidal respirations occur. The latter is related to a change in tension of inspiratory muscles.

YAWNING

Yawning is a reflex act which involves the lungs, blood vessels, lacrimal and salivary glands, respiratory and other skeletal muscles. Once initiated, yawning cannot be suppressed, but its manifestations can voluntarily be modified. The act of yawning begins as an inspiration associated with marked dilatation of the pharynx. At the peak of inspiration there are associated facial movements and the final part of yawning is passive expiration. No area in the central nervous system has been found which induces yawning on stimulation. Because of the relationship of yawning to sleep, it is thought that the brainstem reticular formation is intimately concerned with yawning, but the true physiologic significance of this act has not been established. Very little indeed is known about such a ubiquitous and common reflex. Yawning is accompanied by lacrimation, salivation, reflex vasoconstriction in the skin and usually by stretching. The initiation of lacrimation and salivation by yawning is reflex in origin, but the mechanism by which this is brought about is not understood. Vasoconstriction in skin vessels after yawning is probably similar to reflex vasoconstriction which occurs after a deep breath. Man can voluntarily separate yawning from stretching. In all other animals, however, these occur together. Experimentally, yawning has been produced in animals by the intraventricular administration of ACTH and melanocyte stimulation hormone. The site of action of these hormones in inducing yawning is thought to be on the hypothalamus and probably included connections with descending and ascending fibers to and from the reticular formation in the brainstem. The instillation of zinc, but not of manganese or copper, into the lateral ventricle of rats also produces yawning and stretching behavior, after a latent period of some 40 to 60 min. The mechanism of production of this behavior by the zinc ion, though specific, has not been further elucidated.

PAIN SYNDROMES

Pain syndromes associated with peripheral nerve lesions are common. In areas of incomplete sensory loss due to transection and after surgical repair of a peripheral nerve with partial recovery or in association with neuromas, over-response to stimuli may be seen. Such dysesthesiae occur after lesions of the nerves in the arm or leg. Careful clinical examination usually shows a heightened threshold to ordinary stimuli in association with pain of peculiar and unpleasant quality which is confined to the dermatome of the injured nerve. It is thought that the sensory abnormalities are due to incomplete regeneration of pain fibers in the cutaneous sensory network. Most patients eventually recover and do not require surgery, but excision of neuromas or neurolysis is not usually effective. When the dysesthetic area becomes sensitive

to cold, relief may be obtained by sympathectomy. This condition
is distinguished from causalgia, in which the disorder is not
confined to a single dermatome.

Causalgia is characterized by hyperpathia, trophic changes and
autonomic phenomena. It occurs after peripheral nerve injury and
usually involves either the arm or leg. There is partial nerve
injury, usually, and the hyperpathia is most marked in fingers and
toes. Trophic changes in the skin are marked but are not different
from those seen after peripheral nerve lesions without causalgia.
The pain and dysesthesiae are not confined to denervated dermatomes
but involve a large part of the affected limb. Excessive sweating
and vasodilatation occur and the limb may be either hot or cold,
depending mainly on the amount of sweat. Cool limbs are particularly common in the later stages.

Because movement causes pain, the limb is kept immobile and
joints become stiff. Contact with clothing may be unpleasant and
patients may wrap their limbs in cotton-wool or moistened towels.
Many stimuli applied to other parts of the body, ordinarily well
tolerated, may cause excruciating pain in the affected limb.
Psychologic studies of patients who have recovered from causalgia
show no abnormalities. Pain is the most characteristic feature of
this syndrome, and vasomotor and sudomotor abnormalities are thought
to be secondary to it. The pathogenesis of causalgia is not understood, but it can be successfully treated by sympathectomy in
properly selected patients. Patients respond well if there is
relief of pain by prior sympathetic block and if the pain is aggravated by cold or other environmental factors. Those who have
dysesthesiae or do not have the complete clinical syndrome do not
usually do well after sympathectomy. These other painful conditions are distinguished from causalgia by the absence of burning
pain. They occur after trauma, infections or arthritis without
necessarily direct injury to major nerve trunks. Sympathetic
dystrophies are not only found in young healthy subjects with normal personalities, but occur in those who may have some personality
defects as well.

The syndrome of Algo-neural dystrophies has been described in
middle-aged and elderly women. It occurs after minor trauma or
occasionally without discernible injury. Pain and a reluctance to
move the affected limb are the hallmark of this condition which may
involve the lower or the upper limbs. Swelling is often present and
radiologic examination may show some osteoporosis of the involved
parts. The pathogenesis of this syndrome is not clear, but emotional factors seem to play a large role in its genesis. Avoidance
of surgical procedures in such patients, encouragement to mobilize
the limb again with appropriate strengthening exercises, short
courses with tranquilizers and mood elevators, and some anti-
inflammatory agents seem to lead to improvement in some patients,

but many continue for long periods of time until the limb becomes
atrophic and contractures develop.

Recent neurophysiologic evidence suggests that normally inhibitory influences can abolish stimulus-evoked activity in a
sensory system almost as soon as the stimulus is removed. It has
been proposed that the brainstem reticular formation acts in a way
that allows it to influence this firing pattern by a "central
biasing mechanism". This is achieved by continuous tonic inhibitory
influences on transmission at all levels of the somatic afferent
projection system. This bias or tonic inhibition is maintained, in
part at least, by a continuous sensory input from the skin. Abnormal responses occur in conditions which impair the activity of
the sensory input or of the central biasing mechanism. Some anesthetic substances abolish the inhibitory influence of the central
biasing mechanism so that continuous activity at several synaptic
levels of the skin afferent system can occur. A stimulus, therefore,
which normally has only a transient effect, can result in persistent
activity. Conversely, if there is a loss or decrease in sensory
input from the skin, the activity of the central biasing mechanism
is also decreased. In amputated limbs the sensory afferent fibers
are destroyed and the amount of input to the reticular formation is
markedly decreased. This may result in continuous self-perpetuating
activity in neurone loops at all levels which can be repeatedly initiated by minor noxious or other stimuli from the site of injury
and may be related to the phenomenon of phantom pain. Emotional
stress has the capacity to interfere with the efficacy of the central biasing mechanism also. This may account for the aggravation
of spontaneous burning pains associated with causalgia, for example.

An explanation for the well-known sustained benefit of analgesic blocks in these situations is that the anesthetic agents
break activity in neurone loops. After the block has worn off,
peripheral stimulation triggers sustained activity again, but there
is a time lag for it to spread to a large number of neurones and
this time lag accounts for the pain relief which often outlasts the
action of local anesthetics. Moreover, in conditions such as
causalgia and Algo-neuro dystrophies, the temporary removal of
discomfort allows the limb to be used again which increases the
pattern of impulses from the periphery, particularly from muscles,
which in turn increases the bias in the central biasing mechanism
and also delays the resumption of self-sustaining firing in various
neurone pools.

Sudeck described a post-traumatic dystrophy in which, after
minor trauma, usually in the region of the wrist or ankle joint,
atrophy and spotty decalcification of bone occurs. Pain may be
severe and abnormal vasomotor and sudomotor activity is seen.
Many changes in Sudeck's atrophy are due to disuse because of pain.

This condition is successfully treatable by sympathectomy. Sudeck's atrophy associated with pelvic or lumbar spine lesions has been reported. This condition appears to be more common in females, it is often bilateral, nearly all patients have involvement of both the foot and knee region. Though radiologically the hip joint may show osteoporosis, this is usually clinically silent. Pain of causalgic nature is often present and brings the patient to the attention of the physician. Almost all have had surgical procedures on the back, bone grafts, some were found after hip joint surgery, and a number of cases occurred after infectious spondylitis, metastic carcinoma to the pelvis, or after pelvic surgery. Stiffness of the joints usually involving the ankle is prominent though reflex vasomotor abnormalities are less marked than in Sudeck's atrophy involving the upper limb. The aggravation of symptoms by stress is not very prominent in this type of Sudeck's atrophy, but precipitating traumatic factors are almost universally present. The best treatment for this reflex sympathetic dystrophy is lumbar sympathetic block. Occasionally, local anesthetic infiltration of the femoral artery perivascular nerves plexuses is also helpful. Whether pain in sympathetic dystrophy is conducted via the sympathetic nervous system or is the result of cross-excitation from sympathetic fibers to sensory afferents at the site of minor nerve injuries is not clear. There have been a number of studies to suggest that pain in these disorders is conducted along sympathetic fibers from the limb, though others claim that cross-excitation from sympathetic pain fibers is the likely mechanism.

The shoulder-hand syndrome is another form of reflex sympathetic dystrophy. This occurs commonly after myocardial infarction or hemiplegia. The shoulder becomes painful on movement, the hand may be sweaty with vasomotor changes and finally atrophy, particularly of hand muscles, may be seen. The palmar aponeurosis and the skin of the palm are often thickened in long-standing cases. The painful shoulder in patients with hemiplegia develops within days after the onset of the weakness and this cannot as a rule be prevented by early passive movement of the joint. The cause of the shoulder-hand syndrome is unknown. The pain usually subsides after a variable length of time and sympathectomy is rarely necessary.

Lumbar sympathectomy may lead to neuralgic pain. This usually occurs about 2 weeks after the operation. The pain is localized to the thighs and is deep and boring in character and often disappears spontaneously within 10 days or 2 weeks. A few patients, however, have severe pain which is not relieved by narcotics. A number of such patients were markedly improved by the administration of diphenylhydantoin or carbamazepine. This condition, termed post-sympathectomy neuralgia, has not been satisfactorily explained. The effectiveness of the two drugs in its treatment, both of which alter the excitability of nerve membranes and depress polysynaptic responses, does not help in interpreting the pathogenesis of this syndrome.

REFERRED PAIN

Viscera are not sensitive to ordinary stimuli. However, some stimuli produce pain and they are those to which the viscera are commonly exposed. Distention of the capsule of solid organs like the liver, stretching or crushing of blood vessels, and anoxia of muscles are all painful. Because nerve endings sensitive to pain are not numerous in viscera, the summation of a widespread stimulus appears necessary before pain is felt. The threshold for pain can, however, be lowered by prior irritation of the organ. The pain from viscera is essentially similar to that arising from deep structures such as muscles, ligaments, joints and periosteum. While the site of reference of pain from viscera for a given stimulus is constant for any one individual, it is not always confined to the segment in which stimulation occurs. It is also known that preexistent pain in another segment could change the site of referred pain from one segment to the segment already painful. Experimentally, if the site of referred pain is anesthetized, referred effects after stimulation of deep structures may often be abolished. Peripheral lesions can modify the referral of pain from viscera. For example, after myocardial eschemia, pressure on a painful amputated neuroma on a shoulder stump can produce anginal pain. Occasionally, like in another patient, fracture of an elbow can cause ischemic cardiac pain to be referred to the fracture site. Because of these and other studies, it has been suggested that cutaneous afferent impulses entering a spinal segment facilitate awareness of visceral discomfort if a simultaneous discharge from a viscus occurs in the same segment. If the cutaneous segment is anesthetized, however, visceral pain may still be referred to the segment and anginal pain has, on rare occasions, been referred to a left phantom limb.

Another type of referred pain has also been described. This type is initiated by non-traumatic stimulation of a point on the skin and it is referred to another distant skin area. It appears to be a common phenomenon. Most often this sensation is recognized after "unconscious grooming behavior" such as scraping fingernails over the scalp, plucking of hairs and sometimes by minor skin lesions. The stimulus which elicits the referred sensation causes a normal sensibility on the site of stimulation but in addition there is a localized, often sharp, feeling at a distant point on the skin. These sensations are not very painful and are often followed by an itchy feeling in the referred area.

Though only about half of interviewed normal subjects were able to spontaneously recall this referred cutaneous sensation, the other subjects could repeat this phenomenon subsequent to the inquiry. These referred sensations are always ipsilateral to the stimulus. No feeling can be elicited in the original initiating area by stimulating the referred side and, most importantly, the referred sensation is never in the same dermatome as the stimulus.

Similar sensations have been reported after squeezing of a testicle which causes an abnormal crushing feeling superficially in the region of the nipple. In some patients with dilating abdominal aneurysms, testicular pain may appear and precede a fatal rupture of the aneurysm. These phenomena resemble in some way the experimentally produced, misdirected reflex responses in frogs which have belly skin transplanted to the back. Stimulation of this skin gives rise to a normal reflex directed to the back and a misdirected reflex toward the belly. Whether cutaneous referred sensations arise from abnormal embryonic specification of connections of peripheral nerves or from a temporary abnormality due to abnormal fiber growth is not known. But animal experiments would be necessary to further define the physiology of this rather widespread but not generally recognized phenomenon. Moreover, the findings of referred cutaneous sensation in most subjects suggest that sensory disturbances which are not confined to dermatomal distributions should not be glibly dismissed as hysterical.

Extensive experience with visceral pain has clearly shown that the best way to terminate the pain is by interrupting the splanchnic pathways which mediate impulses from the viscera to the central nervous system. This has also been confirmed at reoperations after splanchnicectomy when a number of normally painful stimuli to the gallbladder or intestines failed to elicit pain. Knowledge of the autonomic innervation of thoracic and abdominal viscera and the pathways which are related to visceral pain has been used in surgical attempts to relieve this pain. Extensive experience with sympathectomies for angina pectoris has shown that such operations are palliative and often very effective in removing the pain, at least temporarily, but they do not affect the course of the underlying disorder, and are not now recommended. Similarly, the surgical relief of pain arising in abdominal viscera, though best achieved by splanchnicectomy, cannot always be carried out effectively. The commonest type of prolonged intractable abdominal pain is associated with malignancy in which invasion of tissues other than the viscera, such as nerves and the abdominal wall itself, is often responsible for the pain. Such sources of pain cannot be influenced by surgery on autonomic nerves or ganglia.

AUTONOMIC SYSTEM REACTIONS CAUSED BY EXCITATION OF SOMATIC AFFERENTS: STUDY OF CUTANEO-INTESTINAL REFLEX*

Kiyomi Koizumi

Department of Physiology, State University of New York

Downstate Medical Center, Brooklyn, New York

Somatic responses in the body are always accompanied by reactions involving the autonomic nervous system. Any active or passive muscle movement is assisted by cardiovascular changes; painful stimuli applied to the skin or the muscle also produce changes in blood pressure and heart rate. These autonomic changes are not limited to cardiovascular changes only but also occur in other organs, such as the bladder, stomach or intestine. Thermal application, massage or gentle rubbing of the skin and the muscle are often used to relieve visceral discomfort, presumably because these sensory inputs from the cutaneo-muscular tissues affect autonomic innervation to the viscera.

These somatoautonomic reflex responses can best be studied by recording the electrical activity of sympathetic or parasympathetic efferent fibers as well as by measuring effector organ response (Koizumi & Brooks, 1972; Koizumi & Brooks, 1974; Sato, 1975; Sato & Schmidt, 1973). Figure 1 illustrates sympathetic reflex responses recorded from a lumbar white ramus following stimulation of the sciatic nerve. It also shows somatic reflex responses simultaneously recorded from the lumbar 7th ventral root. The sympathetic reflex consists of short-latency spinal and long-latency supraspinal response. The somatic reflex shows mono- and polysynaptic components. When stimulus strength to the sciatic nerve is increased, as shown in the middle pair of tracings, autonomic responses increase greatly and the somatic spinal reflex

*A part of the research described in this paper is supported by grants from the U. S. Public Health Service (NS-00847) and the National Science Foundation.

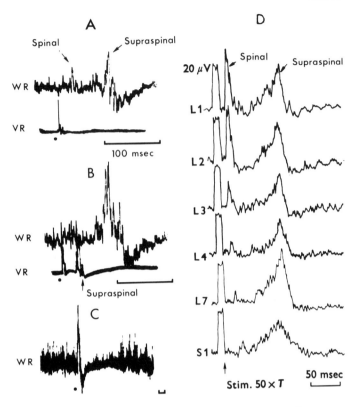

Figure 1. A to C: Sympathetic reflex responses from L_1 white
ramus (WR) and somatic reflex responses from L_7 ventral root (VR)
following stimulations of sciatic nerve (marked by dots) are simultaneously recorded. In A, the sympathetic reflex consists of
short-latency spinal and long-latency supraspinal responses. The
somatic reflex shows mono- and polysynaptic components. In B, a
stronger stimulus is applied to the sciatic nerve. Sympathetic
reflexes are greater and a large somatic reflex (mono- and polysynaptic reflexes fused in initial response) as well as a somatic
supraspinal reflex are evoked. C is taken at slow sweep-speed to
show that the sympathetic reflex response is followed by a long
"silent period" or depression of tonic discharges. All time marks
are 100 msec. D: Sympathetic reflex responses are recorded from
L_1 white ramus but stimuli are applied to spinal nerves at various
segmental levels (L_1 to S_1) at times indicated by arrow. Stimulus
intensity is 50 times the threshold strength of the largest afferent fibers (50 x T). Each record is the average of 10 individual
reflexes. Initial rectangular deflection is 20 μv calibration
pulse. Early spinal reflex tends to be segmental and is reduced
as afferent impulses enter more distant segments, while supraspinal
reflex remains constant. (A to C taken from Koizumi et al., 1968;
D from Sato & Schmidt, 1971.)

also increases, particularly the polysynaptic component, so that
mono- and polysynaptic responses are fused in the initial response.
There appears also a somatic supraspinal reflex.

The right side of this figure (Figure 1D) illustrates characteristics of the two components of the somatosympathetic reflex.
Figure 1D is the sympathetic reflex recorded from the L_1 white
ramus, but stimuli were applied to spinal nerves at various segmental levels. The spinal autonomic reflex from the L_1 white ramus
is largest when the L_1 spinal nerve is stimulated, but it gradually
diminishes in size as the stimulus is given to spinal nerves entering at distant spinal levels, while the magnitudes of supraspinal
sympathetic reflex responses are similar regardless of the different spinal nerves stimulated. Thus, the spinal component of the
somatosympathetic reflex is segmentally organized, as in the case
of the somatic spinal reflex, but the supraspinally-mediated autonomic reflex response is widespread or generalized.

In the parasympathetic system the somatoautonomic reflex responses are more complicated (Koizumi & Brooks, 1972). No distinct
response can be elicited in cardiac vagal fibers when somatic afferents are excited. In sacral parasympathetic nerves, however,
somatic afferents do evoke autonomic discharges.

Sympathetic discharges recorded from a white ramus, as shown
above, or from postganglionic fibers in response to somatic nerve
excitation, in turn produce distinct changes in effector organ responses. It has been reported that in cats and rats stimulation
of the skin evoked changes in the blood pressure (Koizumi & Brooks,
1972; Koizumi et al., 1968), heart rate (Kaufman et al., 1977;
Sato et al., 1976), bladder function (Sato et al., 1975b; Sato et
al., 1977) and gastric and duodenal motility (Sato et al., 1975a;
Sato & Terui, 1976) mainly through the sympathetic system. As an
example of a somatoautonomic reflex, I would like to discuss our
recent study on the small intestine. This illustrates how strongly
cutaneous afferents influence the intestinal motility (Koizumi,
Sato & Terui, 1978).

In anesthetized rats and cats, we recorded intestinal motility
by measuring the pressure of a balloon inserted into the jejunum.
Also, the activity of the extrinsic autonomic nerves innervating
the jejunum was monitored by recording potentials from mesenteric
nerve fibers. The stimulus was applied to various areas of the
skin by pinching with smooth-edged forceps. This stimulus mostly
excited all of group III and some group IV fibers and can be classified as a "painful" or nociceptive stimulus. The advantage of
using this type of "natural stimulus" is that the stimulus produces
good spatial and temporal summation of afferent impulses. If the
same effect is to be produced by afferent nerve stimulation, it is

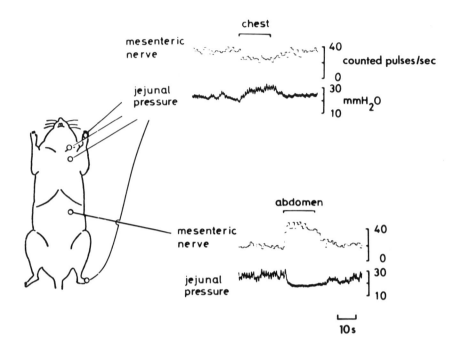

Figure 2. Effects of pinching various skin areas on jejunal motility and mesenteric nerve activity. Pinching abdominal skin evokes
depression of jejunal motility (measured by pressure) and increase
in activity of mesenteric nerve (lower pair of tracings). Pinching other skin areas (neck, chest, fore- or hindlimb) evokes opposite effect (upper pair of tracings). (Modified from Koizumi,
Sato & Terui, 1978.)

often necessary to stimulate more than one nerve with repetitive
pulses.

    Figure 2 shows that pinching the abdominal skin produces pro-
found inhibition of intestinal movement. This is quite a strong
effect and the intestine often becomes completely quiescent. The
afferent impulses from the abdominal skin area enter the spinal
cord at levels where the sympathetic supply to the intestine
leaves the cord; that is, this reflex is segmental. On the other
hand, pinching skin area of neck, chest, fore- or hindlimb (i.e.,
nonsegmental input) produces augmentation of intestinal motility.
Thus, impulses arising from various skin areas can affect intestinal movement; strong depression or augmentation can occur depending
on the site stimulated and whether the reflex is segmental or

nonsegmental. Both reflexes are bilateral, that is, pinching the
right or the left side of the skin as well as the midline area
produces the same effect.

Figure 2 also shows recordings from mesenteric nerve fibers.
Stimulation of abdominal skin produces an increase in sympathetic
fiber activity innervating the intestine, and thereby inhibits the
motility. On the other hand, stimulation of other parts of the
skin, namely, neck, chest, fore- or hindlimb, inhibits sympathetic
activity and therefore intestinal motility is augmented. In this
particular reflex, changes in intestinal motility are brought about
mainly by action of sympathetic fibers to the intestine; vagal contribution seems to be minimal. This conclusion is based on the
following observation. When both vagi are sectioned at the neck,
no detectable changes in reflex response occur. On the other hand,
when the sympathetic nerve supply to the intestine is eliminated by
sectioning bilateral splanchnic nerves, reflex responses disappear.

It is an interesting finding that this somatosympathetic reflex from the abdominal skin is a spinal reflex, while a reflex
originating from the other skin areas (neck, chest and fore- and
hindlimbs) is likely to be a supraspinal reflex. Figure 3 illustrates the result which has enabled us to reach this conclusion.
When typical reflex responses are obtained in our experiments, the
spinal cord is sectioned at C_{2-3}, and the animal is left to recover.
When the abdominal skin is pinched in the spinal animal, the stimulus again produces an increase in sympathetic activity, accompanied by a distinct inhibition of intestinal motility. Such
response is almost the same as before the cord transsection, indicating that this reflex is spinally mediated. On the other hand,
responses to pinching the skin area of neck, chest, fore- or hindlimb, which usually causes inhibition of sympathetic discharges and
augmentation of intestinal motility in a CNS-intact animal, change
after cord transsection; the reflex disappears completely. This
suggests that the latter reflex responses probably are mediated
through supraspinal pathways.

Figure 4 summarizes the result in a schematic diagram. Afferent impulses entering the spinal cord from the abdominal skin area
produce excitation of sympathetic pre- and postganglionic neurons
through segmental pathways. Since action of the sympathetic nerve
supply to the small intestinal musculatures is the inhibiting one,
the result is depression of the intestinal motility. This is quite
a strong spinal reflex and the intestinal wall can become completely
quiescent in our experimental condition. It must be remembered that
these afferent impulses are produced by a particular stimulus,
namely, by pinching the skin. This excites almost all fibers including unmyelinated afferents. Therefore, the stimulus can be said
to be nociceptive. On the other hand, impulses originating from

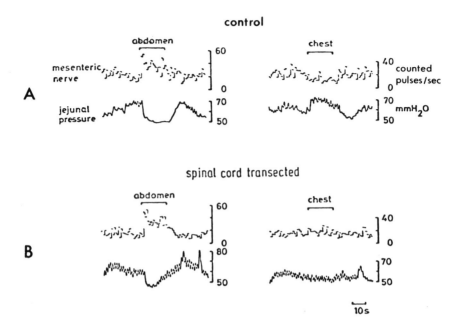

Figure 3.   Effect of cord transsection on cutaneo-intestinal reflex.
A: Control responses. Stimuli (pinching) are applied to abdomen
or chest skin areas. B: After spinal cord transsection at C_{2-3}.
Note that effects produced by abdominal skin stimulation are unaffected, while those evoked by chest stimulus disappear after cord
section. (Modified from Koizumi, Sato & Terui, 1978.)

skin areas of neck, chest, fore- and hindlimbs travel up to the
medulla or higher nervous structures and produce an inhibition of
sympathetic preganglionic neurons. This, in turn, reduces postganglionic sympathetic discharges innervating the intestine and
results in augmentation of intestinal motility. Thus, this is the
supraspinal somatosympathetic reflex. This augmenting reflex action is not as powerful as the inhibitory action due to the spinal
reflex, but it can reverse the inhibition of intestinal motility
caused during the intestino-intestinal reflex. Although Figure 4
shows afferents originating from only one side of the body, these
reflex reactions are bilateral, as stated previously.

Finally, I would like to point out that, in the particular
reflexes which I have just described, control of the effector organ
by the sympathetic nerve supply plays a dominant role. The parasympathetic system through vagal innervation to the intestine, in
this case, seems to contribute very little to this reflex. However,

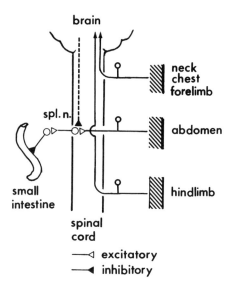

Figure 4.   Schematic summary diagram of cutaneo-intestinal reflex.
Open nerve endings are excitatory, black endings inhibitory.
(Modified from Koizumi, Sato & Terui, 1978.)

in other instances (e.g., in an emotional reaction), vagal control
of the intestinal motility may play an important role. Thus, both
autonomic systems exert extrinsic neural influence on the intestine, but depending on afferent inputs, there seem to be differences in emphasis as to which system exerts dominant control.

In conclusion, I have discussed some of our experimental results in order to indicate the importance of somatic afferents from
the skin for control of visceral functions. In this particular
example, only nociceptive stimuli are employed in evoking autonomic
response in anesthetized animals. It is also important that in
future studies various types of stimulations of the skin, such as
touch, weak pressure or warmth applied to the skin should be tested.

It seems to me that to understand manipulative therapy properly, the relationships between cutaneous and other somatic afferents
and the autonomic responses must be clarified. It is hoped that the
basic physiological study of somatoautonomic reflexes may contribute
to this purpose.

REFERENCES

KAUFMAN, A., A. SATO, Y. SATO, and H. SUGIMOTO. Reflex changes in heart rate after mechanical and thermal stimulation of the skin at various segmental levels in cats. *Neuroscience* 2: 103–109, 1977.

KOIZUMI, K., and C. McC. BROOKS. The integration of autonomic system reactions. *Ergebn. Physiol.* 67:1–68, 1972.

KOIZUMI, K., and C. McC. BROOKS. The autonomic nervous system and its role in controlling visceral activities. In: *Medical Physiology*, 13th ed., edited by V. B. Mountcastle. St. Louis: C. V. Mosby Co., 1974, pp. 783–812.

KOIZUMI, K., A. SATO, A. KAUFMAN, and C. McC. BROOKS. Studies of sympathetic neuron discharges modified by central and peripheral excitation. *Brain Res.* 11:212–224, 1968.

KOIZUMI, K., A. SATO, and N. TERUI. Role of somatic afferents in autonomic system control of the intestinal motility. *Brain Res.* Submitted, 1978.

SATO, A. The somatosympathetic reflexes: Their physiological and clinical significance. In: *The Research Status of Spinal Manipulative Therapy*. NINCDS Monograph No. 15, DHEW Publication No. (NIH)76–998, 1975, pp. 163–172.

SATO, A., Y. SATO, F. SHIMADA, and Y. TORIGATA. Changes in gastric motility produced by nociceptive stimulation of the skin in rats. *Brain Res.* 87:151–159, 1975a.

SATO, A., Y. SATO, F. SHIMADA, and Y. TORIGATA. Changes in vesical function produced by cutaneous stimulation in rats. *Brain Res.* 94:465–474, 1975b.

SATO, A., Y. SATO, F. SHIMADA, and Y. TORIGATA. Varying changes in heart rate produced by cutaneous nociceptive stimulation of the skin in rats at different temperature. *Brain Res.* 110: 301–311, 1976.

SATO, A., Y. SATO, H. SUGIMOTO, and N. TERUI. Reflex changes in the urinary bladder after mechanical and thermal stimulation of the skin at various segmental levels in cats. *Neuroscience* 2:111–117, 1977.

SATO, A., and R. F. SCHMIDT. Spinal and supraspinal components of the reflex discharges into lumbar and thoracic white rami. *J. Physiol.* 212:839–850, 1971.

SATO, A., and R. F. SCHMIDT.   Somatosympathetic reflexes:
    Afferent fibers, central pathways, discharge characteristics.
    Physiol. Rev.   53:916-947, 1973.

SATO, Y., and N. TERUI.   Changes in duodenal motility produced by
    noxious mechanical stimulation of the skin in rats.   *Neurosci.*
    Letters   2:189-193, 1976.

SUSTAINED SYMPATHICOTONIA AS A FACTOR IN DISEASE

Irvin M. Korr

Department of Biomechanics, Michigan State University

East Lansing, Michigan

INTRODUCTION

There is a large though scattered body of clinical and experimental literature that gives the distinct impression of a significant, often critical sympathetic component as a common feature in a large variety of syndromes. Chronic hyperactivity of the innervating sympathetic pathways seems to be a prevailing theme in many clinical conditions, involving many organs and tissues. Whatever the etiological or therapeutic implications, it appears that this widely shared feature of local, regional or segmental sympathetic hyperactivity is overlooked or dismissed because of the barriers erected by specialization. Thus, the ophthalmologist is not ordinarily exposed to the gastroenterological literature, the gastroenterologist to the cardiological, the cardiologist to the gynecological, etc. Each discoverer of a sympathetic component seems, therefore, to regard it as peculiar to this or that disease within his or her area of specialization, rather than as part of a general theme.

My long-time exposure to osteopathic theory and practice and my research experience in related fields have led me to the following hypotheses:

(1) Long-term hyperactivity of particular sympathetic pathways is deleterious to the target tissues and may indeed have a rather general clinical significance.

(2) Clinical manifestations are determined by the organs or tissues which are innervated by the hyperactive sympathetic neurons, each responding in its own way, even to

229

the sympathetically induced vasoconstriction that may be a common factor.

(3)   The high impulse traffic in selected sympathetic pathways may be related to musculoskeletal dysfunction, especially in the spinal and paraspinal area.

It is the purpose of this paper to review the support for these hypotheses in available knowledge of the autonomic nervous system, in experimental findings, including our own, and in clinical literature.

THE SYMPATHETIC ROLE IN MUSCULOSKELETAL ACTIVITY

One of the most important roles of the sympathetic nervous system (SNS), not always emphasized or recognized in textbooks, is part of its "ergotropic" function (Hess, 1954), that of adjusting circulatory, metabolic and visceral activity according to postural and musculoskeletal demand. These adjustments include changes in cardiac output, in distribution of blood flow by regulation of peripheral resistance, in heat dissipation through the skin, and release of stored metabolites. These adjustments are of systemic nature, yet they have a high degree of localization according to the site and the amount of muscular activity. (It is understood of course that autoregulation is also important and often the dominant factor in these adjustments.)

In order for the SNS to perform this role, it must receive, directly (through segmental afferent pathways) and indirectly (through the higher centers), sensory input from the musculoskeletal system. Coote has given us an excellent review of this aspect. It seems safe to assume that the SNS would be similarly informed about strain, injury or malfunction of some part of the musculoskeletal system (e.g., of a joint), and that there would be a major impact locally or segmentally if a segment of the vertebral column was involved.

On this assumption, in the late 1940's, my colleagues and I at the Kirksville College of Osteopathic Medicine undertook studies on human subjects to see if any alteration in sympathetic activity was associated with the vertebral and paravertebral dysfunctions to which osteopathic physicians give attention in diagnosis and therapy

In a series of studies in which we used sudomotor and cutaneous vasomotor activity as physiological indicators of topographical variations in sympathetic activity, we showed the following:

(1) In most individuals, even under cool, resting conditions, there are areas of hydrated skin associated with persistent, low-grade sweat-gland activity (reflected in low electrical skin resistance, hence "low-resistance areas," LRA) and of high vasomotor tone (Wright, Korr & Thomas, 1953; Thomas & Korr, 1957; Thomas, Korr & Wright, 1958; Thomas & Kawahata, 1962).

(2) The segmental patterns of distribution of these aberrant areas varied from subject to subject, but were highly constant and reproducible for each subject over periods of months. This is not to say that the actual shapes and sizes of the aberrant areas were invariable; they were areas in which, at any given time, the probability was very high, as compared with all other areas, that we would find high sudomotor and vasomotor activity. They were areas, for example, in which in the course of cooling the warm, lightly perspiring subject, the sweat-gland activity persisted long after it had subsided in other areas, and were the first to respond with increased activity as the subject was warmed (Korr, Thomas & Wright, 1958; Wright, Korr & Thomas, 1960).

(3) These areas of sympathetic hyperactivity correlated well, in segmental distribution, with existing musculoskeletal strain, trauma, deep and superficial tenderness, electromyographic activity of paraspinal muscles, etc. New areas could be induced experimentally with postural and myofascial insult which were related regionally or segmentally to the site of insult (Korr, Wright & Thomas, 1962; Korr, Wright & Chace, 1964).

(4) Similar signs of sympathetic hyperactivity were found to be associated with visceral pathology, apparently in areas of referred pain and tenderness, segmentally related to the visceral pathology. In a few subjects studied over long periods of time, the aberrant areas appeared in advance of the first symptoms of visceral disease (Korr, 1949).

(5) The sympathetically hyperactive areas of skin _functioned_ differently from the normal areas. Thus, the sudomotor responses of the low-resistance areas to a variety of factors were grossly exaggerated. This was demonstrated in a group of subjects who had asymmetrical patterns, that is, in whom we had found low electrical skin resistance on one side at a given segmental level, while the contralateral area was normal.

As illustrated by Figures 1-3, and as previously shown (Thomas & Korr, 1957; Thomas & Kawahata, 1962), we found that in a low-resistance area, there was conspicuous sweat-gland activity under cool, resting conditions when, as shown by most areas of the trunk (including the contralateral area), there was no evidence of thermoregulatory demand for sweat secretion. That same low-resistance

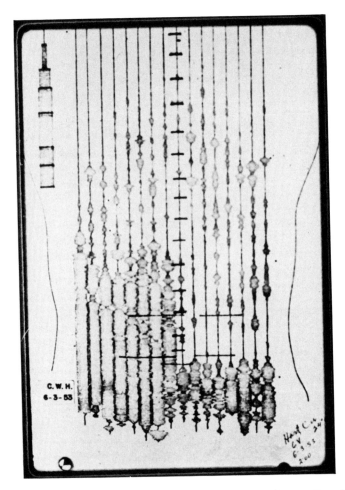

Figure 1. Electrical skin resistance pattern of C.W.H. This
record was made under cool, resting conditions with the pantographic
dermohmeter described by Thomas, Korr and Wright (1958). The lower
the resistance, the larger the oscillation. Segmental areas of
marked asymmetry in resistance between left and right sides from
L 3-5 were chosen for experiments presented in Figures 2 and 3.
Short horizontal lines in midline mark tips of spinous processes.

area also made exaggerated sudomotor responses (earlier and more
rapid recruitment of sweat glands and more copious secretion) to
generalized stimuli (e.g., heating other parts of the body), painful
stimuli, threat of pain and other emotional stimuli. These areas
seemed to be continually in, or verging on, a "cold sweat" (Korr,
Thomas & Wright, 1955).

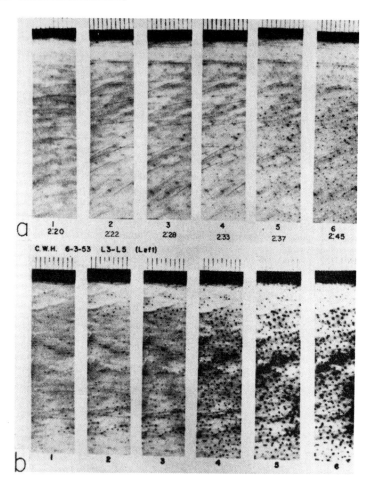

Figure 2.   Comparison of sweating in high- and low-resistance areas.
Subject C.W.H.   (a) Photographs 1-6 are enlargements showing a strip
of skin, 1 cm wide, from the right area.   (b) Photographs 1-6 are
from the left area identified in Figure 1.   Sweat secretion of individual glands was chemically visualized.   Photographs numbered 1
were taken before, and subsequent photographs 2-6, during heating
of the abdomen with electrical hot pad.   Note activity on left side
(b) in the pre-heat period, and the early, rapid recruitment of
additional glands, as compared with the right side.

On the basis of these findings and other considerations, we
concluded that peripheral sympathetic pathways at segmental levels
corresponding to somatic dysfunction in and around the spinal column
are in a state of chronic facilitation similar to that shown by
Denslow and his co-workers for neuromuscular activity (Denslow &

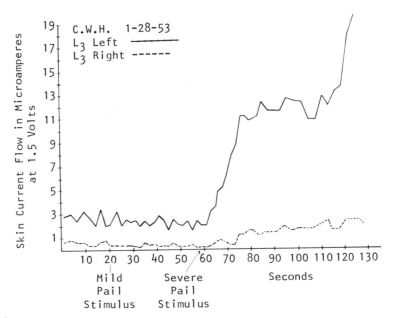

Figure 3. Comparison of response to pain in high- and low-
resistance areas. Subject C.W.H. Sweat-gland activity was recorded
by intermittent measurements of current flow in the two areas identified in Figure 1. Each pain stimulus consisted of a single pinprick to the calf of the right leg. Note the large responses of
the left side (after approximately 40-sec latencies) as compared
with the small response of the right side, which occurred only after
the second stimulus. (Similar responses were obtained to the threat
of pain.)

Hassett, 1942; Denslow, 1944; Denslow, Korr & Krems, 1947). Persistent local, regional or dermatomal elevation in sympathetic activity and predisposition to high activity appear to be related to
spinal and paraspinal motor dysfunction as disclosed by osteopathic
palpatory diagnosis. In general, the concept of chronic segmental
facilitation has been found to be consistent with observations in
osteopathic practice, and helpful in their rationalization. The
concept has recently been reviewed in a broader context (Korr,
1976) and re-examined in terms of conditioning, habituation and
sensitization in spinal reflex pathways (Patterson, 1976).

THE INFLUENCES OF SYMPATHETIC INNERVATION

What is the clinical significance of chronic facilitation and
hyperactivity of sympathetic innervation on various tissues and

organs? Let us review first the physiological influence of sympathetic innervation. This is a great deal more varied than can be
ascribed to the regulation merely of exocrine secretion and of contraction in smooth and cardiac muscle and the metabolic energizing
of these activities, as is widely taught. The literature, some of
it quite old and long ignored, indicates a much larger repertoire,
as illustrated by the following examples.

1.   Skeletal Muscle

The sympathetic innervation of skeletal muscle appears to have
a direct augmentor effect on the energetics of skeletal muscle, possibly similar to the inotropic effect on cardiac muscle ("Orbeli
phenomenon"; see Bach, 1953; Kelly & Bach, 1959). It also appears
to facilitate neuromuscular transmission (Hutter & Loewenstein,
1955; Naseldov, 1960). Sympathetic innervation is also involved
in the development of contractures following trauma to the spinal
cord (Galitskaya, 1965).

2.   Peripheral Sensory Mechanisms

Several types of receptors and sense organs have been shown to
be influenced by sympathetic impulses. In general, the effect of
repetitive sympathetic stimulation is facilitatory, that of increasing the frequency of afferent discharge and lowering the threshold.
In some cases, threshold may be reduced to zero, causing afferent
discharge without direct stimulation of the receptor. In short,
the effect of increased impulse traffic in the sympathetic fibers
innervating receptors is that of exaggerating their discharge,
causing them to report a greater intensity of stimulation than is
actually occurring. The sensory mechanisms in which sympathetic
influence has been demonstrated include: (a) muscle spindle (Hunt,
1960; Eldred, Schnitzlein & Buchwald, 1960); (b) tactile receptors
(Chernetski, 1964a); (c) taste receptors (Chernetski, 1964a);
(d) olfactory apparatus (Tucker & Beidler, 1955); (3) carotid sinus
chemo- and baroreceptors (Koizumi & Sato, 1969; Mills & Sampson,
1969; Sampson & Mills, 1970; McCloskey, 1975); (f) Pacinian corpuscles (Loewenstein & Altamirano-Orrego, 1956); (g) retina
(Mascetti, Marzi & Berlucchi, 1969); and (h) cochlea (Vasil'ev,
1962).

3.   Central Nervous System

Following the demonstration by Bonvallet, Dell and Heibel
(1954) of adrenergic elements in the reticular formation and of
the effect of the SNS thereon and on the reticulospinal system, a

series of studies appeared in the Soviet literature, indicating
strong influence of the superior cervical ganglion on cortical and
subcortical activity. Thus, Karamian (1958) and his co-worker,
Sollertinskaya (1957), found that unilateral removal of the superior
cervical ganglion in rabbits resulted in behavioral changes, including lowered intensity and even total disappearance of established
positive food-conditioned motor reflexes. These effects were accompanied by profound changes in spontaneous cortical electrical
activity and in responses to peripheral stimulation. The effects
were more marked in the ipsilateral hemisphere. After removal of
both left and right ganglia followed by adrenal demedullization,
the EEG voltage became very unstable and changes in behavior and
response to peripheral stimulation also took place. Subcutaneous
injection of adrenalin produced a transient return to normal
activity.

Tay-An (1960) demonstrated that ganglionectomy also affected
electrical activity of the hypothalamus. In a later study, Tay-An
and Gelehkova (1961) studied the effects on the recruitment reaction in the ipsilateral hemisphere of stimulating one cervical
sympathetic nerve in cats. (The recruitment reaction is the increase in cortical electrical activity produced by stimulation of
non-specific thalamic nuclei.) In most cases, sympathetic stimulation reduced the amplitude of the reaction in the ipsilateral hemisphere. Occasionally, usually on repeated stimulation, there was an
increase. Intravenous adrenalin more consistently weakened the recruitment reaction. In contrast, there seemed to be little sympathetic influence on the primary responses of the auditory cortex to
stimulation of the specific nucleus, the medial geniculate body.

Changes in electrical activity of the visual regions of the
cerebral cortex following unilateral extirpation of the superior
cervical ganglion in rabbits support Zagorul'ko's conclusion (1965)
that the sympathetic innervation primarily influences the mechanisms
responsible for the generation of the background electrical activity
the "rhythm assimilation reaction" (reproduction of various fre-
quencies of flashing light) and the secondary components of the
induced responses to light.

Aleksanyan and Arutunian (1959) observed diffuse electrical
activation on stimulation of the cervical sympathetic nerve, and
concluded that the sympathetic effect is on the total brain, including the reticular formation, and that the cortical effect is not
necessarily mediated by the reticular formation. Ganglionectomy
also produced electrical changes in both cortical and subcortical
structures, of such a nature as to indicate diffuse inhibition.
Observations of Veselkin (1959) on the pigeon indicate that the
cerebellum is similarly under direct influence of the sympathetic
innervation.

The work of Skoglund (1961) and of Chernetski (1964b) indicates
that the facilitatory influence of the SNS may also extend to the
spinal cord. In the cat, Skoglund showed that threshold doses of
noradrenalin converted single-spike responses (to single afferent
volleys) to repetitive discharges, set up discharges in initially
silent cells and increased the frequency of prevailing activity.
In the frog, Chernetski showed that sympathectomy markedly reduced
intersensory facilitation of the leg flexion reflex. He attributed
the depression to reduced central nervous responsiveness in the
absence of the sympathetic influence.

To what extent these SNS-related changes are based on vasomotor
changes is difficult to determine, especially in view of conflicting
reports regarding the role of SNS innervation on circulation through
the CNS. Whether the observed changes are of indirect vasomotor
origin or are the more direct effects on neuronal excitation or
metabolism, such as that described by Hunter and Stefanik (1975),
the influence of the sympathetic innervation on CNS function seems
an important and neglected area of neurophysiology, despite the
obvious importance of the catecholamines in brain function and
dysfunction.

4.   Collateral Circulation

Bardina (1956) showed that, following experimental occlusion
of the lingual artery, interruption of the sympathetic innervation
of the tongue greatly accelerated the development of collateral
circulation. Similarly, Dansker (1957), using the Clark-Chamber
rabbit-ear technique, found that unilateral sympathectomy increased
the development of arteriovenous anastamoses, both in number and
diameter.

5.   Bone Growth

Sympathetic innervation has been found to exert an important
influence on longitudinal bone growth (Kottke, Gullickson & Olson,
1958). Other influences, e.g., on the response of bone to estrogens
(Rosenfeld et al., 1959), and on the activity of bone cells, possibly in collagen elaboration and matrix formation (Chiego & Singh,
1974), have also been reported.

6.   Adipose Tissue

It is now well established that adipose tissue may also be regarded as a true effector organ making its own specific responses
to stimulation of its sympathetic innervation. The sympathetic

innervation is requisite for the rapid lipolysis (release of free
fatty acids and glycerol) that takes place in cold exposure and for
the slower lipolysis in starvation. Sympathetic blockade or sympathectomy (the latter usually done unilaterally, the contralateral
fat pad serving as control) prevents the adaptive response (Paoletti
& Vertua, 1964; Hull & Segall, 1965). Sympathectomized adipose
tissue increases in fat content, suggesting a tonic influence on
the balance between release and mobilization.

Electrical stimulation of the nerve supply to adipose tissue
causes the release of free fatty acids and glycerol. Obviously,
sympathetic excitation, either experimentally or as part of an
adaptive response such as that to cold, involves the rapid activation of several enzyme systems. The noradrenalin content and
metabolism in adipose tissue is the same as in other organs with
adrenergic innervation (Fredholm, 1970).

The lipolytic effect of sympathetic stimulation with accompanying glycogenolysis and increase in O_2 consumption are not
dependent on the concurrent vasomotor responses to nerve stimulation. Indeed, the metabolic response is delayed by the accompanying vasoconstriction. The independence is further substantiated
by the fact that the adipocyte responses to sympathetic stimulation
are blocked by adrenergic β-receptor antagonists, whereas the vasomotor responses involve α-receptors (Fredholm, 1970; Fredholm et al.,
1975; Rosell & Belfrage, 1975).

7. Reticuloendothelial System

In 1953 Kuntz summarized the evidence then available that sympathetic innervation has important influences not only on blood
flow through the blood-forming tissues, but also on such specific
functions and factors as the phagocytic activity of the reticuloendothelial cells of bone marrow, on erythropoiesis and on the
release and distribution of leucocytes and on endothelial permeability. Linke (1953) showed that prolonged, low-frequency stimulation of the splanchnic nerves, lumbar sympathetic trunks and sympathetic nerves to the liver (but not to the spleen) caused large
increases in circulating reticulocytes and normoblasts. The increases lasted for periods of 80 min to 30 h, depending on the
nerves stimulated. Responses to stimulation of the sympathetic
nerves were unchanged by clamping of the adrenal blood vessels.

In a more recent study on the marrow of the rat femur, DePace
and Webber (1975), using electrostimulation and morphological
methods, have extended these older observations. They found
abundant adrenergic fibers terminating on arteries and fibers
coursing through parenchyma close to many marrow cells, but no

evidence of terminations on these cells. Stimulation of lumbar sympathetic trunks triggered the release of large numbers of reticulocytes and neutrophils into the circulating blood. The changes affecting other cells were somewhat variable. The mechanism governing the release of blood cells from the bone marrow following sympathetic stimulation seems to be a selective one apparently involving the sinusoidal wall. On the basis of cited electron micrographic evidence and the studies of numerous other investigators, the authors conclude that the transmitter released at sympathetic terminals increases the (apparently active) passage of selected white blood cells through cells of the sinusoidal wall, in a manner similar to that described for erythrocytes.

8.   Endocrine Systems

One of the most interesting examples of sympathetic control is that on the pineal body and, through the pineal, on other endocrine systems, particularly those related to sexual development and reproduction. (For reviews, see Wurtman, Axelrod & Kelly, 1968; Wolstenholme & Knight, 1971.) The pineal controls the release of releasing factors for luteinizing hormone, follicle stimulating hormone and prolactin inhibiting and releasing factors. This pineal control of releasing factors is mediated by the elaboration and secretion of melatonin and other polypeptide hormones which exert antigonadal action.

The synthesis of melatonin is under the control of the sympathetic innervation of the pineal, from the superior cervical ganglion. Synthesis is augmented in the dark and reduced in the light, the optic pathways somehow being involved in the regulation of impulse traffic in the sympathetic branch to the pineal (Brooks, Ishikawa & Koizumi, 1975). This accounts for the impaired growth and sexual development of rats raised in the dark and for diurnal behavioral phenomena related to photoperiodicity. These behavioral phenomena also reflect the influence of the pineal on functions of the higher centers of the brain. Section of the sympathetic innervation of the pineal obliterates the diurnal fluctuation of melatonin synthesis and related diurnal changes, and blocks the antigonadal and growth-inhibiting influence of the pineal in the dark.

Other, more direct, influences of the sympathetic innervation on secretion of hormones by endocrine have long been known, e.g., on the thyroid (Friedgood & Cannon, 1940; Comsa, 1963; Lowe, Ivy & Brock, 1949; Melander et al., 1974), on the adrenal cortex (Jung & Comsa, 1958), on the secretion of insulin by the pancreas (Porte, 1971; Shevchuk, Sandulyak & Rybachuk, 1970) and the testicle (Khodorovski, 1964). Koizumi and Brooks (1972) have summarized

recent confirmation and extension of these older observations on
the sympathetic control of endocrine function.

9. Others

There are many other examples of sympathetic influence on
various functions and processes, e.g., on enzyme activity (Nordenfelt, Ohlin & Stromblad, 1960), on mitosis and RNA and DNA synthesis
(Schneyer, 1973) and on growth and development of the salivary
glands (Wells, Handelman & Milgram, 1961) and of the kidney (Hix,
1966). Additional examples will be found in the review by Koizumi
and Brooks (1972). Still others, including the sympathetic conditioning of tissue responses to other factors, e.g., to parasympathetic stimulation, hormones, etc., are evident in connection with
clinical and pathological manifestations of sympathetic hyperactivity discussed in the next section. The examples discussed
above, however, will serve to illustrate the diversity of sympathetic influences which cannot be explained merely on the basis of
regulation of secretion and contraction (including that of blood
vessels).

The diversity of the effects of stimulating various peripheral
sympathetic pathways is not in the influences of the sympathetic
neurons, but in the responses of the innervated tissues and organs.
The responses are as varied as the tissues and organs which are
innervated -- virtually every tissue in the body. Sympathetic
stimulation introduces no new qualities, but modifies (increases
or decreases, accelerates or retards, stimulates or inhibits) the
inherent functional properties of the target tissue, each, therefore, responding in its own manner.

CLINICAL IMPACT OF SYMPATHETIC HYPERACTIVITY

It should not be surprising, in view of these diverse organ
and tissue responses, that sympathetic hyperactivity, sustained
over long periods of time, may tend to produce pathological changes
in the target tissues, the clinical impact varying with the tissue
and its role in the body. Evidence for sympathetic components in
a variety of clinical disturbances is reviewed in this section.
The evidence is in four categories: (a) the manifestations, that
is, signs, symptoms and pathophysiology; (b) the effects of chronic
experimental stimulation; (c) the effects of therapeutic or experimental interruption or reduction of sympathetic activity; and
(d) morphological changes in sympathetic components.

Since sympathetic vasomotor fibers are contrictor in most
areas, ischemia of various degrees is often a common consequence

of sympathetic hyperactivity. The reduced blood flow would, in turn, alter the functional properties of the tissues and their responses to other factors, e.g., parasympathetic or endocrine influence. It may also render them vulnerable to various agents (such as normal digestive secretions, infectious agents and toxins) and less able to recover from insult. In some of the following examples of the pathogenic influences of sympathetic hyperactivity, the vasomotor component is clearly evident; in others it is of minor importance or is obscured by other sympathetic effects.

1. Neurogenic Pulmonary Edema

A dramatic example of the pathogenic influence of intense sympathetic discharge is neurogenic pulmonary edema. Severe pulmonary edema, with marked vascular congestion, atelectasis, intra-alveolar hemorrhage and protein-rich edema fluid, appears very rapidly after severe, often fatal blows to the head and other severe injuries to the central nervous system (CNS). It occurs quite independently of underlying pulmonary or cardiac disease. It has been produced experimentally in various species by blunt head trauma, electrolytic lesions in various parts of the brain, sudden large increases in cerebrospinal fluid pressure (see Theodore & Robin, 1976, for references), hyperbaric oxygen (Johnson & Bean, 1957), injection of chloramine (Rudin, 1963) and localized pulmonary infarction (Kabins et al., 1962). Of great interest is the fact that pulmonary edema, with its associated changes, is also produced by stimulation of the stellate ganglia. Conversely, treatment of animals with various adrenergic blocking agents or extirpation of stellate or other sympathetic ganglia prior to administration of any of the above forms of trauma and stimuli completely prevents the appearance of pulmonary edema.

It seems to be assumed by most workers in this field that the SNS-induced pulmonary edema is due to vascular responses and hemodynamic changes in the pulmonary circulation, perhaps including constriction of pulmonary veins (Kadowitz, 1975); other factors such as changes in capillary permeability have also been postulated (Theodore & Robin, 1976). In the course of their extensive studies on pulmonary edema produced by head trauma, high oxygen pressure and stellate ganglion stimulation, Beckman and his collaborators (Beckman & Houlihan, 1973; Droste & Beckman, 1974; Beckman, Bean & Blaslock, 1974; Sexton & Beckman, 1975) have implicated another, non-vascular, factor. They have demonstrated, under these circumstances, a large, abrupt decrease in lung compliance, accompanied by a large increase of minimum surface tension and of cholesterol content of the wash fluid. The changes in compliance and surface tension are tentatively ascribed to increased (intra-alveolar) cholesterol. In monkeys and cats these changes in lung compliance

occurred independently of, or in advance of, any signs of lung
injury such as congestion or edema.

Whatever the mechanisms eventually disclosed, it is well
established that severe lung damage may be produced by intense
sympathetic bombardment of the lungs, triggered in various ways.

2.   Peptic Ulcer and Pancreatitis

Sympathetic components have been identified in peptic ulcer
(e.g., DeSousa-Pereira, 1959) and in pancreatitis. Gage and Gillespie (1951) and Walker and Pembleton (1955) showed the therapeutic effects of conduction block in pancreatitis. Gilsdorf et
al. (1965), on the other hand, demonstrated that sympathetic stimulation converted mild, non-lethal, bile-induced pancreatitis to
the hemorrhagic, necrotizing and lethal form. That this sympathetic
effect may be ascribable to vasoconstriction is indicated by an
earlier study by Block, Wakim and Baggenstoss (1954). In their
experimental study, obstruction of the flow of pancreatic juice,
even when permitted to mix with bile, produced only non-necrotic
changes in the parenchyma of the pancreas. When, however, brief
ischemia was superimposed on obstruction of the pancreatic duct,
parenchymal necrosis developed which varied in severity with the
degree of arterial obstruction. Lesions comparable to acute
hemorrhagic pancreatitis in man were occasionally produced by
ischemia alone.

3.   Arteriopathy

Gutstein, LaTaillade and Lewis (1962) produced the histological
features of arteriosclerosis in the aorta by sustained stimulation
of the splanchnic nerve in unanesthetized rats. Sympathetic stimulation apparently produced some change in the arterial wall that
favored the development of arteriosclerotic lesions. A tendency
toward thrombosis seems to have been a factor. It is interesting
in this connection that in studies on experimental thrombosis in
the rabbit ear, denervation of the ear markedly accelerated thrombolysis (Fowler, 1949; Cho, 1967).

4.   Cardiovascular-Renal Syndromes

Hypertension. It has long been suspected, on the basis of
physiological, pharmacotherapeutic and behavioral considerations,
that high activity of the peripheral SNS is an important contributing factor in at least some forms of arterial hypertension. This
has been difficult to establish, by direct means, in patients.

Recent studies of Wallin, Delius & Habgarth (1973), in which they
recorded multiunit sympathetic activity in skin and muscle nerves,
have yielded preliminary support for this hypothesis. In a more
quantitative study on spontaneously hypertensive rats, Iriuchijima's
studies (1973) indicated a much higher efferent impulse traffic in
the splanchnic nerves of hypertensive than of normotensive rats.

Heart Disease. Among the most threatening and often fatal
complications following myocardial infarction are ventricular
fibrillation and other arrhythmias. The recent work of several
investigators indicates that heightened discharge through the sympathetic innervation of the heart may be a most important factor.
In an experimental study on transient coronary occlusion in cats,
with the use of direct recording techniques, Malliani, Schwartz and
Zanchetti (1969) showed an increased discharge in most of the fibers
tested (in the third thoracic ramus communicans). The reflex, which
the authors characterized as a sympathetic cardio-cardiac reflex,
occurred also in the spinal animal, did not depend on the baroreceptors, on vagal reflexes or on direct anoxic stimulation of
preganglionic neurons.

Others have found that experimental coronary occlusion lowers
the ventricular fibrillation threshold (determined by repetitive
electrical stimulation of the ventricle) and increases the incidence
of ectopic discharges and arrhythmias. Adrenergic blockade and ablation of the stellate ganglia protected the heart against these manifestations and even prevented them, especially during the first few
hours of occlusion (Harris, Bocage & Otero, 1975; Kliks, Burgess &
Abildskov, 1975). Conversely, stimulation of the stellate ganglia,
even in the absence of coronary occlusion, markedly lowered the
fibrillation threshold. When ganglionic stimulation was superimposed
on occlusion, the threshold was depressed far below that following
occlusion alone. The conclusion that postinfarction sympathicotonia
is a critical factor in the triggering of ectopic activity and fibrillation is further supported by the demonstration that cardiac sympathectomy prior to occlusion protects against these complications
and lowers the mortality rate (Fowlis et al., 1974).

A study with unilateral stellectomy or reversible cold block
of individual stellate ganglia revealed significantly different influences of the right and left ganglia on cardiac excitability,
perhaps comparable to the well established differences with respect
to inotropic and chronotropic influences (Schwartz, Snebold & Brown,
1976). Thus, left sympathetic denervation of the heart raised the
ventricular fibrillation threshold 72 + 35 percent above control
values, whereas right-sided denervation lowered the threshold 48 +
14 percent. The authors believe that these observations help explain the pathogenesis of ventricular arrhythmias and fibrillation
(e.g., in the so-called long Q-T syndrome) associated with increased
sympathetic activity. They recommend left stellectomy as a logical

measure in patients at high risk from such arrhythmias, when medical therapy has not been effective.

Schwartz (1976) has further proposed, on the basis of these observations and studies on infants, that the Sudden Infant Death Syndrome is due to the long Q-T syndrome brought on by an abrupt sympathetic discharge taking place through asymmetrical cardiac sympathetic innervation in which the right side is, for some reason (congenital?), subnormal in activity.

At any rate, it seems clear that the increased sympathetic discharge to the heart which accompanies myocardial infarction (Malliani et al., 1969) greatly imperils the effective function of the heart and the survival of the patient. There is not only the hazard of ectopic activity and fibrillation, but also cardio-acceleration and increased oxygen demand. Also to be considered is the probability that the increased sympathetic discharge to the heart includes that of the α-receptor sympathetic coronary con-strictors (Szentiványi & Juhasz-Nágy, 1963a, 1963b; Feigl, 1975) which would contribute to intensification and spread of the myo-cardial ischemia. Indeed, it is possible that hyperactivity of these neurons would contribute to coronary arteriospasm implicated in acute myocardial ischemia and angina pectoris. The apparent in-hibitory influence of the sympathetic innervation on the development of collateral circulation, previously discussed, may also have important implications for the patient with coronary artery disease.

Other examples of sympathetic components in cardiovascular disease are the following:

(a) Dietzman et al. (1973) found heightened SNS activity during cardiogenic shock in dogs. Renal and intestinal vascular beds were most affected. Reduction of SNS influences lengthened the survival period. These studies support the concept that the SNS plays a lethal role in cardiogenic shock in dogs.

(b) Raab (1963) and Kaye, McDonald and Randall (1961) have shown that hyperactivity of cardiac sympathetic pathways may produce severe cardiac lesions.

(c) Barger (1960) found that retention of Na and water in con-gestive heart failure is ascribable to increase in sympathetic ac-tivity in the kidney. As a matter of fact, the renal sympathi-cotonia is evident before the development of heart failure. Blocking the adrenergic nerves produced diuresis and natriuresis. In patients with ureteral calculi and during experimental stimulation of the ureter in humans and dogs (by ureteral catheterization), Hix (1970) found the renal sympathetic pathways markedly facilitated on the affected side. In these subjects superimposed emotional stimuli

caused unilateral, abrupt reduction in glomerular filtration and
renal blood flow. In dogs, Kottke, Kubicek and Visscher (1945)
produced arterial hypertension by chronic renal artery-nerve
stimulation.

It is of interest in this connection that Anselmino (1950)
found that novocaine blockade of the renal innervation reduced
arterial blood pressure in most eclamptic patients, improved diuresis and, in some, stopped coma and convulsions. Blockade of the
stellate ganglia in these patients improved diuresis, stopped coma
and convulsions in some and improved subjective manifestations
including headache, ocular disturbances and nausea.

5.   Posttraumatic Pain Syndromes

"The expected response to trauma in an extremity after
proper treatment is orderly and predictable healing of the
wound, return of function, return of circulatory dynamics,
and gradual cessation of pain. Occasionally this predictable response reacts in a bizarre fashion despite adequate
treatment and the absence of any obvious factors detrimental
to prompt healing. Pain may become severe and unrelenting,
with a marked disparity between severity of pain and the
apparent injury. Sympathetic dysfunction, usually overactivity, becomes evident. Trophic changes usually ensue
to varying degrees, and if the process is left unattended
for any length of time they become irreversible."

This is the way that the surgeon-authors of a contribution to
the management of posttraumatic syndromes introduce their paper
(Thompson, Patman & Persson, 1975). The paragraph is a synopsis
of an assortment of causalgia-like syndromes affecting the extremities, in which, at least from the therapeutic viewpoint,
hyperactivity of the sympathetic innervation is a critical feature.

The manifestations (and the inciting factors) of these syndromes occur in such great variety, with respect to intensity and
quality of the pain, motor dysfunction, sympathetic dysfunction and
trophic disturbances, that many different terms have been invented
reflecting not only these variations but also the special interests,
emphases and viewpoints of the observers. Among the terms for these
"entities" are the following: minor causalgia, reflex sympathetic
dystrophy, Sudek's atrophy, painful osteoporosis, acute atrophy of
bone, shoulder-hand syndrome (following myocardial infarction or
stroke), chronic traumatic edema, posttraumatic pain syndromes,
sympathetic neurovascular dystrophy, traumatic angiospasm, post-
traumatic spreading neuralgia, sympathalgia, peripheral tropho-
neurosis, and others. The most favored in current literature seem

to be reflex (or posttraumatic) sympathetic dystrophy and post-traumatic pain syndromes (Patman et al., 1973; Thompson et al., 1975; Genant et al., 1975; Kozin et al., 1976; Kleinert et al., 1973; Omer & Thomas, 1974). The terms "mimocausalgia" (proposed by Thompson et al.) and "minor causalgia", however, would seem to be most useful, especially for those familiar with causalgia through clinical experience or through the classical descriptions of causalgia by S. Weir Mitchell and associates, in reports of their experience with gunshot wounds in the American Civil War, and in more recent reviews (Richards, 1967).

The pain may vary from the extremely severe, burning, unrelenting, personality-destroying type of full causalgia to the equally chronic but more tolerable pain of the "minor" causalgias. Hyperesthesia may be so exquisite that the patient cannot tolerate the weight of clothing on the extremity, the gentlest touch or the slightest air current. Paroxysms of even more intense pain are often triggered by any of the above and by such minor disturbances as noise, change in ambient temperature or movement of the limb. The limb is held as immobile as possible. The patient is, therefore, extremely resistant to therapy.

The manifestations of sympathetic dysfunction include vasospasm and hyperhidrosis, cold and wet skin, cyanosis and chronic edema. In some cases, however, or temporarily in an early stage, the skin may be hot and dry as well as edematous, possibly due to the release of vasoactive agents and irritants from sensory endings by antidromic impulses (discussed later).

The most bizarre manifestations are those in the "trophic" category. They include change in the thickness, texture and other qualities of the skin, changes in the nails and hair growth, shortening of tendons, atrophy of musculature, osteoporosis and other degenerative changes in bones, joints (which become stiff and even frozen) and juxta-articular tissues. The arthropathies and other skeletal changes have recently received thorough study by Genant et al. (1975) and Kozin et al. (1976) with fine-detail radiography, radionuclide techniques and mineral analyses.

The degenerative changes in bone, "frozen" joints, muscle atrophy, etc., have been ascribed by some to immobilization of the affected limb by the patient, and this is almost certainly a factor. However, the distribution of pathological changes bespeaks a central neural mechanism. Whether the trophic manifestations are due to circulatory changes, some other influences of sympathetic impulse activity or the non-impulse mechanisms discussed by others in the Workshop remains to be investigated.

Another feature difficult to explain is the gross disparity
between the response, on the one hand (the severity, persistence
and progressive nature of the pain and other manifestations), and
the injury, on the other. In some cases the injury may not only
be non-penetrating but so slight that it would ordinarily be dismissed as a superficial bump or a bruise; in other cases it may be
a small fracture, a minor surgical procedure, a laceration, a tool
dropped on the foot.

One of the most remarkable common features of these syndromes
and their variants is their responsiveness to interruption of impulse traffic in the sympathetic innervation of the affected extremity. In many cases, the pain and autonomic manifestations may
be immediately relieved by blockade of the appropriate ganglia
(ipsilateral stellate or lumbar). The relief may outlast by several hours or days the usual anesthetic action of the agent injected
around the ganglia. The relief may even be permanent following a
single block or a series of blocks. When, as is more usual, and if
the ganglionic blockade has given temporary relief outlasting anesthetic action, then permanent relief and "cure" may be obtained with
surgical interruption of the sympathetic pathway to the extremity.

Ganglionic blockade and sympathectomy are much less likely to
be effective if diagnosis and effective treatment have been too
long delayed. Most authors urge early recognition and treatment
of the syndrome not only because delayed interruption of the local
sympathicotonia is less likely to be effective (which, in turn,
often prevents examination of the extremity and application of sup-
portive measures such as physical therapy), but because the trophic
and degenerative changes may become so advanced as to be irreversible. Under such circumstances, even were the pain and vasomotor
changes eventually relieved, the patient would be left with a dis-
figured and disabled extremity and often with severe emotional
disturbances.

No hypothesis has yet been offered that satisfactorily explains
reflex sympathetic dystrophy. In general, three mechanisms (Sternschein et al., 1975) seem to have won adherents:

(1) Increased excitability (facilitation) of internuncial
neuronal pools at the involved cord levels, presumably incited by
aberrant sensory input from the injured site. Sensory, motor and
sympathetic pathways are thought to be affected by the enhanced
central excitatory state. The increased sympathetic discharges
produce changes in the periphery which incite secondary afferent
discharges, thus initiating and sustaining vicious, autogenic cycles
of impulses.

(2) Excitation of ectopic impulses in pain fibers by impulses passing in neighboring sympathetic postganglionic fibers (inter-axonal "cross-talk", lateral or ephaptic transmission, "artificial synapse"). The antidromic (as well as orthodromic, afferent) impulses triggered in this manner are thought by some to release vasoactive agents and irritants at the endings.

(3) Various adaptations of the gate-control theory of pain.

While hypotheses (2) and (3) may possibly contribute to under-standing of the pain components of the syndromes, they offer none regarding the signs of sympathicotonia (which the first hypothesis does) or of the trophic manifestations (which are referrable, at least in part, to the sympathicotonia). This seems a worthy area for investigation, perhaps in an animal model which simulates the causalgia-like syndromes. The preparation described by Kennard (1950) may be a promising one with which to begin.

6. Other Skeletal Disorders

In 1957 Herfort first reported excellent results following lumbar sympathectomy in patients bedridden by arthritic pain in weight-bearing joints. The extirpation of the lumbar ganglionic chain affected the rheumatoid activity only in the denervated ex-tremities, and equally good results were obtained in rheumatoid and osteoarthritic disease. Neurons and neuroglial supporting cells in sympathetic ganglia surgically removed from patients with chronic polyarthritis showed morphological signs of prolonged preganglionic stimulation (Kuntz, 1958).

Coujard (1960) reported a variety of osteodystrophies produced in the guinea pig by irritation of the sympathetic fibers in the sciatic nerve (and by diencephalic lesions). The bony manifesta-tions included various arthropathies mimicking those of tabes and syringomyelia, alteration of calcium fixation, and heterotopic osteogenesis, such as spicules on the periosteum and tumor-like outgrowths of bone.

Kottke et al. (1958) studied longitudinal bone growth in chil-dren who had paresis of one leg and nearly normal strength in the other after acute anterior poliomyelitis. The average rate of growth of the bones of paretic legs was substantially less than that of normal legs; total extremity length was 82.9 percent of normal. Treatment with a sympatholytic drug restored growth to the rate of the normal leg. The authors attributed the retarded bone growth to reflex hyperactivity of SNS in response to cold, which results in vasoconstriction in the extremity and inhibits epiphyseal bone growth. They cite an earlier study in which chronic unilateral stimulation of the lumbar sympathetic chain in puppies substantially reduced growth of the hind limb on the stimulated side. Coujard (1957), however, reported evidence that the sympathetic innervation influenced the sensitivity of bone and other tissues to morphogenetic hormones.

We may also include in this category many clinical reports on the painful joint syndrome known as shoulder-hand syndrome, occasionally a distressing sequel to myocardial infarction and stroke, which is often dramatically responsive to stellate block. Some of these studies are cited in the references of the foregoing section on reflex sympathetic dystrophy.

7.   Shock

Pre-treatment of experimental animals to be subjected to traumatic shock (Levy, North & Wells, 1954; Ross & Herczeg, 1956) or hemorrhagic shock (Berger, 1965) with adrenergic blocking agents at certain critical dose ranges or with sympathectomy protects them against the lethal effects. Apparently, as is true in other clinical situations, ". . . . the sympathetic discharge is a protective mechanism, but initiates processes which are detrimental to survival" (Levy et al., 1954).

8.   Hepatotoxicity

This principle is again illustrated in liver pathology produced by administration of carbon tetrachloride. According to the evidence of Calvert and Brody (1960), the characteristic hepatic changes are the result of massive discharge of the peripheral SNS. This leads to hepatic ischemia, hypoxia and necrosis around the central vein of the hepatic lobule and certain changes in enzyme activities. As discussed in an earlier section of this paper, the sympathetic discharge also releases fatty acids from the peripheral fat pads and the consequent deposition of lipids in the liver.

9.   The Uterus

On the basis of their own experimental work with animals and review of clinical and research literature, Shabanah, Toth and Maughan (1964) concluded that many unexplained obstetrical and gynecological conditions involving disturbances in uterine contractility may be ". . . . related to abnormal neurohumoral causative factors reflected in a final picture of autonomic imbalance-- sympathetic hyperactivity."

A study by Miller and Marshall (1965) on rabbits lends support
to this conclusion. They found that stimulation of the hypogastric
nerve inhibited spontaneous uterine contractions in rabbits treated
with estrogen + progesterone. This effect was abolished by adrenergic blocking agents, but was unchanged by atropine or hexamethonium.

    10. The Eye (as a Model Illustrating Sympathetic Influences
              on Tissue Responses to Other Factors)

The role of the innervation of the eye in such disorders as
glaucoma has long been under study, but no clear picture has emerged
despite evidence for an important sympathetic influence on intraocular pressure, through influences on formation or drainage of
aqueous humor or both. Sympathetic influence on the permeability
of the blood-aqueous barrier to protein, and therefore outflow resistance, may also be a major factor (Langham, 1958).

The detrimental influence of the sympathetic innervation on
the responses of the eye to other factors is much clearer. For
example, when the trigeminal nerve was interrupted, corneal ulcer-
ations developed in all of the animals (cats). Prior stellectomy
prevented the lesion in almost all of the animals, and permitted
healing if the lesion did appear (Baker & Gottlieb, 1959).

Howes and McKay (1972) demonstrated the protective effect of
sympathectomy in quite a different kind of situation. Systemic
bacterial endotoxin in rabbits produces a marked increase in
ocular vascular permeability, primarily in the iridial portion of
the ciliary process. The initial consequence is edema, followed
by hemorrhages and thrombi. Postganglionic sympathectomy (extirpation of the superior cervical ganglion) reduced the severity of the
ocular response to systemic endotoxin. This effect required several hours to appear, and at 4 h after administration of the toxin
to the unilaterally sympathectomized rabbit there was a decrease
in the altered vascular permeability as measured by ^{125}I-serum
albumin, in stromal hemorrhages and in small-vessel thrombi in the
sympathectomized eye as compared to the contralateral or sham-
operated eye.

The apparent exacerbating influence of the sympathetic innervation in conjunction with systemic endotoxin is by no means peculiar to the eye. As is evident, for example, from the reports of
other investigators cited by Howes and McKay, sympathetic denervation and α-adrenergic blocking agents are known to suppress or prevent other reactions to endotoxins (local and generalized Schwartz-
man reaction). As far as the eye alone is concerned, it would
certainly seem important to investigate, from the etiological and
therapeutic, as well as pathophysiological, viewpoints, the role

of the sympathetic innervation in such common and damaging disorders
as uveitis or iritis.

11.   Other Examples

Other clinical situations may be cited in which a contributing,
exacerbating and often critical role of the sympathetic innervation
has been implicated, but which are only mentioned here without docu-
mentation in the interest of space. These include colitis, mega-
colon, peripheral vascular disease, ulcers of the legs, dermatitis,
postsurgical paralytic ileus, various diseases of the kidney,
Dupuytren's contracture and "pelvic congestion" in women.

A mass of clinical evidence, beyond the scope of this paper,
much of it empirical, indicates an important role of the peripheral
autonomic nervous system, and particularly the SNS, in determining
reactivity, resistance and responses of individual tissues - and
therefore the defenses of the entire organism - to infectious,
toxic, antigenic and irritative agents. These influences apparently extend to such processes as inflammation, immune reactions,
anaphylaxis, allergic manifestations and "physical allergies".
There is even evidence for sympathetic influences on the response
of tissues to carcinogenic agents and on immunobiologic mechanisms
that determine tumor "take" in experimental implants. (See, for
example, Stein-Werblowsky, 1974.) These interfaces between neuroscience and immunology and microbiology would be worthy areas of
investigation, from scientific and clinical viewpoints.

The "normal" influences of sympathetic innervation on various
endorgans, discussed in an earlier section, may also be expected
to be deleterious when the impulse activity is intensified and
sustained. For example, falsely exaggerated reports from sympathetically bombarded receptors, especially baro- and chemoreceptors,
would certainly have a disturbing effect on reflex regulatory mechanisms. This would be true also of SNS influences on CNS functions.
The effects of sympathetic hyperactivity on the reticuloendothelial
system, fat metabolism, enzyme activity, endocrine systems and
others may also be expected to be harmful over long periods of time.

Finally, it is important to mention again that any clinical
disturbance or augmented tissue vulnerability in which ischemia is
a contributing factor often may be related to sympathetic hyperactivity in view of the strong constrictor influence of sympathetic
vasomotor fibers.

12. Other Kinds of Evidence for a General SNS Role
in Disease Processes

(a) Neuropathological. Profound morphological alterations are
exhibited by ganglion cells in ganglia removed surgically in the
treatment of patients with various diseases and at autopsy. There
is also marked proliferation of neuroglial supporting cells. The
changes are such as to indicate overstimulation of the ganglion
cells, and indeed many alterations seen in surgically removed ganglia
and their cellular components have been induced experimentally by
prolonged preganglionic stimulation (Kuntz, 1958; Schilew, 1965).

(b) Irritative Lesions. Prolonged irritation, with various
agents and injuries, of peripheral sympathetic structures (e.g.,
collateral or paravertebral ganglia, splanchnic nerve) or of sensory
fibers in spinal nerves produces many types of lesion and dysfunction
of visceral and somatic structures, often lethal, which simulate
naturally occurring pathology (Mosinger, 1957; Reilly et al., 1955).

MECHANISMS

In considering the participation of the SNS in disease processes, we are confronted with an apparent paradox. On the one hand,
thanks especially to the pioneering studies of W. B. Cannon, we have
reason to be impressed with the important role of the SNS in organizing adaptive, moment-to-moment responses of the total organism
to changes in environment, posture and physical activity, and to
injury and emergencies. As adaptive responses, they are protective
and appropriate to the situation (or to what is perceived to be the
situation). On the other hand, we have many examples of harmful and
even life-endangering effects of sympathetic activity which is
focused too intensely and for too long on individual tissues and
organs.

The roles of the higher centers, including the cerebral cortex,
in initiating and organizing somato-autonomic response patterns are
now fairly well understood. However, in a prevailing emphasis on
these whole-body patterns, which are based on the capacity of the
SNS to discharge as a whole and to broadcast its influences throughout the body, there is a tendency to overlook the high degree of
local and regional control that is essential to proper execution of
the responses, as they change from moment to moment. Much of the
capacity for localization resides of course in some of the higher
centers, which can direct descending impulses (e.g., via cortico-
spinal fibers) to appropriate neuron pools. But the precise modulation of the local and regional components of the total pattern is
based on sensory signals from participating and affected tissues and

organs and on specificity and selectivity of connections, through segmental pathways, between afferents and sympathetic neurons.

These two moieties of the total patterns seem to correspond to what neurophysiologists, recording from sympathetic efferents at various spinal levels, as they stimulate selected somatic afferents, have designated as "late" (supraspinal) and "early" (spinal) somato-sympathetic reflexes (Koizumi & Brooks, 1972). All or nearly all of the total SNS neuron pool can be activated in this way via the supraspinal pathways. Only a fraction of the pool, however, is activated by the same afferent stimulation via the spinal pathways; and some somatic afferents (Group I) seem to have no access, normally, to sympathetic neurons via segmental pathways. The fraction of the efferent (preganglionic) neuron pool that is activated via spinal pathways by stimulation of selected somatic afferents is concentrated at the corresponding spinal level, the number of responding neurons declining sharply with increasing segmental interval (reviewed by Koizumi & Brooks, 1972, and by various authors in Sato, 1975). In other words, the "early" and most direct impact of impulses entering via a given dorsal root (and hence coming from a given dermatome, myotome or viscerotome) is mainly focused on the neurons whose axons emerge through the corresponding ventral roots (conveying motor and sympathetic impulses to organs and tissues in the same body "segments").

I suggest that the clinical disturbances which are apparently based on hyperactivity in related sympathetic pathways, described in the previous section, are aberrations of these local and regional feedback mechanisms. They appear to be triggered by unusual patterns of afferent impulses originating in part in injured, strained, impaired or chemically altered tissues or at sites of injury in nerves or roots. The aberration appears to be sustained (and intensified) by either (1) secondary afferent discharges from tissues bombarded by the sympathetic impulses, (2) facilitatory changes in the spinal cord, or both. While the initial trauma need not be painful to launch the vicious cycle, pain may be brought on by the sympathetic discharge (e.g., in ischemia) and by lateral (ephaptic) transmission at sites of nerve deformation, from sympathetic post-ganglionic axons to neighboring unmyelinated sensory fibers.

The aberration may also begin as a component of a total response pattern. The patterns are adaptive and protective when initiated by circumstances likely to occur in daily animal life, such as environmental extremes, exertion ("fight or flight"), injury by external forces, threat of injury and death, hypoxia, etc. When confronted with circumstances unlikely to have been encountered in the course of evolution of these adaptive sympathetic patterns, the responses may not only be inappropriate, but even harmful and detrimental to survival. Thus, while reflex vasoconstriction (and accompanying cardiovascular and other systemic changes) may be appropriate for, let us say, a painful laceration of an extremity, sympathetic hyperactivity with resultant ischemia is totally inappropriate and definitely "contraindicated" for a joint which is painfully irritated or inflamed. The ischemia itself causes pain which further intensifies the sympathetic discharge. The vicious cycle set up in that manner aggravates the pathological state (Kuntz, 1958). For similar reasons, heightened sympathetic discharge to a heart already laboring under impairment by myocardial ischemia can only, as we have seen, further impair and burden the heart and decrease the probability of survival. Bodily responses to anoxia, a common hazard in terrestrial life, are the adaptive product of evolution, which become destructive and lethal when evoked by a circumstance as unlikely as high O_2 tension (Ramey & Goldstein, 1957).

Similar, spinally organized reflexes seem to operate in the therapeutic application of hot packs, cold packs and counterirritants (e.g., rubefacients) to the skin in the region of inflamed, congested, ischemic, edematous or injured viscera and joints. When, however, the skin over apparently healthy organs is chilled, the responses may be such as to predispose to infection or other illness, as, for example, in the upper respiratory tract (Ralston & Kerr, 1945), gastrointestinal tract (Richins & Brizzee, 1949) or kidney (Nedzel, 1956).

One of the most interesting and clinically significant features of these aberrant, spinally organized somatosympathetic reflexes is the making of synaptic connections that are not ordinarily in use. This is similar to the experimental situation in which Group I afferents, which do not have access to sympathetic neurons via the "early", spinal pathways, are able, through the opening of "potential" pathways, to activate these neurons when the spinal cord is moderately cooled (Koizumi & Brooks, 1972). The result in the clinical situation is to link, reflexly, somatic and visceral structures which are not functionally coupled in any normal bodily activity or adaptive response pattern. In the clinical situation, they become linked only by virtue of the segmental proximity of their innervating neurons. Not only is this reflex "entanglement" nonadaptive and harmful to each of the structures involved in this aberrant reflex coupling, but it is disruptive of the adaptive reflex patterns in which these organs and tissues are called on to participate.

Dysfunctional, segmental coupling is clearly illustrated in patterns of referred pain and associated phenomena, of both visceral and somatic origin. Not only is the distribution of referred pain (e.g., from ischemic myocardium to chest wall, upper back, left shoulder and arm) unrelated to any normal functional pattern,

but the same is true of the reflex motor and sympathetic (sudomotor
and vasomotor) responses in the reference zones. The reflex responses to the initiating insult are not only useless, but secondary
pathology may be instigated in the reference zones (as in postinfarction shoulder-hand syndrome). The affected tissues may in turn become secondary sources of abnormal afferent bombardment that helps
sustain, intensify and spread the sympathetic hyperactivity. Although referred pain and reflex patterns of visceral origin have
been more thoroughly investigated and described, it is important to
point out that similar and even indistinguishable patterns may be
initiated from deep somatic structures (Lewis & Kellgren, 1939;
Kellgren, 1940; Travell & Rinzler, 1949). Reflex activity through
sympathetic pathways seems to be elicited with equal facility by
painful somatic or visceral afferent stimulation (Kuntz, 1958), and
with no fundamental difference in the manifestations.

RELATION TO MANIPULATIVE THERAPY

In accordance with the objectives of the Workshop, I venture
to offer for exploration hypotheses which purport to link the clinical and experimental material just reviewed and their apparent
mechanisms to those at work in manipulative therapy. In view of
the rich access of somatic afferents, via spinal and supraspinal
pathways, to sympathetic neurons, it would be truly amazing if
even relatively minor disturbances in motion of intervertebral or
other joints, which are amenable to manipulative therapy, did not
have autonomic and, therefore, circulatory, metabolic and visceral
repercussions of some degree. It would be equally surprising if
the cost did not increase with time and with the superimposition
of other detrimental factors in the patient's life.

On the basis of available data and my observations of the
skillful practice of manual medicine over a third of a century as
a physiologist, I suggest that:

1. Local musculoskeletal dysfunctions, especially in and
around the axial and weight-bearing parts of the skeleton, are
clinically significant not only because of the motor impairment
and the pain that are sometimes present, but also because they
instigate or contribute to the sustained sympathicotonia which is
a common feature in so many syndromes. Like those syndromes, they
also appear to be aberrant versions of the spinal ("early")
somatosympathetic reflexes discussed above.

2. The disturbance in the cord is due to distorted patterns
of afferent impulses from (a) the affected musculoskeletal tissues
and/or (b) irritative lesions of nerves, roots and ganglia, such
that adaptive, appropriate responses are not possible. (In view

of the sharply delineated dermatomal bands showing sympathetic
hyperactivity, often encountered in our studies, it is likely that
part of the segmental sympathicotonia may be due to irritation of
sympathetic ganglia.)

3.   Effective manipulation is that which results in the re-
establishment of coherent patterns of afferent input such that
local adjustive reflexes are once more appropriate and harmoniously
integrated in the total, supraspinally directed patterns of activity and adaptive response. The most critical effect, clinically,
is the subsidence of sympathetic hyperactivity and its pathogenic,
pain-producing influences.

4.   Improvement in the afferent input is accomplished by appropriate adjustment of articular, interosseus relationships,
muscle lengths and muscular, fascial and ligamentous tensions that
enable these tissues once more to report in coherent proprioceptive
patterns; and, in the same process, by relieving mechanical
deformation or irritation of neural structures.

5.   The mechanisms are the same when the primary perturbation
of the cord is of visceral origin, and the musculoskeletal involvement is of secondary, reflex origin, as occurs in association with
referred pain. The therapeutic effect (among others) of manipulation is still to slow the vicious cycle and reduce the sympathetic
discharge to the visceral and somatic structures which have become
reflexly coupled to their mutual detriment.

6.   The impairing effects of biomechanical insult to nerve on
the transfer of information (and material), explored in a later
section of the Workshop, are also part of the proposed mechanisms
in manipulative therapy, as reflected in our earlier publications
(Appeltauer & Korr, 1975, 1977; Korr, 1972; Korr & Appeltauer, 1974;
Korr, Wilkinson & Chornock, 1967).

REFERENCES

ALEKSANYAN, A. M., and R. S. ARUTUNIAN. The effect of sympathetic
     nerves on the electrical activity of the brain. *Proc. Acad.
     Sci. USSR, English Transl.* 125:236, 1959.

ANSELMINO, K. J. Neue Wege der Eklampsie und Praeklampsiebehand-
     lung: Die Blockade des Nierenbereichs und des Ganglion
     stellatum. *J. Suisse Med.* 80:1373-1377, 1950.

APPELTAUER, G.S.L., and I. M. KORR. Axonal delivery of soluble,
     insoluble and electrophoretic fractions of neuronal proteins
     to muscle. *Exptl. Neurol.* 46:132-146, 1975.

APPELTAUER, G.S.L., and I. M. KORR. Further electrophoretic studies
    on proteins of neuronal origins in skeletal muscle. *Exptl.
    Neurol.* 57:713-724, 1977.

BACH, L.M.N. Brainstem facilitation of the knee jerk and the
    Orbeli effect. *Am. J. Physiol.* 171:705, 1953.

BAKER, G. S., and C. M. GOTTLIEB. The prevention of corneal ulcera-
    tion in the denervated eye by cervical sympathectomy: An ex-
    perimental study in cats. *Proc. Staff Meet. Mayo Clinic* 34:
    474-478, 1959.

BARDINA, R. A. Effect of injury of the CNS on collateral circula-
    tion. *Arkh. Anat. Gistol. Embriol., English Transl.*   33:
    55-58, 1956.

BARGER, A. C. The kidney in congestive heart failure. *Circulation*
    21:124-128, 1960.

BECKMAN, D. L., J. W. BEAN, and D. R. BLASLOCK. Head injury and
    lung compliance. *J. Med. Prim.* 3:244-250, 1974.

BECKMAN, D. L., and R. D. HOULIHAN. Hyperbaric oxygen and alveolar
    surfactants. *Aerospace Med.* 44:422-424, 1973.

BERGER, R. L. Surgical and chemical denervation of abdominal viscera
    in irreversible hemorrhagic shock. *Ann. Surg.* 162:181-186,
    1965.

BLOCK, M. A., K. G. WAKIM, and A. H. BAGGENSTOSS. Experimental
    studies concerning factors in the pathogenesis of acute pan-
    creatitis. *Surg., Gynecol. Obstet.* 99:83-90, 1954.

BONVALLET, M., P. DELL, and G. HIEBEL. Tonus sympathique et
    activité électrique corticale. *EEG Clin. Neurophysiol.* 6:
    119-144, 1954.

BROOKS, C. McC., T. ISHIKAWA, and K. KOIZUMI. Autonomic system
    control of the pineal gland and the role of this complex in
    the integration of body function. *Brain Res.* 87:181-190,
    1975.

CALVERT, D. N., and T. M. BRODY. Role of the sympathetic nervous
    system in CCl_4 hepatotoxicity. *Am. J. Physiol.* 198:669-676,
    1960.

CHERNETSKI, K. E. Sympathetic enhancement of peripheral sensory
    input in the frog. *J. Neurophysiol.* 27:493-515, 1964a.

CHERNETSKI, K. E.   Facilitation of a somatic reflex by sound in Rana Clamitans: Effects of sympathectomy and decerebration. *Zeitschr. f. Tierpsychol.*   21:813-821, 1964b.

CHIEGO, D. J., Jr., and I. J. SINGH.   An autoradiographic study of H^3-proline utilization by denervated bone. *Anat. Rec.*   178: 326-327, 1974.

CHO, M.-H.   Neurogenic control of thrombolysis. *Am. J. Physiol.* 212:431-435, 1967.

COMSA, J.   Folgen der einseitigen cervicalen Sympathektomie auf die Schilddrüse der Ratte. *Pflügers Archiv*   277:16-22, 1963.

COUJARD, R.   Ostéodystrophies par lésions du système neurovégetatif. *Acta Neuroveg.*   21:177-184, 1960.

COUJARD, R.   Le sympathique regulateur de croissance et d'equilibre tissulaire. *Acta Neuroveg.*   16:32-47, 1957.

DANSKER, V. L.   Effect of sympathectomy on arterio-venous anastomoses in rabbit ear. *Doklady, Biol. Sci., Transl.*   113:203-205, 1957.

DENSLOW, J. S.   An analysis of the variability of spinal reflex thresholds. *J. Neurophysiol.*   7:207-216, 1944.

DENSLOW, J. S., and C. C. HASSETT.   The central excitatory state associated with postural abnormalities. *J. Neurophysiol.*   5: 393-402, 1944.

DENSLOW, J. S., I. M. KORR, and A. D. KREMS.   Quantitative studies of chronic facilitation in human motoneuron pools. *Am. J. Physiol.*   105:229-238, 1947.

DePACE, D. M., and R. H. WEBBER.   Electrostimulation and morphologic study of the nerves to the bone marrow of the albino rat. *Acta Anat.*   93:1-18, 1975.

DeSOUSA-PEREIRA, A.   Sympathetic innervation in peptic ulcer. *Proc. World Congr. Gastroent.*   1:405-418, 1959.

DIETZMAN, R. H., L. H. ROMERO, C. B. BECKMAN, C. H. SHATNEY, and R. C. LILLEHEI.   The influence of the sympathetic nervous system during cardiogenic shock. *Surg., Gynecol., Obstet.* 137:773-783, 1973.

DROSTE, D. L., and D. L. BECKMAN. Pulmonary effects of prolonged
    sympathetic stimulation. *Proc. Soc. Exptl. Biol. Med.* 146:
    352-353, 1974.

ELDRED, E., H. N. SCHNITZLEIN, and J. BUCHWALD. Response of muscle
    spindles to stimulation of the sympathetic trunk. *Exptl.
    Neurol.* 2:13-25, 1960.

FEIGL, E. O. Control of myocardial oxygen tension by sympathetic
    coronary vasoconstriction in the dog. *Circulation Res.* 37:
    88-95, 1975.

FOWLER, E. P., Jr. Capillary circulation with changes in sympa-
    thetic activity. I. Blood sludge from sympathetic stimulation.
    Proc. Soc. Exptl. Biol. Med. 72:592-594, 1959.

FOWLIS, R.A.F., C.T.M. SANG, P. M. LUNDY, S. P. AHUJA, and H. CAL-
    HOUN. Experimental coronary artery ligation in conscious dogs
    six months after bilateral cardiac sympathectomy. *Am. Heart J.*
    88:748-757, 1974.

FREDHOLM, B. B. Studies on the sympathetic regulation of circula-
    tion and metabolism in isolated canine subcutaneous adipose
    tissue. *Acta Physiol. Scand. Suppl.* 354, 1970.

FREDHOLM, B. B., B. LINDE, R. L. PREWITT, and P. C. JOHNSON. Oxygen
    uptake and tissue oxygen tension during adrenergic stimulation
    in canine subcutaneous adipose tissue. *Acta Physiol. Scand.*
    97:48-59, 1976.

FRIEDGOOD, H. B., and W. B. CANNON. Autonomic control of thyroid
    secretion. *Endocrinol.* 26:142-152, 1940.

GAGE, M., and G. GILLESPIE. Acute pancreatitis and its treatment.
    South. Med. J. 44:769-775, 1951.

GALITSKAYA, N. A. Role of the sympathetic nervous system in the
    development of contractures arising in the presence of spinal
    cord traumas. *Fiziol. Zh. SSSR IM I M Sechenova, Transl.*
    51:506-512, 1965.

GENANT, H. K., F. KOZIN, C. BEKERMAN, D. J. McCARTY, and J. SIMS.
    The reflex sympathetic dystrophy syndrome. A comprehensive
    analysis using fine-detail radiography, photon absorptiometry,
    and bone and joint scintigraphy. *Radiol.* 117:21-32, 1975.

GILSDORF, R. B., D. LONG, A. MOBERG, and A. S. LEONARD. Central-
    nervous system influence on experimentally induced pancreatitis
    (in cats). *J. Am. Med. Assoc.* 192:394-397, 1965.

GUTSTEIN, W. H., J. N. LaTAILLADE, and L. LEWIS. Role of vasocon-
    striction in experimental arteriosclerosis. *Circulation Res.*
    10:925-932, 1962.

HARRIS, X. S., A. J. BOCAGE, and H. OTERO. Role of sympathetic
    excitation in generating arrhythmias in early and late phases
    of ectopic responses after coronary arterial occlusion in dog
    heart. *Recent Adv. Stud. Card. Struct. Metab.* 5:315-321, 1975.

HERFORT, R. A. Extended sympathectomy in the treatment of chronic
    arthritis. *J. Am. Geriat. Soc.* 5:904-915, 1957.

HESS, W. R. *The Diencephalon - Autonomic and Extrapyramidal Func-
    tions.* New York: Grune & Stratton, 1954.

HIX, E. L. Continued studies of the trophic function of renal nerves
    The Physiologist 9:205, 1966.

HIX, E. L. Viscerovisceral and somatovisceral reflex communication.
    In: *The Physiological Basis of Osteopathic Medicine (Symposium,*
    edited by I. M. Korr, K. A. Buzzell, and E. L. Hix. New York:
    Postgraduate Institute of Osteopathic Medicine, 1970.

HOWES, E. L., Jr., and D. G. McKAY. Effect of cervical sympathec-
    tomy on the ocular response to systemic endotoxin. *Proc. Soc.
    Exptl. Biol. Med.* 137:839-844, 1972.

HULL, D., and M. M. SEGALL. Sympathetic nervous control of brown
    adipose tissue and heat production in the new-born rabbit. *J.
    Physiol.* 181:458-467, 1965.

HUNT, C. C. The effect of sympathetic stimulation on mammalian
    muscle spindles. *J. Physiol.* 151:332-341, 1960.

HUNTER, J., and P. STEFANIK. Sympathetic nervous system effects on
    rat brain metabolism. *Life Sci.* 17:1381-1386, 1975.

HUTTER, O. F., and W. R. LOEWENSTEIN. Nature of neuromuscular
    facilitation by sympathetic stimulation in the frog. *J.
    Physiol.* 130:559-571, 1955.

IRIUCHIJIMA, J. Sympathetic discharge rate in spontaneously hyper-
    tensive rats. *Jpn. Heart J.* 14:350-356, 1973.

JOHNSON, P. C., and J. W. BEAN. Effect of sympathetic blocking
    agents on the toxic action of O_2 at high pressure. *Am. J.
    Physiol.* 188:593-598, 1957.

JUNG, A., and J. COMSA. Conséquences de l'extirpation du ganglion cervical supérieur droit sur l'état fonctionnel de la cortico-surrénale chez le rat. *Ann. Endocr.*, *Paris* 19:17-21, 1958.

KABINS, S. A., J. FRIDMAN, M. KANDELMAN, and H. WEISBERG. Effect of sympathectomy on pulmonary embolism-induced lung edema. *Am. J. Physiol.* 202:687-689, 1962.

KADOWITZ, P. J., P. D. JOINER, and A. L. HYMAN. Influence of sympathetic stimulation and vasoactive substances on the canine pulmonary veins. *J. Clin. Invest.* 56:354-365, 1975.

KARAMIAN, A. I. Influence of the sympathico-adrenal system upon reflex activity at higher levels of the central nervous system. *Sechenov Physiol. J. USSR, Transl.* 44:285-295, 1958.

KAYE, M. P., R. H. McDONALD, and W. C. RANDALL. Systolic hypertension and subendocardial hemorrhages produced by electrical stimulation of the stellate ganglion. *Circulation Res.* 9: 1164-1170, 1961.

KELLY, H. B., Jr., and L.M.N. BACH. Blocking interactions between brain-stem reflex facilitation and sympathetic reflex enhancement. *Am. J. Physiol.* 196:669-673, 1959.

KELLGREN, J. H. Somatic simulating visceral pain. *Clin. Sci.* 4:303-309, 1940.

KENNARD, M. A. Chronic focal hyper-irritability of sensory nervous system in cats. *J. Neurophysiol.* 13:215-222, 1950.

KHODOROVS'KYI, H. I. The effect of disturbance of the sympathetic and parasympathetic innervation of the testicles on their structure and function. *FIZIOL. ZH. AKAD. NAUK. UKR.RSR, Transl.* 10:674-677, 1964.

KLEINERT, H. E., N. M. COLE, L. WAYNE, R. HARVEY, J. E. KUTZ, and E. ATASOY. Post-traumatic sympathetic dystrophy. *Orthop. Clin. N. Am.* 4:917-927, 1973.

KLIKS, B. R., M. J. BURGESS, and J. A. ABILDSKOV. Influence of sympathetic tone on ventricular fibrillation threshold during experimental coronary occlusion. *Am. J. Cardiol.* 36:45-49, 1975.

KOIZUMI, K., and C. McC. BROOKS. The integration of autonomic system reactions. *Ergebn. Physiol.* 67:1-68, 1972.

KOIZUMI, K., and A. SATO. Influence of sympathetic innervation on carotid sinus baroreceptor activity. *Am. J. Physiol.* 216: 321-329, 1969.

KORR, I. M. Skin resistance patterns associated with visceral disease. *Fed. Proc.* 8:87, 1949.

KORR, I. M. The trophic functions of nerves and their mechanisms. *J. Am. Osteop. Assoc.* 72:163-171, 1972.

KORR, I.M. The spinal cord as organizer of disease processes: Some preliminary perspectives. *J. Am. Osteop. Assoc.* 76: 35-55, 1976.

KORR, I. M., and G.S.L. APPELTAUER. The time-course of axonal transport of neuronal proteins to muscle. *Exptl. Neurol.* 43: 452-463, 1974.

KORR, I. M., P. E. THOMAS, and H. M. WRIGHT. Symposium on the functional implications of segmental facilitation. *J. Am. Osteop. Assoc.* 54:265-282, 1955.

KORR, I. M., P. E. THOMAS, and H. M. WRIGHT. Patterns of electrical skin resistance in man. *Acta Neuroveg.* 17:77-96, 1958.

KORR, I. M., P. N. WILKINSON, and F. W. CHORNOCK. Axonal delivery of neuroplasmic components to muscle cells. *Science* 155: 342-345, 1967.

KORR, I. M., H. M. WRIGHT, and J. A. CHACE. Cutaneous patterns of sympathetic activity in clinical abnormalities of the musculo-skeletal system. *Acta Neuroveg.* 25:589-606, 1964.

KORR, I. M., H. M. WRIGHT, and P. E. THOMAS. Effects of experimental myofascial insults on cutaneous patterns of sympathetic activity in man. *Acta Neuroveg.* 23:329-355, 1962.

KOTTKE, F. J., G. GULLICKSON, Jr., and M. E. OLSON. Studies on the disturbance of longitudinal bone growth: II. Effect of the sympathetic nervous system on longitudinal bone growth after acute anterior poliomyelitis. *Arch. Phys. Med.* 39:770-779, 1958.

KOTTKE, F. J., W. G. KUBICEK, and M. B. VISSCHER. The production of arterial hypertension by chronic renal artery-nerve stimulation. *Am. J. Physiol.* 145:38-47, 1945.

KOZIN, F., D. J. McCARTY, J. SIMS, and H. GENANT. The reflex sympathetic dystrophy syndrome. I. Clinical and histological

studies: evidence for bilaterality, response to corticosteroids and articular involvement. *Am. J. Med.* 60:321-338,
1976.

KUNTZ, A. The autonomic nervous system in retrospect. *Acta
Neuroveg.* 17:200-210, 1958.

KUNTZ, A. *The Autonomic Nervous System.* Philadelphia: Lea &
Febiger, 1953, pp. 267-268, 462-465.

LANGHAM, M. E. Aqueous humor and control of intra-ocular pressure.
Physiol. Rev. 38:215-242, 1958.

LEVY, E. A., W. C. NORTH, and J. A. WELLS. Modification of traumatic
shock by adrenergic blocking agents. *J. Pharmacol. Exptl.
Therap.* 112:151-157, 1954.

LEWIS, T., and J. H. KELLGREN. Observations relating to referred
pain visceromotor reflexes and other associated phenomena.
Clin. Sci. 4:47-71, 1939.

LINKE, P.-G. von. Beeinflussung der Erythropoese durch Reizung
vegetativer Nervenstämme in der Bauchhöhle des Hundes.
Zeitsch. f. Biol. 106:292-305, 1953.

LOEWENSTEIN, W. R., and R. ALTAMIRANO-ORREGO. The refractory state
of the generator and propagated potentials in a Pacinian Cor-
puscle. *J. Gen. Physiol.* 41:805-824, 1958.

LOWE, G. H., A. C. IVY, and S. BROCK. The effect of bilateral
cervical sympathectomy on thyroid activity. *Endocrinol.* 36:
130-136, 1949.

MALLIANI, A., P. J. SCHWARTZ, and A. ZANCHETTI. A sympathetic reflex elicited by experimental coronary occlusion. *Am. J.
Physiol.* 217:703-709, 1969.

MASCETTI, G. G., C. A. MARZI, and G. BERLUCCHI. Sympathetic influences on the dark-discharge of the retina in the feely moving
cat. *Archiv. Ital. Biol.* 107:158-166, 1969.

McCLOSKEY, D. I. Mechanisms of autonomic control of carotid chemo-
receptor activity. *Resp. Physiol.* 25:53-61, 1975.

MELANDER, A., L. E. ERICKSON, F. SUNDLER, and S. H. INGBAR. Sympathetic innervation of the mouse thyroid and its significance
in thyroid hormone secretion. *Endocrinol.* 94:959-966, 1974.

MILLER, M. D., and J. M. MARSHALL. Uterine response to nerve stimulation; relation to hormonal status and catecholamines. *Am. J. Physiol.* 209:859-865, 1965.

MILLS, E., and S. R. SAMPSON. Respiratory responses to electrical stimulation of the cervical sympathetic nerves in decerebrate, unanesthetized cats. *J. Physiol.* 202:271-282, 1969.

MOSINGER, M. Sur la Pathologie d'origine neuro-splanchnique et solaire dans le cadre de la Pathologie neurogène en général. *Acta Neuroveg.* 16:130-135, 1957.

NASELDOV, G. A. Influence of the sympathetic nerve on the passage of excitation from the motor nerve to muscle. *Sechenov Physiol. J. USSR, Transl.* 46:1462-1471, 1960.

NEDZEL, A. J., and J. BROWN. Effects of body chilling upon the blood vessels of denervated and intact kidneys in dogs and rabbits. *J. Aviat. Med.* 27:236-238, 1956.

NORDENFELT, I., P. OHLIN, and B.C.R. STRÖMBLAD. Effect of denervation on respiratory enzymes in salivary glands. *J. Physiol.* 152:99-107, 1960.

OMER, G. E., and S. R. THOMAS. The management of chronic pain syndromes in the upper extremity. *Clin. Orthoped.* 104:37-45, 1974.

PAOLETTI, R., and R. VERTUA. Drugs affecting the sympathetic regulation of lipid transport. In: *Comparative Neurochemistry, Proc. Fifth Inter. Neurochem. Symp.*, edited by D. Richter. Elmsford, N.Y.: Pergamon, The Macmillan Company, 1964.

PATMAN, D., J. E. THOMPSON, and A. V. PERSSON. Management of post-traumatic syndromes: Report of 113 cases. *Ann. Surg.* 177: 780-787, 1973.

PATTERSON, M. M. A model mechanism for spinal segmental facilitation. *J. Am. Osteop. Assoc.* 76:62-72, 1976.

PORTE, D., Jr. Neural regulation of insulin secretion. *Diabetes* 20 (Suppl.): 340, 1971.

RAAB, W. Neurogenic multifocal destruction of myocardial tissue (pathogenic mechanism and its prevention). *Rev. Canad. Biol.* 22:217-239, 1963.

RALSTON, H. J., and W. J. KERR. Vascular responses of the nasal mucosa to thermal stimuli with some observations on skin temperature. *Am. J. Physiol.* 144:305-310, 1945.

RAMEY, E. R., and M. S. GOLDSTEIN. The adrenal cortex and the sympathetic nervous system. *Physiol. Rev.* 37:155-159, 1957.

REILLY, J., A. COMPAGNON, P. TOURNIER, and H. DUBUIT. L'irritation neurovegetative et son role en pathologie. *Vie Medicale, Transl.* May 19, 1955, pp. 6-12.

RICHARDS, R. L. Causalgia: centennial review. *Arch. Neurol.* 16: 339-350, 1967.

RICHINS, C. A., and K. BRIZZEE. Effect of localized cutaneous stimulation on circulation in duodenal arterioles and capillary beds. *J. Neurophysiol.* 12:131-136, 1949.

ROSELL, S., and E. BELFRAGE. Adrenergic receptors in adipose tissue and their relation to adrenergic innervation. *Nature* 253: 738-739, 1975.

ROSENFELD, R., J. ŠIMÍČEK, and A. ROSENFULDOVÁ. The effect of oestrogens on the weight of innervated and denervated bone in rats. *Physiol. Bohemosl.* 8:30-35, 1959.

ROSS, C. A., and S. A. HERCZEG. Protective effect of ganglionic blocking agents on traumatic shock in the rat. *Proc. Soc. Exptl. Biol. Med.* 91:196-199, 1956.

RUDIN, E. P. The effect of extirpation of stellate ganglia on the development of acute pulmonary edema. *Patolog. Fiziolog. Eksper. Terap. USSR, Transl.* 7:55-58, 1963.

SAMPSON, S. R., and E. MILLS. Effects of sympathetic stimulation on discharges of carotid sinus baroreceptors. *Am. J. Physiol.* 218:1650-1653, 1970.

SATO, A., editor. Symposium: Central organization of the autonomic nervous system. *Brain Res.* 87, special issue, No. 2/3, 1975, 448 pp.

SCHILEW, P. G. Histopathological studies on the sympathetic endings in the superior cervical ganglion and in the thoracic ganglion of the human sympathetic trunk. *Z. Mikroskop. Anat. Forsch* 73:20-31, 1965.

SCHNEYER, C. A. Mitotic activity and cell number of denervated parotid of adult rat. *Proc. Soc. Exptl. Biol. Med.* 142:542-547, 1973.

SCHWARTZ, P. J. Cardiac sympathetic innervation and the sudden
    death syndrome. *Am. J. Med.* 60:167-172, 1976.

SCHWARTZ, P. J., N. E. SNEBOLD, and A. M. BROWN. Effects of uni-
    lateral cardiac sympathetic denervation on the ventricular
    fibrillation threshold. *Am. J. Cardiol.* 37:1034-1040, 1976.

SEXTON, H. D., and D. L. BECKMAN. Neurogenic influence on pulmonary
    surface tension and cholesterol in cats. *Proc. Soc. Exptl.*
    Biol. Med. 148:674-681, 1975.

SHABANAH, E. H., A. TOTH, and G. B. MAUGHAN. The role of the
    autonomic nervous system in uterine contractility and blood
    flow. I. The interaction between neurohormones and sex
    steroids in the intact and isolated uterus. *Am. J. Obstet.*
    Gynec. 89:841-859, 1964.

SHEVCHUK, I. A., L. I. SANDULYAK, and I. M. RYBACHUK. The effect
    of the peripheral region of the sympathetic nervous system on
    the morpho-functional state of the insular apparatus of the
    pancreas. *Byull. Eksp. Biol. Med., Transl.* 70:9-12, 1970.

SKOGLUND, C. R. Influence of noradrenaline on spinal interneuron
    activity. *Acta Physiol. Scand.* 51:142-149, 1961.

SOLLERTINSKAYA, T. N. The effect on the electrical activity of the
    cerebral cortex of removal of the superior sympathetic cervical
    ganglia. *Doklady, Biol. Sci., Transl.* 112:145-147, 1957.

STEIN-WERBLOWSKY, R. The sympathetic nervous system and cancer.
    Exp. Neurol. 42:97-100, 1974.

STERNSCHEIN, M. J., S. J. MYERS, D. B. FREWIN, and J. A. DOWNEY.
    Causalgia. *Arch. Phys. Med. Rehab.* 56:58-63, 1975.

SZENTIVÁNYI, M., and A. JUHÁSZ-NAGY. The physiological role of the
    coronary constrictor fibres. I. The effect of the coronary
    vasomotors on the systemic blood pressure. *Quart. J. Exptl.*
    Physiol. 48:93-104, 1963a.

SZENTIVÁNYI, M., and A. JUHÁSZ-NAGY. The physiological role of the
    coronary constrictor fibres. II. The role of the coronary
    vasomotors in metabolic adaptation of the coronaries. *Quart.*
    J. Exptl. Physiol. 48:105-118, 1963b.

TAY-AN, V. Changes in the electrical activity of the cortex and
    hypothalamus following ablation of the superior and inferior
    cervical sympathetic ganglia in the rabbit. *Sechenov Physiol.*
    J. USSR, Transl. 46:957-965, 1960.

TAY-AN, V., and M. G. GELEKHOVA. The influence of the cervical sympathetic nerve and the effects of some pharmacological substances on the "recruitment reaction". *Sechenov Physiol. J. USSR, Transl.* 47:18-29, 1961.

THEODORE, J., and E. D. ROBIN. Speculations on neurogenic pulmonary edema (NPE). *Am. Rev. Resp. Dis.* 113:405-410, 1976.

THOMAS, P. E., and A. KAWAHATA. Neural factors underlying variations in electrical skin resistance of apparently non-sweating skin. *J. Appl. Physiol.* 17:999-1002, 1962.

THOMAS, P. E., and I. M. KORR. Relationship between sweat gland activity and the electrical resistance of the skin. *J. Appl. Physiol.* 10:505-510, 1957.

THOMAS, P. E., I. M. KORR, and H. M. WRIGHT. A mobile instrument for recording electrical skin resistance patterns of the human trunk. *Acta Neuroveg.* 17:97-106, 1958.

THOMPSON, J. E., R. D. PATMAN, and A. V. PERSSON. Management of post-traumatic pain syndromes (causalgia). *Am. Surg.* 41: 599-602, 1975.

TRAVELL, J., and S. H. RINZLER. Pain syndromes of the chest muscles: resemblance to effort angina and myocardial infarction, and relief by local block. *Can. Med. Assoc. J.* 59:333-338, 1948.

TUCKER, D., and L. M. BEIDLER. Autonomic nervous system influence on olfactory receptors. *J. Neurophysiol.* 18:362, 1955.

VASIL'EV, A. I. The role of the sympathetic nervous system in the functioning of the peripheral end of the auditory analysor. *Z. Ushnykh, Nosovykh, Gorlovykh Boleznei, USSR, Transl.* 22: 9-12, 1962.

VESELKIN, N. P. The effect of unilateral cervical sympathectomy on cerebellar electrical activity in the pigeon. *Doklady, Biol. Sci., Transl.* 124:129-131, 1959.

WALKER, T., and W. E. PEMBLETON. Continuous epidural block in treatment of pancreatitis. *Anesthesiol.* 14:33-37, 1953.

WALLIN, G., W. DELIUS, and K.-E. HAGBARTH. Comparison of sympathetic nerve activity in normotensive and hypertensive subjects. *Circulation Res.* 23:9-21, 1973.

WELLS, H., C. HANDELMAN, and E. MILGRAM. Regulation by sympathetic nervous system of accelerated growth of salivary glands of rats. *Am. J. Physiol.* 201:707-710, 1961.

WOLSTENHOLME, G.E.W., and J. KNIGHT, editors. *The Pineal Gland, Ciba Foundation Symp.* London: Churchill Livingston, 1971.

WRIGHT, H. M., I. M. KORR, and P. E. THOMAS. Regional or segmental variations in vasomotor activity. *Federation Proc.* 12:161, 1953.

WRIGHT, H. M., I. M. KORR, and P. E. THOMAS. Local and regional variations in cutaneous vasomotor tone of the human trunk. *Acta Neuroveg.* 22:33-52, 1960.

WORTMAN, R. J., J. AXELROD, and D. E. KELLY. *The Pineal.* New York: Academic, 1968.

ZAGORUL'KO, T. M. On the influence of the cervical sympathetic nerve and adrenalin on the induced responses of the visual system of the rabbit. *Sechenov Physiol. J. USSR, Transl.* 44:54-64, 1965.

DISCUSSION OF IMPULSE-BASED MECHANISMS

Horace W. Magoun, Chairman

DR. HORACE W. MAGOUN: This period is for summaries, discussion, comments and supplemental information, as you wish, regarding impulse-based mechanisms in relation to manipulative therapy.

DR. P. W. NATHAN: I would like to ask Sir Sydney to explain why he thinks that ischemia causes pain.

DR. SYDNEY SUNDERLAND: I don't think we know how ischemia causes pain. Two hypotheses have been offered. An article in the *Journal of Physiology* some years ago reported that with the onset of anoxia, fibers commence to discharge spontaneously in a manner which suggested that this could be a nocifensor response to the anoxia itself. The other hypothesis, of course, is that since the large-caliber fibers are the more susceptible to anoxia, they are the first to be eliminated, and with the elimination of the large-diameter fibers, their inhibitory influence on small-fiber activity is lost. As a consequence, the gating mechanism in the posterior column is opened, allowing the ascending passage of pain impulses. I think that there are many gaps in this hypothesis.

DR. MAGOUN: Dr. Sunderland, you have provided an explanation for the involvement of the posterior ramus, as a cause of back pain, about which yesterday's morning discussion centered. Would you comment about the possible involvement of the preganglionic outflow of the sympathetic system in the thoracolumbar cord, as the basis for the disorders of visceral function which Dr. Korr and others talked about yesterday afternoon? May I just amplify for a moment. We have heard so far at this meeting the proposed basis for two major foci of emphasis of osteopathic therapy with respect to the spinal nerves and their exit from the vertebral canal. One of these emphases is the back-pain syndrome. The other is, as proposed, those disorders of visceral function which have been given an unusual emphasis so far in the program, and which I think merit all possible further discussion.

269

You have proposed a basis for the involvement of the posterior rami as getting the fine myelinated and unmyelinated fibers involved in the genesis of back pain. What is the analogous basis for the possible involvement of the fine myelinated preganglionic sympathetic fibers, exiting from the thoracolumbar roots, to the postganglionic supply to the viscera from the thorax down into the pelvis? It seems to me that if there is any basis for osteopathic conceptions of the genesis of visceral disorders of the kind that involve everything that has been included in psychosomatic medicine, you need to point to how that can happen from your malaligned vertebrae.

DR. SUNDERLAND: Yes, I think that that is an important point. Let me show again Figure 4 (p. 143) of my paper, where the anterior and posterior nerve roots come together to form the spinal nerve and, initially, the spinal nerve is composed of a single funiculus. Now, the posterior roots are two to three times larger than the ventral so that sensory fibers will predominate in the single funiculus of the spinal nerve. But as regards the ventral roots, remember that between the eighth cervical and the second lumbar and, conceivably, even the third lumbar, the anterior nerve root also contains outgoing preganglionic fibers. These fibers will pass into the spinal nerve, and leave it quite soon to pass to the sympathetic ganglia. So that in the case of the eighth cervical to, say, the second (occasionally the third) lumbar segments, the anterior part of the spinal nerve will have a concentrated component of preganglionic nerve fibers. And therefore, if you are looking at any situation or any pathology which will implicate the spinal nerve itself, then there is quite clearly the possibility of affecting those preganglionic fibers between the eighth cervical and the second lumbar.

There are no preganglionics in the fourth and fifth lumbars and first sacral. When you get down to the second, third and fourth sacrals, of course, you are dealing with the parasympathetic outflow into the pelvis. And the fourth and fifth lumbar and the first sacral nerve roots are often the ones involved in intervertebral disc prolapses. But when you get up into the cervical region, there is a heavy concentration of preganglionic fibers in the eighth cervical and the first thoracic, which are going to pass out into the lower trunk of the brachial plexus. And this is evidenced if you are dealing with a severe trophic disturbance in this region. Remember, I did indicate in my paper that the eighth cervical and first thoracic nerves have no particular attachment to a transverse process. They unite to form the lower trunk, and therefore, in severe traction injuries of the upper extremity, particularly if the arm is drawn violently upward, the eighth cervical and the first thoracic nerve roots are not torn, but are avulsed from the spinal cord. And of course, evidence of that type of avulsion is the appearance of Horner's syndrome, an indication of complete sympathetic denervation of the head and neck on that side. This illustrates that the preganglionics are an important component of the ventral nerve roots; they are still concentrated in the spinal nerve at the foramen and just beyond it, but soon after they leave to pass to the ganglionated sympathetic trunk.

DR. MAGOUN: Your response to my question provides a focus for its further discussion. I simply wanted to get the two components of the spinal nerves around which most of this Conference discussion is centered; namely, the pain fibers in the dorsal root and the preganglionic sympathetic fibers in the ventral root. And I thank you very much for making this so beautifully clear.

DR. IRVIN M. KORR: I think you'll find in osteopathic and chiropractic literature, repeated references to the sinu-vertebral or recurrent meningeal nerve--sometimes called Luschka's nerve. Would you comment on that and its possible involvement in pathological situations?

DR. SUNDERLAND: Yes, this is really the first branch of the system, and it appears to be distributed entirely anteriorly. It certainly innervates the dura and the posterior longitudinal ligament; there is some debate as to whether or not it actually innervates the disc tissue itself. The interesting thing is that it appears to be, as I have just mentioned, confined to an anterior distribution, because posteriorly the dura appears to be insensitive, as illustrated in a lumbar puncture. Penetration of the posterior dura is painless.

Now, the question is whether the pathology in this region could be responsible for affecting the sinu-vertebral nerve and whether that could be the genesis of the pain. You don't need many fibers to fire to give you intense pain. The sinu-vertebral nerve can be demonstrated microscopically and dissected. I have never counted the fibers in it, but it is obviously a nerve of some substance. In its immediate proximity to the posterior longitudinal ligament and to the annulus fibrosis of the disc--it passes into the tissue in this region--it would be the first structure to suffer in disc herniation. One might ask, would not this be the factor responsible for the pain?

I think the point is that you do get pathology in this region, as in spondylosis. But where the lesion has obviously been there a long time, and the lesion is a painless one, it will very often show up at the periphery as loss of sensory acuity and weakening of muscles; in other words, as failing conduction. I don't think that one can be absolutely convincing on that point.

DR. RONALD GITELMAN: I just want to point out the remoteness of the possibility of compression syndromes occurring in the dorsal spine, because of the limitation of mobility in that region due to the thoracic cage.

DR. SUNDERLAND: In this region, then, one gives up the idea now of nerve root compression and speaks rather in terms of nerve root dysfunction.

DR. SCOTT HALDEMAN: Dr. Sunderland, you mentioned that in your opinion the primary factor in conduction block caused by compression was ischemia. I would like you to comment on the work of Seth Sharpless at the University of Colorado-Boulder, who has found that small amounts of pressure (in the neighborhood of 5 to 10 mm Hg) directly on the root are capable of causing significant conduction block. He has stated that this is insufficient to cause ischemia and has, therefore, felt it necessary to postulate a mechanical factor in the conduction block.

DR. SUNDERLAND: Yes, I didn't want to create the impression that all compression lesions are due to ischemic anoxia. I did want to emphasize that with slowly developing compression, the more chronic lesion, ischemia, is unquestionably a factor. I am equally convinced that with very rapid deformation such as with a cuff or an ill-fitting plaster across the lateral popliteal nerve, that it's not an ischemic lesion. First, the blood is squeezed out of the area, this then is ultimately converted into a physical deformation of the fibers. This was beautifully shown by the group at Queen Square in London, where they demonstrated that rapid and high-level deformation produced an intussusception at the node-- actually at each of the margins of the compression. One node was intussuscepted into another and there is no doubt about the deformation which occurs. Under those circumstances, of course, it then takes considerable time after the mechanical force is removed for recovery to occur, because a structural defect in the nerve fiber must be corrected.

There is no doubt that there are conditions and circumstances under which mechanical deformation will give rise to a conduction block. But there is also the type of lesion, and I think it's the more slowly developing lesion, where the vascular factor becomes important. In the carpal tunnel syndrome, incidentally, the vascular factor is operating only initially. If you follow it through to its conclusion you finish up with a segment of nerve which contains no nerve fibers at all--only fibrous tissue. Fibrous tissue has replaced all elements in the nerve fibers. That is because of the edema and proliferation of fibroblasts; also involved are the breakdown of the various membranes protecting the nerve fiber, Wallerian degeneration, and finally, the loss even of Schwann cells. The process culminates in relatively avascular fibrous tissues.

DR. HALDEMAN: It's not quite the point I was asking. In Sharpless' experiments, they used very light pressures acutely, only 5 to 10 mm Hg, not like a cuff or a traumatic type of compression. And whereas in the peripheral nerves, one requires 200 mm Hg usually to cause a conduction block, they found these light pressures on the root could cause a significant block. And there was no obvious interruption of blood flow or blood supply in that area.

DR. SUNDERLAND: Well, they would have to prove that convincingly, but there is another point here and that is, as I mentioned, that the fibers in the nerve roots have really no significant connective-tissue protection. Each fiber has only a light endoneurial sheath and the bundles are loosely held together. Also, it has been shown that the endoneurium of the posterior root fibers is much finer than the endoneurium of peripheral nerve fibers; that the collagen fibrils which are the basic component of the endoneurium were much finer in the case of nerve roots than in the case of peripheral nerves. So one would expect the nerve root to fail much earlier than the peripheral nerve.

DR. ALFRED BUERGER: Would you comment on a recently published study from the Neurosurgery Service at the University of California-San Francisco? It was one of the few recent double-blind studies that I know of done in neurosurgery. They made purely muscular lesions in the back without, as they showed, damaging the medial branch of dorsal ramus. They were working on patients who had pain radiating down the leg in all cases, and foot-drops in some. All appraisals were done by a surgeon who did not know the nature of the operation that had been performed on that individual patient. Nevertheless, they found a statistically significant tendency for these patients to show decreased pain radiation and, in at least one case, the loss of foot drop--although, at least in their opinion, there had been no neural intervention.

Tentatively, they ascribe their findings to some kind of reflex phenomenon involving both the paraspinal musculature and the muscles of the leg innervated by the same spinal segment. This is analogous to the kinds of effects obtained when hypertonic saline is injected into the paravertebral muscles, producing pain that radiates down the leg in a nondermatomal pattern.

DR. SUNDERLAND: Were they then attributing this to a peripheral factor rather than a central one?

DR. BUERGER: They feel that it is absolutely a reflex phenomenon, but it follows the reflex distribution of the kind found by Lewis and Kellgren, as opposed to the dermatomal distribution.

DR. SUNDERLAND: Where were they placing the lesion?

DR. BUERGER: In the muscle . . .

DR. SUNDERLAND: In the muscle, just posteriorly. Yes, and
the assumption is that what changes had taken place in the muscles
did not have a neurogenic basis; that it would be primarily a muscular lesion, a myogenic lesion.

DR. BUERGER: Yes, their opinion that they did not reach the
branch of the medial nerve is based on cadaver experiments and
radiographic analysis of the surgery while it was in process.

DR. SUNDERLAND: Yes, I think it would be difficult under those
circumstances to exclude a possible implication of the posterior
primary ramus. As you know, an operation has been designed to
divide the posterior primary ramus where it is on the transverse
process. There is a tissue plane that goes down the back between
the multifidus muscle system medially, in the longissimus system
laterally. It is quite a clear one and it takes you down to the
transverse process and it takes you to the exact point where that
posterior primary ramus is dividing into its lateral and medial
divisions. Indeed, there is a neurosurgeon in Australia who has
made a fortune in a few years by occasionally relieving back pain
in his consulting rooms with a well-placed stab wound in the back.
It is suspected that what he is in fact doing is dividing, just by
chance, the posterior primary ramus, and is denervating the epiphyseal joint system and the muscles in that region. Now, of
course, as you say, this could be a myogenic lesion, because if
the pathway over which the reflexes are going to be served is
divided, well, then, it would presumably have the same effect.

DR. BUERGER: Yes, I think that is the point: When the surgeons looked at the tissue they were cutting they found that they
were not reaching the nerve, but were cutting only muscle.

DR. SUNDERLAND: Yes, whether the surgical trauma is acting
in the form of a counterirritant, it's difficult to say. These
findings are open to many interpretations. Although this shifting
of attention away from the intervertebral foramen to the back,
toward the epiphyseal joint and the muscles which are innervated
by those nerves is interesting, we've still got to think in terms
of the spinal nerve in the intervertebral foramen, because there
are lesions that do develop in these regions which affect the spinal
nerve, and which produce the characteristic symptomatology seen, for
example, in the field of the sciatic nerve, or of the affected root.

DR. KAREL LEWIT: Yesterday, we were quite satisfied that most
back pain is not due to nerve compression. Now, we have returned

to nerve compression in the form of the posterior medial rami. In this Conference, we have to deal with the mechanisms of manipulative therapy. What we know is that in the conditions where we give treatment, we find, say, in the lumbar spine, that there is a loss of mobility, and if we achieve normal mobility, then pain, if this is the cause, subsides. The nerve plays the role only of the cable which brings the information from the receptor. It is not the cause of the pain. Otherwise, as I pointed out in my paper, what would be the use of the nervous system if it signaled pain only when it has become the object of the lesion. I think even here there is no exception. The posterior ramus conveys information that there is something wrong in the tissues, and if function--and that's the most important thing--in the tissue normalizes, then they have nothing to signal. While I do not believe that an entrapment syndrome is involved here, it should be said again that entrapment, if it exists, does not give pain primarily, but dysesthesia. If there is an entrapment syndrome of the carpal tunnel, then neurological examination reveals dysesthesia and discomfort, but not real pain. And in my opinion, these neurosurgeons did with a knife the same thing that Janet Travell--and I do it very largely too--did with a needle. Inserted at the most painful place, it seems to act as a counterirritant by irritation of the receptors.

DR. SUNDERLAND: Well, my initial comment would be that patients in Czechoslovakia must differ significantly from patients in Australia, because with their carpal tunnel syndrome, the presenting symptom of Australian patients is pain. It's only as the lesion develops that the median area becomes numb. But there is no doubt that what worries the patient is pain. And he or she will tell you that at around two o'clock in the morning they are suddenly awakened with an incapacitating pain in the median field. And what do they do to relieve it? They get up and walk around the room. One interpretation is that movement relieves the venous congestion that has developed as a result of the immobility of the limb during sleep. Now, Dr. Lewit would seem to place the initial disturbance out at the periphery in terms of the receptors, and say that there is no involvement of the nerve. Well, that may be the case, but I doubt very much if that could be responsible for the majority of cases in which we know there is a lesion in the nerve.

Now, I suppose this takes us back again to another physiological phenomenon investigated in great detail, and beautifully, by Adrian in the 1930's of the after-discharges, the injury discharges, which follow injury to the nerve. That work has been repeated more recently by Wall and others, who showed that if the lesion is complete, you get these injury discharges for only a short time after the injury occurs. You can prolong them by dehydrating the nerve, and treating it in other ways. But they maintain that the only occasion when injury discharges can continue is when other nerve

fibers in the vicinity are in continuity with the receptors, or
even the injured nerve fiber is still in anatomical continuity with
the receptor in the periphery. But they clearly demonstrate that
you must have a lesion of the nerve to have the receptor producing
the effects centrally which it does in those cases.

DR. JOHN J. COOTE: I don't know how relevant it is, but Sir
Sydney mentioned this possibility of atrophy of muscle, and I just
remembered some work in the early 1960's showing that in atrophied
muscles the input from small sensory fibers increases considerably.
So, you know, this is another contributing factor, although one
can't see how you could relieve this by some manipulation, in the
short term, anyway.

DR. ROBERT E. KAPPLER: In keeping with the purposes of the
Conference, I would like to review some of the axioms that the
clinicians of various disciplines seemed to agree on yesterday.
The first is, that pain in itself is not an indication for manipulative treatment. Restriction of joint motion is. Pain may well
be associated with restricted motion. Joints which are unstable,
hypermobile, traumatized, are painful joints; direct manipulation
of these joints is generally contraindicated. Manipulation of adjacent areas of restriction may be indicated. Manipulative treatment does not, per se, treat diseases. We treat patients who have
problems as identified in the physical examination; the problems
include restriction of joint motion. How joint motion is related
to the patient's overall problems remains a matter for speculation.

The effects of joint manipulation are related to the skills of
the operator: skills, first, in the diagnosis and assessment of
the joint motion, then in overcoming the restrictions, and in avoiding side effects which may be produced by the manipulative procedure.
Side effects are a matter of concern when unskilled operators use
excessive force. Compression of nerves, we agreed, is a relatively
rare phenomenon as it relates to manipulative treatment. Compression
of nerves does exist. We have discussed this and how nerves may be
affected by traction, entrapment, ischemia, friction fibrosis, trauma
and so forth.

There is another area in question which I would like to see
this Conference discuss, and that falls outside of the realm of back
pain. Dr. Greenman identified in his paper the prognostic implications of the physical examination identifying tissue texture change.
This tissue texture change involves all layers, not just muscle.
It involves skin and subcutaneous tissue. He feels, as I do, that
irrespective of whether manipulative treatment is used, these palpable findings reflect what is going on within that patient physiologically. This has great implications for me, as a clinician,
because I use it. I apologize perhaps for anecdotal reporting and

inadequate hypothesis testing, but this is the kind of thing that is a very real part of my assessment of a patient's condition. Dr. Greenman reported the same thing. I have to speculate that there are changes within the autonomic nervous system which may be responsible for mediating some of these tissue texture changes. I would like to hear some speculation or questions as to how joint restriction, which is also an identifiable part of the physical examination, relates to the patient's problem, perhaps through autonomic dysfunctions.

DR. MAGOUN: Dr. Korr, did you have a comment?

DR. KORR: I am in complete accord with Dr. Kappler's remarks. This morning's emphasis on nerve entrapment has been valuable, but at the cost of the much more common--and, I think, more manipulable --problems of disturbed afferent input and its reflex manifestations, including the autonomic.

DR. PHILIP E. GREENMAN: I would like to ask Dr. Coote a question, similar to one asked of Dr. Sunderland by Dr. Magoun, because I was fascinated by Dr. Coote's conceptualizations of the summation effects through the sympathetic fibers. Is it a reasonable hypothesis that the somatic dysfunctions Dr. Kappler just mentioned could impact the ventral root and its contained preganglionic fibers, with the summating effect that Dr. Coote described? Those are the kinds of things that we seem to observe in the clinical realm. Wherein does this somatosympathetic linkage occur, and what is the basis for it?

DR. COOTE: All that one can say is that if there is damage to the sympathetic motor supply to an organ, then of course, there is going to be some dysfunction as far as the sympathetic system is concerned. And you may, as a consequence, get altered sensory input to the nervous system from the viscera.

I would like to emphasize that if you record from sympathetic neurons, about 40% of them are quite silent--they're doing nothing. The other 60% show various sorts of activity. But if you try to activate them reflexly through the segmental nerves, either visceral or somatic, only about 20 to 25% of all the sampled preganglionics can be reflexly activated. That has been consistent over a period of years. Yet intracellular recording shows that they are all receiving an input, because you can show the EPSP's, which is what I tried to show yesterday.

Now, the point that this must bring home to us is that the input to the preganglionic sympathetic neurons is just providing a background level of excitation with which other inputs may summate. Let's conceptualize the situation just at the segmental

level, omitting, for the sake of simplicity, the descending inputs.
Imagine the sympathetic preganglionic neuron on which converge two
inputs, neither of which is sufficient to discharge it: a somatic
segmental input with a slow discharge rate, and a visceral input,
also with a low activity which is out of phase with the somatic.
The likelihood of summation under these conditions is very low indeed. But we could increase the input in the visceral afferent so
that there is the possibility of synchronization with the somatic
input, and then we may get a summation. Now this could be happening at several segmental levels and might be a consequence of a
change in either the somatic or the visceral input.

DR. GREENMAN: Clinically, the somatic things that we treat
by restoration of function might well be reduction in the amount
of somatic input into that preganglionic neuron, thus reducing the
possibilities of the summative effect from viscera.

DR. COOTE: That's right. But I think one has to be careful
that there may even be altered activity as a consequence of damage
to the visceral structure, which is not going to be changed by
this procedure. You may change the output from the sympathetic
preganglionic neuron as a consequence of decreasing somatic input,
but you may not, thereby, necessarily alter the dysfunction in the
visceral organ, because then there may be some local factor involved, rather than being due to an exaggerated outflow in the
sympathetic innervation of that structure.

DR. GREENMAN: Then how does the pathology in that viscus
occur in the first place, that starts the visceral input into that
system? Can these clinically observable somatic changes contribute
to the vicious cycle that sustains the output to the viscus and, in
turn, its input?

DR. COOTE: That's fine, yes.

DR. HARRY GRUNDFEST: I'd like to pursue further the question
raised by Dr. Magoun: Where is the beginning of all of this? Are
the preganglionic sympathetics being irritated, and setting up
changes in the viscera, that now cause a feedback from them? Is
this the point that Dr. Magoun was questioning?

DR. MAGOUN: I think we both want to ask you, Dr. Coote, if
you have explored experimentally the degree to which somatic or
visceral afferent stimulation is able to set up continuing activity
in preganglionic sympathetic neurons. You have diagrammed exactly
what we are talking about here; could you tell us more about what
your experimental findings were?

DR. COOTE: We have done no experiment to see whether changes
occur in an organ as a consequence of altering the somatic input.
That would directly answer your question. The question that I have
been involved in, and referred to in Dr. Korr's paper, is the question of hypertension, and the possibility that there is an increased sympathetic activity in certain types of hypertension. We
have to be careful about the sort of hypertension we are dealing
with, and make a critical appraisal of the numerous papers on the
subject, because some of the data are questionable. Nonetheless,
I think there is evidence of an increased sympathetic activity to
vascular beds in certain types of hypertension. In our own studies
on the spontaneously hypertensive rat, we find increased sympathetic
outflow to the kidney.

Now, the problem is, why does that increase occur? And this
relates particularly to your question. In such animals it seems
to be a genetic factor and there is possibly some change in the
central nervous system. Other investigators have reported the development of hypertension in experimental animals--monkeys--with
inputs from the periphery, such as sporadic painful stimuli. But,
other than that, all that has been done is to stimulate a somatic
nerve and look at the effect on an organ, shall we say the muscle
vascular beds, and it is demonstrated that sustained vasoconstriction can be produced by prolonged stimulation. Intense stimulation
of a somatic nerve with reflexly produced increase in the sympathetic outflow to the kidney may decrease the blood flow dramatically, almost to zero. It holds there for a while, but it then
begins gradually and slowly to come back.

DR. MAGOUN: Would that be analogous to a manipulation treat-
ment--or something more intense?

DR. COOTE: I think it would be something more intense.

DR. MAGOUN: I see. Did any of your experiments involve
somatic stimulation comparable or analogous to manipulative
therapy?

DR. COOTE: No, because I knew little about manipulative
therapy when I did the experiments.

DR. KORR: But, John, I know that you have stimulated the
muscle and joint receptors and studied sympathetic responses.
Could you tell us about that? I think that is what we are looking
for here.

DR. COOTE: When muscles are caused to contract isometrically,
by stimulating the ventral roots, one can show an increase in activity in the small afferent fiber population coming from the

muscle, and that these reflexly produce an increase in blood pressure, heart rate and respiration. The stimulus to those receptors is probably a metabolite produced during isometric contraction. So, I suppose one might imagine that sustained contraction is comparable to that in patients, reported by Dr. Greenman and our other clinical colleagues. You do see muscles in spasm in some patients, is that not right? In such circumstances, one might expect the input from those muscles to the central nervous system to increase, and that it would be in these small fibers.

Now, as to stimulation of joint receptors: The brain of the cat is sectioned at an appropriate level, and, with the cat on its back, the legs are then affixed to a bicycle-like device. The muscles are denervated while leaving innervation to the joints intact. The legs are then passively moved, while the cardiovascular and respiratory responses to input from the joints are studied. One can show that those responses are abolished by cutting the nerves to the joints.

Most studies of sensory reporting on joint motion and position have been done on the large-fiber population from the joint, because they are easiest to work from, and because these are the ones thought to be conveying proprioceptive signals from the joints. In our studies on the autonomic responses, however, we found that it is the small-fiber population only that seems to be involved. These small fibers, myelinated and unmyelinated, had not previously been implicated in reporting of the joint angles. So again, we come back to this finding, that it is only small myelinated and unmyelinated afferents that make the sorts of connections in the cord that can influence sympathetic preganglionic neurons.

DR. KIYOMI KOIZUMI: Our purpose is to try to understand what manipulative therapy does to the somatoautonomic reflexes, ordinarily responding to normal inputs. Now, we have evidence that somatic input as well as visceral input produces reflexes in the autonomic system as well as in the somatic system, in the physiological range. In the abnormal situation, with abnormal input, we produce the abnormally strong flexor reflex; in the autonomic system, we produce the changes in cardiac rate, vasoconstriction, changes in gastrointestinal movement and so on. This may produce a vicious cycle of autonomic and somatic reflexes and their manifestations. Perhaps manipulative therapy can break this vicious cycle, and then start to change the abnormal reflex manifestation or gradually change it to normal. But I think we should not forget that there may be an effect on the trophic action of the nerve, to be discussed later.

Another factor may be hormonal responses to stressful stimuli involving, for example, the familiar defense response which releases hormones from the hypothalamus to the pituitary gland. But if the stimuli last too long it would be harmful for the body. So that there may be painful factors or humoral factors for us to consider in relation to long-term changes.

DR. GREENMAN: I would like to ask Dr. Coote another question. In some of the old osteopathic literature and among the older osteopathic practitioners, there are reports, with respect to manipulation, of stimulating treatment and of inhibiting treatment. Would you comment on inhibition of sympathetic preganglionic neurons by somatic stimulation, perhaps through a long pathway involving descending inhibitory neurons?

DR. COOTE: Well, one of the things that has puzzled a lot of people in the last fifteen years is that if you stimulated a somatic nerve electrically (admittedly, a very artificial way of doing things), you would see first of all an excitatory response in the sympathetic preganglionic neuron outflow, and then a period of inhibition. Recent evidence, from intracellular recording, has shown that what you are doing is stimulating a particular group of afferent fibers that produce pure inhibitory effects on the sympathetic neurons. Furthermore, it looks very much as though the profound inhibition resulting from stimulating the somatic afferent nerve is due to a long-circuited reflex, involving a pathway ascending to the brainstem, and a descending pathway in the ventral part of the lateral funiculus. Hence, it's possible that there may be some sort of therapy which will stimulate only those sorts of receptors. The problem, for those of us who are basic scientists, is first to find out what is the meaning in normal physiology of that inhibitory input, which is quite difficult.

DR. MAGOUN: Are the descending inhibitory and excitatory pathways in any way related to the depressor and pressor centers of the vasomotor system? May I comment also that in the autonomic nervous system you have not only the Sherringtonian spinal mechanism of inhibition of an excitatory component in the spinal cord, but additionally, you have a reciprocal innervation directly to the peripheral visceral organ. Hence, you have a double way of reducing input to the visceral structures. Do you want to comment on this in relation to your own work?

DR. COOTE: In my opinion, the concept of pressor and depressor vasomotor centers is much in question, and further discussion would be a digression from the theme of this workshop. As to your other comment, perhaps I should have mentioned that the somatic input which can inhibit sympathetic preganglionic neurons through this descending pathway, may also affect the effector organ by influencing the parasympathetic outflow as well. That is certainly a possibility, yes.

DR. HALDEMAN: Dr. Coote, there was a recent report that
ablation of the area of the inferior olive selectively eliminated
the inhibitory component of the somatovisceral reflex, and that
ablation of a small area in the floor of the fourth ventricle, I
think, selectively eliminated the excitatory components. The suggestion was that the inhibitory and excitatory effect of the somatovisceral reflex was in effect mediated or determined by brainstem
factors, rather than a direct spinal inhibitory or excitatory
reflex.

The question I would like you to address follows on Dr. Greenman's. Are there specific excitatory and inhibitory inflows, or is
it simply that the sympathetic comes in and is modified, the output
being excitatory or inhibitory depending on what else is happening
in the nervous system?

DR. COOTE: I think simply one could say that an input into a
segment of the spinal cord can excite sympathetic neurons at that
segment, that they are functionally distinct in that they may be
destined for a particular effector organ. The one in which the
"synaptic potency" is most powerful is the sympathetic group of
neurons going out to the gastrointestinal tract, as Dr. Koizumi
showed in her presentation, which are part of a reflex pathway involving the G.I. tract. In my review, I talked about this as
being, apparently, a segmental reflex.

Now, as far as the pressor responses are concerned, then it
seems that this segmental pathway cannot be utilized. It is present, but inhibited by the descending system. This is where the
significance of these descending systems comes in and they, of
course, are activated by specific ascending limbs of the long
reflex pathway. You can get a small amount of inhibition at the
segmental level through some interneurons in the cord, but only in
specific reflexes related to particular organs. It seems that for
long-circuit inhibition, the profound inhibition that I was just
talking about, you need again to activate some region that
Dr. Magoun likes to call the depressor region of the brainstem.

According to the conceptualization that I presented regarding
the excitatory states of preganglionic neurons, the input from the
segmental level is going to be interacting with the descending inputs, which will be inhibiting and exciting neurons in the way that
I have described. But the excitatory pathway will also be contributing to the possibility of getting synchronization in the sympathetic neuron. I have tried to simplify the situation schemati-
cally, but there are all these other factors. The sympathetic
preganglionic neuron is an integrative neuron. There is fractiona-
tion of the inputs coming to it and it is interaction of the
effects of those inputs in the neuron that determines the output
of the neuron.

DR. MICHAEL M. PATTERSON: My question is in regard to the
vicious cycle, mentioned by Dr. Koizumi and frequently occurring
in the osteopathic literature.   In the vicious cycle of feedback,
the spinal cord, of course, is acting as a transmitter, both from
somatic to visceral and visceral to somatic structures and reflex
pathways.   But it seems to me that the cord may also act in an
active role, sometimes protecting against the vicious cycle and
sometimes contributing to it in terms of plasticity in the reflex
pathways, by sensitization and habituation processes--and possibly,
long-term changes analogous to conditioning.

We know that this occurs probably at the synaptic level in
invertebrates, and in vertebrates, most likely in the spinal cord,
where it is an interneuron phenomenon.   One of your diagrams
seemed to have a component of habituation in it, in terms of blood
pressure effects.   There is a strong possibility then, it seems to
me, that habituation would act against the occurrence of a vicious
cycle, but if certain types or strengths of inputs occurred, the
opposite, sensitization, may take place.   I was wondering if you
have seen evidence for a sensitization process in somatovisceral
reflex pathways?

DR. COOTE: Of course, it's always difficult to equate responses that one describes as sensitization or habituation with
the neurophysiological responses that we see when we are looking
at single units.   I don't know if one can say that the facilitation
one observes, for example, might be equivalent to some form of
sensitization, but it's a possibility.   There is bound to be some
sort of increased possibility of summation as a consequence of
sensitization.   But experimentally you could see this only as
facilitation.   It is interesting that the really marked facilitation comes on only when you knock out the descending inhibitory
pathways, leaving the descending excitatory pathways active, and
then you can produce a response with a segmental input which previously had no effect at all.   Now it produces a really marked
response, recruiting lots of neurons, with repetitive stimulation.
Whether that is related to sensitization, I don't know.

Just one final point: The observation about the blood flow
to the kidney that I mentioned is not really an habituation.   What
we are seeing there is a local autoregulation of the blood vessels
themselves, which is actually contributing to this decrement   of
the response, and this is something else that one has to be careful
of in evaluating data.

DR. LYNNE C. WEAVER: I would like to make a comment that I
think also bears on this.   We have talked about the various overlapping inputs to a given preganglionic motor neuron, some excitatory, some inhibitory.   Something that can be seen often in the

literature is the fact that some of these inputs may be relatively quiescent most of the time, and others relatively active. However, when one eliminates one of these inputs, for example, an inhibitory input, from the carotid sinus sensors, there is temporarily an increased rate of discharge of preganglionic neuron. But this is only an acute effect. There is not yet good evidence that there is a long-term hyperexcitability of the sympathetic nerves after carotid sinus denervation; the resulting hypertension is only temporary. As a matter of fact, after such a procedure, other inhibitory inputs, those from the vagal afferents, for example, begin to have a greater influence. So perhaps a secondary or an additional system now has a greater influence, after one input has been removed.

Therefore, one has to question the potential influence of alteration of one input to this complex system, because it is likely that through plasticity--if I can use that word--the final output of the sympathetic nervous system might not be altered on a long-term basis.

DR. KOIZUMI: I don't know if my comment is related to habituation or sensitization, but in the somatosympathetic reflex pathway, it's very easy to get the facilitation due to repetitive stimulation; it's called posttetanic potentiation. In this reflex path, the potentiation can occur much more easily that in the normal somatic motor pathways.

I would like to comment further on the spinal reflex that I mentioned yesterday. I don't want to give you the impression that the spinal reflex involving the small intestine is inhibitory; it is excitatory to the sympathetic system, but the sympathetic outflow to the small intestine is inhibitory to its motility. Hence, the spinal reflex as far as my work is concerned is always excitatory. However, when the higher centers are involved, whether in G.I. reflexes or in cardiac reflexes, such as those from atrial stretch receptors, then their influence on the sympathetic neurons may be either excitatory or inhibitory.

DR. COOTE: I think we have to be very careful not to confuse people. You're giving your own results, while I am trying to give a critical appraisal of all results. There are some very good experiments, by Malliani and his group, which show in the spinal animal that you can get inhibition, with natural stimulation of receptors, in the cardiac field. But the point is that this inhibition, as far as the neurons are concerned, is the short-lasting type. When you bring in the brainstem, then you get this long-lasting, powerful effect. And I think that the important thing to get home to you all is the principle of the system, the organization of the system.

DR. GRUNDFEST: There seems to be a confusion about which is
the horse and which is the cart in this discussion.   If Dr. Korr's
thesis is valid, that manipulation relieves certain kinds of abnormal somatovisceral entities, then the horse must be the injury
or the activity of the efferent preganglionic sympathetics.   Otherwise, there would be no effective manipulative therapy.   And then,
the afferent part of the cycle must be the cart.   I've gotten the
impression that emphasis has been given to the afferent part, as
the first cause in this little system.

DR. COOTE: I take your point, but if you get damage to
muscles, you get an increased activity in small afferent fibers.
Therefore, there is the possibility that you will get an increased
outflow over the sympathetic preganglionic neurons to certain
effector organs.   And this in itself may be damaging in the long
term; if you are getting, say, ischemia of an organ, it may well
be damaging to its function.

DR. MAGOUN: Thank you very much, Dr. Coote.   Dr. Korr, in the
remaining discussion time, or part of it, would you like to comment
on the relevance of this discussion to your proposals?

DR. KORR: Only to say that the reports and the comments of
Dr. Coote and Dr. Koizumi clearly reinforce the central hypothesis
proposed in my paper: it is evident (1) that mechanisms and pathways exist by which certain patterns of somatic afferent input may
initiate aberrations in sympathetic output; and (2) that the resulting feedback from affected visceral structures may contribute
to the establishment of self-sustaining cycles of impulses, through
the spinal cord, between soma and viscus.

DR. GRUNDFEST: I would like to comment on the causalgic syndromes that both Dr. Appenzeller and Dr. Korr talked about.   The
general impression was left that it is due to, or involves, a disturbance of the autonomic system.   There seems to be an entity
like causalgia, in which the autonomic system is not involved.   If
one transsects a nerve (either a purely sensory nerve or a mixed
nerve), one gets a warm limb, a vasodilatation, for about two or
three weeks; and then, as the vessels constrict, the hand becomes
cold.   As long as there is no innervation or re-innervation, there
is no pain.   Once innervation occurs, you get the extreme causalgia
with all of its nasty symptomatology.   It seems to me that that
kind of causalgia implicates some effects on the vascular system,
and perhaps is due to the dorsal root vasodilators.   I was wondering whether there is any evidence for this.

DR. OTTO APPENZELLER: I think there has been a great deal of
confusion about what is called causalgia, and therefore, also a
great deal of controversy on how to treat causalgia.   I think

we have to stick with the definition as proposed by Dr. White in his book on pain: a diffused, nondermatomal pain following a nerve injury and associated with excessive autonomic discharge. This type of causalgia is the one that is treatable by sympathectomy. There are numerous other pain syndromes and some vascular symptoms such as you have mentioned, but they are not causalgia and do not respond to sympathectomy. If there is no excessive sympathetic discharge, they do not respond; if the pain is confined to a single dermatome, sympathectomy is not indicated. The type of disorder that you refer to would not ordinarily be classed as a causalgic syndrome, and may have the pathogenesis that you suggested. It is not one that would be treated by sympathectomy.

DR. GRUNDFEST: But these denervation syndromes do resemble causalgia in that they are extremely painful and have all the signs of causalgia and the extreme sensitivity to mechanical and thermal stimuli. They are really some of the most disturbing features of denervation injuries.

DR. APPENZELLER; May I offer something in quite another area? As an allopathic physician and neurologist, I often have great difficulty in recognizing what is meant by osteopathic physicians when they talk about texture and temperature of the skin, which are difficult to recognize for anyone not skilled in these things. But there are natural experiments which give us some idea that this must have something to do with the autonomic nervous system. Here (projected on screen) is the face of a patient with lepromatous leprosy. And I'd like to draw your attention to the distribution of the lesions in the ears, eyebrows, and here across the cheek. And you will see in the accompanying thermogram of this same patient's face these areas are the coldest in this person's face. And this is the distribution in which the Hansen's bacillus actually thrives. The bacillus does the same texture experiment, I suppose, as the osteopathic physician does, and selects the areas that are most useful for its multiplication--the cold areas of the face. In short, the temperature of the skin which is controlled by the autonomic nervous system determines the distribution of the lepromatous lesions in this individual's face.

DR. GEORGE W. NORTHRUP: I am what has been loosely referred to as one of Dr. Greenman's older colleagues. My perspective, of course, is simply one of clinical observation over a period of some 35 years. And I realize that clinical observation is no substitute for research evaluation and study, but also, on the other hand, I don't believe it's necessarily a lost or false art. From a practicing physician's standpoint, when we refer to manipulation, what we are primarily talking about is joint mobilization--restoration of intersegmental joint motion. In the "passive" movement of synovial joints, as a mobilatory procedure, clinical observations

indicate that the apophyseal joint of the posterior spinal joint is
where the action is.

The question that has always intrigued me as a clinician, is
to discover the origin and nature of the immobilization that
we can detect in a palpatory way. We have seen cineradiography of
the cervical spine showing restriction of motion, and restoration
of motion following joint mobilization by manipulation. But this
still does not satisfy the basic question which seems to be <u>why</u> the
joint lock (or whatever you want to call it). Within the normal
range of joint motion, of course, as you all know, it's not "a
joint out of place". Our observations indicate that something
happens within the range of the physiological motion of that joint,
but we don't know what. It also occurred to me that maybe there is
something within this joint-lock mechanism that holds a key to the
manner in which some of the associated symptoms are manifest.

One clinical problem that I am interested in is the mimicking
of visceral diseases by what are essentially musculoskeletal
lesions--I am interested in what happens in the thoracic column
that will mimic chest disease. This, too, comes back to the same
question: what is this mechanism and does it possibly have something to do with this joint-lock mechanism? What is it? Why is
it? One possibility, of course, is to look at the joint itself.

Dr. Haldeman warned us, particularly us clinicians, not to
grab pieces of research here and there and embrace them to support
our own fantasies. And perhaps we have done this--but to my mind,
basic research, in a certain measure, is sort of a "to-whom-it-
may-concern", and if it does seem relevant, I think that at least
we should look at it and start to think. From taking several
thousand case histories and doing what I consider to be an adequate physical examination, we have made some conclusions. The
first thing is that we believe from our observations that where
the joint lock occurs, there has been, first, joint compression.
And we believe that there may be something within the hydrodynamics
of the synovial fluid that is worth close study. As many of you
know, the so-called joint click has been investigated and marked
changes in the synovial fluid are indicated.

Another feature worth looking into: Dr. Greenman has discussed the importance of symmetry and asymmetry, and it is interesting that so many of the patients who come in and complain
of "joint lock" in the back, do so on a basis of eccentric motion.
In one way or another, the patient says, "I tied my shoelace, or I
picked up a pin, and I couldn't straighten up." If you examine
several hundred of these, you'll find that rarely do they get
"caught" going down. It's almost always on the way back. And
rarely--unless the person is trying to lift a very heavy weight,

do you find them going straight down and lifting straight up. What they do is bend forward, rotate, go off to one side and then, as in pulling on a stuck drawer in an oblique manner, they come back. And it is in the return motion, it has been our observation, where this joint lock occurs.

I would like to suggest in our study for possible mechanisms by which this sort of musculoskeletal lesion occurs that we keep another emphasis in mind: It's not a thing; it's a complex process, a lesion of motion, not something that you can section or biopsy or see on the autopsy table. It's a functional disorder; it is a dysfunction. We are particularly interested in the work of the Bioengineering Group for the Study of Human Joints at the University of Leeds, published in 1971 in the *Annals of Rheumatic Diseases*. They go into considerable detail on the hydrodynamics, the gas exchanges, the interchange of the biochemicals, etc., within the joint. This brings us back to manipulation again. You've heard about the wide variety of manipulative procedures. The thing that has always intrigued me is how such apparently diverse manipulative procedures can produce anything resembling results. In analyzing these procedures, we find that almost without exception, they have one thing in common, which often is not mentioned when the procedure is described, and that is, joint distraction--intersegmental traction. Studies on these mechanisms may also help us understand not only the spontaneous types of pain, but also the palpation-elicited types of pain where, with your finger in the vicinity of the joint, you find areas that the patient will say are tender, but which symptomatically they do not complain of.

One final note: one of the simplest nonspecific manipulative techniques frequently used in severe low back problems is the straight single leg-pull. The workers at Leeds showed that you get considerable joint separation with tension up to 5 kg. Beyond that, you get the "click". But the result is the same. In the joint separation, it is not too hard for me to see that, in that period, there was a restriction of motion due to some compressive factors. This might be the moment of removal of the restriction, the lock. It may fit into what Dr. Lewit talked about--the meniscoid hypothesis of joint lock.

Nonimpulse-Based Mechanisms

Chairman: Fred E. Samson

DR. FRED E. SAMSON: "Nonimpulse-based mechanisms" covers a lot of ground.   In the wisdom of the organizing committee they decided to emphasize axoplasmic transport and the trophic actions of neurons.   There are three distinctive features of nonimpulse-based mechanisms that I would like to point out before we start.   One is that the time-frames are different; these are generally slower, long-lasting kinds of events; secondly, traditional circuitry may or may not be meaningful in terms of the inferences to be drawn; and thirdly, research orientation in this area is strongly chemical and ultrastructural.

It is my assignment to review axonal transport in the antero-grade direction.   Dr. Thoenen will review the transport of materials retrogradely--back to the cell, and influencing its synthetic machinery.   Dr. Sjöstrand will lead discussion, which will include brief presentations by himself, by Dr. Ochs and by Dr. Worth.   Discussion of trophic functions will be initiated with a short review by Dr. Singer.   As part of my own presentation, I would like to show you a videotape of axoplasmic transport of organelles and particles in frog sciatic fibers.   The tape was prepared by David Forman and George Siggins.*

---

*"Movements of Organelles in Living Nerve Fibers," script by David S. Forman; 16 mm black and white sound film, running time 12 minutes. Available for purchase or rental from Order Section, National Audiovisual Center, Washington, D.C. 20409.   Cat. #008425.

AXONAL TRANSPORT: THE MECHANISMS AND THEIR SUSCEPTIBILITY TO DERANGEMENT; ANTEROGRADE TRANSPORT

Fred Samson

Ralph L. Smith Research Center, University of Kansas

Medical Center, Kansas City, Kansas

Among the nonimpulse-based mechanisms of the neuron, axoplasmic transport (or better termed <u>neuroplasmic</u> transport for it is not limited to axons) is one of the neuronal processes of potential significance to disease conditions. Further, axoplasmic transport is a special case of the general phenomena of intracellular movements - important to the normal functioning of all types of cells - and is not limited to neurons. Experimentation has shown that transport is vulnerable to derangement and such derangement may be the basis of certain neurological disorders.

Although the movements of the constituents within cells may, on first glance, appear to be random in character, they are highly controlled, and the concept that is emerging is that the cell is non-random down to the molecular level. Indeed, intracellular membranes, granules, vesicles, and organelles segregate functionally related molecules. Further, if these assemblies are scrambled, the cell has a dramatic capability for sorting them out again. What this amounts to is a segregation of "unit processes" into increasing levels of organization and performances. To coordinate these levels, the traffic within the cell must move under a high degree of control. This paper will examine what is known about the mechanisms and how they may be deranged.

In a recent review, Allen (1974) classifies cytoplasmic movements into three basic types: (a) bulk cytoplasmic transport that accompanies pseudopodia formation and ameboid locomotion; (b) bulk cytoplasmic transport that is unrelated to cell locomotion and serves to circulate cytoplasm; (c) selective transport of cytoplasmic constituents (such as nuclear movements) unrelated to any bulk transport.

291

Allen points out that the endoplasm of cells is variably resistant
to the displacement of particulates within it, behaving as a gel of
cross-linked polymers undergoing sol $\rightleftharpoons$ gel transformations.

Neurons as a class of cells have a great range in size, from a
few microns to greater than several meters long (in the giraffe,
for example) and an enormous heterogeneity of shapes. They are
characterized by a high degree of functional segregation (Palay &
Chan-Palay, 1972) with the spatial separation, for example, of impulse reception, action potential conduction, and synaptic transmitter release. The segregation of particular importance is the
almost complete restriction of protein synthesis and many types of
organelles to the perikaryon and large dendrites. The axon itself
is entirely lacking in ribosomes and with increasing distance from
the cell body the ribosomes selectively disappear in dendrites
(Palay & Chan-Palay, 1972). Therefore, those neurons with long
axonal processes, which depend upon components manufactured in the
perikaryon, make accessible for study the traffic that moves within
them. These movements of cytoplasmic components within the neuron
are referred to as axoplasmic transport (AXT) or less correctly,
axoplasmic flow, and more correctly as neuroplasmic transport. Although the neuron is specialized in its own way, it seems reasonable
to assume that the general principles of intracellular movement (ICM)
in neurons are essentially the same for all eukaryotic cells.

There are a number of excellent reviews of axoplasmic transport
(Barondes & Samson, 1967; Grafstein, 1969; Heslop, 1974; Lasek, 1970;
Lubinska, 1964; Ochs, 1974; Weiss, 1967), an overview of the effect
of drugs upon axoplasmic transport (McClure, 1972) and axoplasmic
transport in motor neuron pathology (Griffin & Price, 1976; Price &
Griffin, 1976). The movement of axoplasmic components from the cell
bodies to the terminals is an old concept but the classical studies
of Weiss and Hiscoe (1948) gave the first direct demonstration. A
major breakthrough was provided by Droz and Leblond's demonstration
that the movements of proteins could be traced by labeling them
with radioactive precursors (Droz & Leblond, 1963) and recently a
number of nonradioactive markers have been developed. The subject
may be summarized as follows: a wide variety of transported materials have been identified (enzymes, proteins, phospholipids,
catecholamine-containing granules, glycoproteins, 5-hydroxytryp-
tamine, dopamine-β-hydroxylase, etc.). The most extensively studied
are labeled proteins, some of which move at rates in the order of
1 mm/day (slow transport) and another group that move about
400 mm/day (fast transport). However, there is a wide spectrum
of rates reported for various types of cytoplasmic components (see
Lasek, 1970, for summary). Among the most rapidly moving components
reported are the neurosecretory granules of the preoptic nucleus,
calculated to move 2000 mm/day (Jasinski et al., 1966).

The transport processes bring not only materials for maintenance and renewal of the axon, but also some of the molecules
released at the terminals. Recently the important trophic action
that nerves have on striated muscles was shown to be related to
axoplasmic transport (Albuquerque et al., 1974; Fernandez &
Ramirez, 1974).

The movements of intracellular particles have been studied in
a wide variety of cells with specialized light microscope techniques, and there is a large literature on the subject (Allen &
Kamiya, 1964; Jahn & Bovee, 1969; Symposia Soc. Exp. Biol., 1974).
There is an increased interest in the use of dark-field microscopy
and the optical sectioning quality of Nomarski optics in observing
the movements within axons (Cooper & Smith, 1974; Kirkpatrick et
al., 1972), and computer analyses of the movements have been carried
out (Forman et al., 1974). The particles visualized by these techniques appear to move in channels in a saltatory fashion. They
move in directions both toward and away from the cell body. The
particles have a range of velocities with the gastest ones moving
at speeds comparable with fast axonal transport (FAXT). This
method is limited in that only the visible particles can be studied,
but it provides another important window to the events of intra-
axonal movements.

MECHANISMS OF AXOPLASMIC TRANSPORT

The mechanism(s) underlying axoplasmic transport (AXT) are no
doubt the work of complicated machinery. There are two major considerations with regard to the mechanisms: one, what are the
chemo-mechanical energy coupling components that harness metaboli-
cally generated energy to drive them and, two, what are the components that give specificity such that certain cytoplasmic constituents are moved to particular intracellular locations? The implicated
structures are extended surfaces such as the plasma membrane; tubular
organelles such as the endoplasmic reticulum and microtubular channels; and linear fibrillar elements such as actomyosin, microfilaments, neurofilaments, and microtubules (external surface of MT).
It is possible that each plays a part in some of the various types
of movements.

The movements are not driven by diffusion and require meta-
bolically generated energy. Therefore, drugs that interfere with
the flow of free energy in the cell generally will arrest the movements. For example, fast axoplasmic transport depends on a local
supply of energy: anoxia, dinitrophenol, and other energy flow
inhibitors have been shown to inhibit FAXT (Kirkpatrick et al.,
1972; Ochs, 1971a, 1971b, 1971c). Important to manipulative
therapy, this local energy flow requirement implies a demand for

a continuous blood and tissue fluid replenishment. There are
indications that fast transport is more susceptible to hypoxia
than the action potential.

RELATED CELLULAR STRUCTURAL ELEMENTS

Plasma Membrane

The movements of the plasma membrane and, in particular, the
peristaltic waves shown by Weiss to sweep periodically down the
axonal membranes (Weiss, 1967), have been proposed to have a role.
There are reasons, however, that might rule out this proposition.
The movements observed in "skinned" amoeba (plasma membrane removed) by Allen and his colleagues show that at least the class
of movements studied required neither a plasma membrane nor hydrostatic pressure generated by an ectoplasmic tube (Allen, 1974; Edds,
1973). In myelinated nerves, the analysis of axoplasmic movement
and myelin movement revealed no evidence to support the idea that
axoplasmic transport results from peristalsis in the myelin cover-
ing the axon (Johnson et al., 1969). Further, it is difficult to
see how peristalsis could provide the specificity or sufficient
intracellular hydrostatic pressure for the movements within the
axoplasm of, say, large invertebrate axons.

Endoplasmic Reticulum

In some cell localities, proteins, lipids, and probably
other materials are known to be distributed via the endoplasmic
reticulum (ER). These substances may accumulate within the ER and,
in addition, often are modified while within the ER. The path of
secretory material from the polysome to the lumen in exocrine cells
and the packaging of material for transport involve the ER. The
smooth ER frequently seen in axons may be involved in axoplasmic
transport but it is still not clear whether the ER is entirely
continuous along the axon length and thus serves as a channel.

Microtubule Channels

The internal diameter of microtubules (MTs) is about 15 nm and
could accommodate sizable molecules. When appropriately stained,
dense particles, which some authors have interpreted as macromolecules, are revealed in the central core of the MT (Tani & Ametani,
1970). Whether this is a stationary structure or material in
transit is unknown.

Actomyosin

Actin has been shown to exist in a wide variety of nonmuscle cells (Pollard & Weiking, 1974) and is probably a universal constituent of eukaryotic cells. The properties of the actin in nonmuscle cells are remarkably similar to those of muscle actin, and this actin is probably involved in the cellular movements, intracellular, and other mechanical events. Where contractile systems are known in detail an interaction of actin with myosin is involved. Myosins, in contrast with actins, are more diverse in their properties. It is now clear that myosin also is present in a number of nonmuscle vertebrate cells (Pollard & Weiking, 1974). Actomyosin complexes have been identified in brain (Berl et al., 1973). Further, the related protein tropomyosin has been identified in nervous tissue (Fine et al., 1973). An attractive, unifying concept is the idea that actomyosin is universal in eukaryotic cells and, with some individual modification or specialization, underlies most, if not all, of the movements, both cellular and intracellular. The evidence is compelling although the details of the activation of the force generation are less well known in nonmuscle cells than in striated muscle (Allen, 1974; Pollard & Weiking, 1974). In particular, the class of ICM described as bulk cytoplasmic transport by Allen (1974) is probably motivated by actomyosin.

Microfilaments

Microfilaments are identified as a class primarily on the basis of their size (about 4 to 5 nm). They are a heterogeneous class; for example, some are clearly actin-like (bind heavy meromyosin) and some are not, and some are cytochalasin-β sensitive. Those that are actinoid probably are part of an actomyosin system.

Neurofilaments and Other 10 nm Filaments

The 10 nm filaments may be a distinct class of filaments that occur in a number of types of cells. The neurofilaments are typically abundant in myelinated axons and less abundant in unmyelinated axons, and the component protein has been characterized by Davison and Winslow (1974). Neurofilaments may be involved in axoplasmic transport; however, there is no experimental evidence and the functions of 10 nm filaments is a mystery. There is an increase in neurofilaments or structures which resemble neurofilaments ultrastructurally in a variety of neuropathies. Their origin and relationship to the neuropathic condition is unknown.

Microtubules

Microtubules are proteinaceous, intracellular tubular structures that are found in varying numbers in almost every type of
animal and plant cell. They have a characteristic tube structure
with an outside diameter of 25 nm and an inside diameter or channel
of 15 nm. They are abundant in neurons, where they may run un-
branched in dendritic and axonic processes for several micrometers.
They are the principal fibrous protein of the mitotic spindle and
dominant components of cilia and flagella. They often occur in
highly ordered arrays. Indeed, as methods improve it seems likely
they will be revealed in axons as components of larger systems in
which a number of MTs are linked and function in a coordinated way.
Recently research on MT has rapidly advanced and this research has
enlarged the understanding of many cellular functions, and there
are a number of excellent reviews that cover the various aspects
of the biochemistry (Bryan et al., 1974; Olmstead & Borisy, 1973)
and biology (McIntosh et al., 1974; Soifer, 1974) of microtubule
protein.

Among the functions proposed for MTs, which now constitute a
sizable list, the most convincing has been their role in the development and maintenance of an isometric cell form (Porter, 1966)
and in intracellular movements. The evidence implicating MTs as
a necessary component of the biological machinery that moves
chromosomes and other cytoplasmic constituents in Allen's class 3
type of movements may be outlined as follows: the MTs are often
oriented in the right way for transport, especially in extended
processes such as axons; their location with respect to large cellular inclusions (such as pigment granules and mitochondria) reveals
that they at least act as guides in the propulsion; their characteristic, universal presence in motile processes such as flagella
and sperm tails suggests that chemomechanical energy coupling is
part of their physiological function. But among the best arguments
are the findings that pharmacological agents that have a strong
affinity for the MT protein subunits, and in many cases that
disrupt MTs, arrest cytoplasmic translocations.

A number of papers on the function of MT in a wide variety of
cells add up to the conclusion that the MTs do not provide the
impelling force but rather the directionality and the scaffold for
the other components of the axoplasmic transport machinery.

Given that MTs are involved in transport, the question is
"how". The actinoid character of tubulin has not been overlooked
and it has been proposed that the mechanism is similar to the
sliding filaments of actin and myosin of muscle contraction, with
tubulin behaving akin to actin, interacting with a myosinoid protein
associated with the particulates (Schmitt & Samson, 1968). Bridges

directly connecting vesicles and MTs have been illustrated in several preparations (Smith et al., 1970).

Another mechanism that has been proposed takes into account the layer of anionic polyelectrolyte, which ensheaths axonal MTs and also extends to form a network through the axoplasm (Samson, 1971). This material is associated with MTs in axons and stains with alcian blue (Hinkley, 1973), ruthenium red, alkaline bismuth (Burton & Hinkley, 1974), and lanthanum (Burton & Fernandez, 1973). These methods under the conditions used have some specificity for mucopolysaccharides, or at least for polyanionic molecules with high charge density. In this minimal model, the MTs are the anchor points of a network composed of macroanionic molecules (macroions). The branching molecular units specifically attach to the transported molecules or organelles. It is well known that linear flexible macroions characteristically extend and contract with small ionic changes in their immediate environment (Oosawa, 1971). The expansion-contraction movements of the anionic polyelectrolyte network might be expected to be discontinuous and generate the saltatory character of cytoplasmic movements.

DERANGEMENT OF AXOPLASMIC TRANSPORT

Anti-Microtubule Drugs

Certain antimitotic drugs are now known to block mitosis by interfering with the movements of the chromosomes. Further, the molecular mechanism of the blockade is the disruption of the micro-tubules of the mitotic spindle by the binding of the drug to the microtubule protein (Taylor, 1965). The drugs for which this mechanism is best established are colchicine and some of its de-rivatives, and the vinca alkaloids (vinblastine and vincristine). The importance of these findings should not be underestimated for they have led to substantial advances in a wide spectrum of re-search from biochemistry to medicine. The interaction of these drugs with microtubule protein has been comprehensively reviewed by Wilson et al. (1974).

Colchicine. Because colchicine binds specifically to tubulin, the protein subunit of the spindle microtubules, it can be con-sidered a prototype of a class of antimitotic drugs known as spindle poisons (Shelanski & Taylor, 1967; Weisenberg et al., 1968).

Colchicine blocks intracellular movements in addition to those of chromosomes in a wide variety of cells. It has been shown to block the axoplasmic transport of axoplasmic constituents such as acetylcholinesterase in sciatic nerve (Kreutzberg, 1969), amine storage granules (Banks et al., 1973; Hokfelt & Dahlstrom, 1971), proteins (Boesch et al., 1972; Fernandez & Davison, 1969; James et al., 1970), and sulfated mucopolysaccharide protein (Elam, 1970). Further, colchicine blocks the movements of pigment granules in chromophore cells (Malawista, 1971), nuclear migrations in fused cells (Holmes & Choppin, 1968), in other words, a wide variety of cytoplasmic movements. Although some work suggests that colchicine blocks only the rapidly transported axonal constituents, a greater number of studies show that the slow transport (1 mm/day) is also blocked (Fernandez & Davison, 1969; Heslop, 1974; James et al., 1970; Karlsson & Sjöstrand, 1968).

Colchicine also blocks the retrograde transport of horseradish peroxidase (LaVail & LaVail, 1975), nerve growth factor (Hendry et al., 1974), and optically observed particulate movements (Kirkpatrick et al., 1972). In many preparations the blockade of transport is associated with a disappearance of the microtubules.

An increasing variety of cellular responses affected by colchicine (and also by the vinca alkaloids) are appearing in the literature. Included in these are the glucose-stimulated release of insulin (Lacy et al., 1968); nerve-stimulated release of norepinephrine and dopamine-β-hydroxylase from sympathetic nerves (Thoa et al., 1972); TSH-stimulated release of thyroxin (Williams & Wolff, 1972); acetylcholine-stimulated release of catecholamines from the adrenal medulla (Poisner & Bernstein, 1971); release of histamine from mast cells (Gillespie et al., 1968) and leukocytes (Levy & Carlton, 1969); release of growth hormone and prolactin induced by prostaglandin E (Labrie et al., 1973). The inference drawn from these experiments generally is that the MTs are involved in the mechanical movements leading to release of the secretory products contained in granules. Still other intracellular events such as the conversion of proparathyroid hormone to parathyroid hormone (Kemper et al., 1975) have been shown to be influenced by colchicine (and the vinca alkaloids). The stimulation of steroid secretion by colchicine and other antimicrotubular agents has been interpreted by Temple & Wolff (1973) to mean that access of cholesterol to the mitochondria is ordinarily restricted by the MTs and that stimulation occurs when this restriction is removed by the antimicrotubular agents.

The antimicrotubular agents have been shown to affect plasma membrane topographical responses (Yin et al., 1972). These agents reverse the inhibition by concanavalin A of patch formation and immunoglobulin receptor mobility in lymphocytes (Edelman, 1975). Also, lymphocyte mitogenesis induced by the binding of antigen to the cell surface receptors is inhibited by colchicine at a step prior to spindle formation. It is not known whether the colchicine-binding protein in this case is tubulin, but the similarity of effects of a variety of antimicrotubular drugs suggests that it is.

The hypothesis proposed by Edelman postulates a subsurface protein (tubulin?) in association-dissociation equilibrium with certain cell receptors that anchors the receptors and modulates their mobility. Further, he proposes that this protein assembly may be involved in a signaling process for mitogenesis (Edelman, 1975).

The question of the specificity of colchicine for microtubule protein in some responses continues to be raised (Trifaro et al., 1972). In an attempt to resolve this, Zweig and Chignell (1973) have suggested that a stronger case for the participation of MTs in these processes could be made if the effect were directly related to the ability of a given analog to bind to tubulin. To illustrate their approach, they have compared the ranking of the binding of 17 colchicine analogs, podophyllotoxin, and vinblastine to tubulin with the ranking in the mouse sarcoma test and an anti-inflammatory activity (Zweig & Chignell, 1973). They found a good correlation between the binding of these drugs and their efficacy as both anti-mitotic and antigout agents. This supports the theory of Malawista (1968) that the binding of colchicine to tubulin is responsible for its antigout as well as its antimitotic activities. The lumicolchicines are useful tools for such studies since these derivatives do not bind to tubulin (Wilson et al., 1974) and are not antimitotic. Lumicolchicine does not affect FAXT under conditions where colchicine does (Price & Griffin, 1976).

The blockade of transport by the tubulin-binding drugs is sometimes reported as occurring without detectable changes in the ultrastructure of MTs. However, the sample of tissue in electron microscopy is small and flaws in the MTs could escape attention. Furthermore, the ultrastructural appearance of the MTs may not always be a reliable index of their functional integrity. This would be particularly true if the dynamic polymerization-depolymerization of pool subunits and MTs is necessary for functioning. Colchicine binds to the tubulin subunits and with a much lower affinity to the polymerized MT itself, so it causes the disappearance of the MT only when there is an ongoing polymerization-depolymerization by drawing the equilibrium away from the polymerized state.

Vinca Alkaloids. The interaction of the vinca alkaloids with tubulin depolymerizes the microtubules and gives rise to highly regular crystalloid structures (Bensch & Malawista, 1969). The chemical properties of the vinca alkaloids that bind to tubulin and the crystalloids that are formed have been studied in some detail (Soifer, 1975). However, it should be cautioned that the vinca alkaloids interact and can precipitate a number of acidic proteins and nucleic acids in addition to tubulin (Wilson et al., 1970). In particular, the vinca alkaloids interact with actin. There is little question that vinblastine sulfate and vincristine sulfate are potent blocking agents of axoplasmic transport – more so than colchicine – on both the fast and slow types of axoplasmic transport (Fernandez et al., 1971; Karlsson et al., 1971), and the retrograde transport as well (Bunt & Lund, 1974).

The antimitotic activity of several of the vinca alkaloids derivatives have been studied and it is noteworthy that the interaction of these derivatives with tubulin parallels the antimitotic activity (Wilson et al., 1974).

Maytansine. A novel ansa macrolide isolated from *Maytemus buchananii* and *M. serrata* inhibits the growth of experimental tumors and is under clinical trials as an antileukemic agent.

Maytansine inhibits the in vitro polymerization of tubulin and appears to share a common binding site with vincristine. We have found that maytansine inhibits FAXT in vitro in concentrations at 20 μM. Further, the extent of inhibition at increasing concentrations correlates with a decreasing number of axonal microtubules.

Nocodazole. _Nocodazole {methyl [5-2-thienylcarbonyl)-1H-benzimidazol-2-Y1] carbamate (R17934, Aldrich Chemical Co., Inc., U.S.A.} is a new synthetic microtubule inhibitor chemically unrelated to the microtubule-disintegrating agents colchicine, the vinca alkaloids, rotenone and podophyllotoxin. In our experiments with Nocodazole we found a partial blockage of FAXT with 2 h of incubation and a complete blockage within 4 h. Nocodazole appears to be a more potent inhibitor of FAXT than the antimicrotubule agents maytansine, vincristine, vinblastine and vindesine. We conclude that the blockade of FAXT by Nocodazole is a consequence of its interaction with microtubules. We have also found that Nocodazole prevents the in vitro polymerization of tubulin and partially depolymerizes in vitro preformed microtubules.

NEUROPATHOGENS

A wide variety of agents have been described as neuropathogens. There are good reasons for believing that some neuropathogens have among their actions the disruption of axoplasmic transport.

The industrial revolution has produced an incredible number of chemical agents, widely used in industry, agriculture and medicine, which by various routes reach the human nervous system and induce neurotoxic effects. Since very few of these substances have one single metabolic action, it has been difficult to sort out which agents induce their untoward actions via derangement of axoplasmic transport. However, many of the axonal pathologies suggest involvement of axoplasmic transport derangement. Neuropathies induced by

acrylamide, triorthocresyl phosphate, η-hexane and the vinca alca-
loids are of a character that axoplasmic transport involvement is
a major consideration. Although the experimental evidence is not
clear cut, the slow 1 mm/day AXT was reported to be disrupted in
cats with acrylamide neuropathy but not in triorthocresyl phosphate
neuropathy (Pleasure et al., 1969). On the other hand, Bradley and
colleagues concluded that both the fast and slow axonal protein
transport waves in cats suffering from neuropathies induced with
vincristine, acrylamide, and triorthocresyl phosphate were normal
(Bradley & Williams, 1973), but they point out that the complexi-
ties involved in transport studies make interpretation of the data
difficult. The design of these experiments is such that the transport in unaffected fibers would dominate and poor transport would
be revealed only if it were pronounced and not close to the site of
precursor injection. Although it is evident that a degenerated
axon would fail to transport proteins, the question is whether a
"causation" is derangement of the transport mechanism. Obviously
it would be valuable to study the relationship of axoplasmic transport perturbation to the neuropathogens with better-designed
experiments.

There are also naturally occurring chemicals which if taken in
sufficient quantities cause paralytic and neuronal pathologies of a
kind that suggest axoplasmic transport involvement. The most important of these diseases is lathyrism, consequent to the ingestion
of peas in the lathyrus species by animals or humans during famines.
The toxic substances in the peas have been shown to be β-amino-
propionitrile and related compounds. Chou and Hartman (1965) concluded from their extensive studies that stagnation of axoplasmic
transport is the cause of the lesions.

MONOAMINE OXIDASE INHIBITORS

The monoamine oxidase inhibitors (MAOI) pargyline and phenel-
zine have unusual effects on fast axoplasmic transport as shown by
Boegman, Wood and Pinaud (1975). Rats were given pargyline (75 mg
Kg^{-1}) daily for up to 7 days, and the FAXT in sciatic nerve was
studied. The rate of the leading front of the transported protein
in the control was in the range of other studies, but the rate of
the leading front in the pargyline-treated rats increased fourfold
(200 mm/day). The authors also related this change in FAXT to a
myopathy, which results from the pargyline treatment. Their report
is brief but is important enough to deserve comment. The design of
the experiments did not permit a discrimination of the following
possibilities: (a) an increase in uptake and incorporation of the
labeled precursor and hence an earlier release from the cell bodies
of the labeled protein, (b) the faster front being composed of proteins other than the control FAXT proteins, and (c) whether the

innervated muscle played a role - to mention only a few possibilities. Since these findings have a bearing on the regulation of
axoplasmic transport, the trophic actions of neurons and possibly
on certain myopathies, they warrant more study.

In a preliminary series in our laboratory, rats were given
pargyline (75 mg/kg) daily for 3 days and control rats an equivalent volume of saline. The fast transport velocity in the control
ventral horn motor neurons was 336 mm/day whereas the ventral horn
motor neurons in pargyline-treated rats had a peak at 650 mm/day
in front of a peak moving at the normal rate. We have explored
this MAOI effect further and found that the velocity of fast axoplasmic transport did not increase in all types of nerves. For
example, the afferent fibers from the dorsal root ganglion appeared
unaffected. Also, sectioning the motor neuron from the innervated
muscles did not eliminate the abnormal faster peak. This suggests
that the muscles which show the myopathic changes were not inducing
the fast axoplasmic transport velocity change.

REGULATION OF AXOPLASMIC TRANSPORT

The regulation of the composition, velocity and the destination of transported materials is largely unknown. Although one
opinion is that it is an "all-or-none" type of phenomenon, this is
highly unlikely in view of the dynamic responsiveness of neurons.
It is known that an individual cell at any one time expresses only
a limited portion of its full genetic capability and that different
types of proteins are synthesized by a cell in response to hormonal
stimulation and other changes in physiological states. One is
forced to the conclusion that the composition of the transported
material differs within different types of neurons and with different physiological states. There have been attempts to identify
differences in the transported material out the centrally directed
process from those out the peripherally directed process in uni-
polar neurons, but these experiments have been inconclusive,
largely because of the great heterogeneity of the transported
material.

CONCLUSION

The intracellular movements of cellular constituents are
largely non-random organized events by which molecules and higher
order aggregates are relocated within the cell. The locations of
origin or synthesis of cellular constituents are usually not the
intracellular locations of function and ongoing metabolism is
associated with continuous translocation. The high degree of
segregation of functions in neurons results in a great demand on

intracellular transport systems and may, indeed, make them particularly vulnerable to derangement. Some of the molecules delivered by axoplasmic transport are needed for transmitter
metabolism and for trophic action on innervated cells; other
molecules no doubt perform equally essential roles. With the
present state of knowledge, the impact that nerve compression,
stretching, angulation or other deformations may have on the
neurochemistry of axonal transport is not known but can reasonably
be inferred to be significant. In view of the trophic actions
which neurons have on cells they innervate, subtle changes in the
transported materials may have a profound influence on the state
of well being of the innervated tissues as well as the neuron
itself. It is clear that any extensive perturbation of the above
mentioned kinds interferes with the amount of material transported.
We can see at least a possibility that the basis of some of the
therapeutic effects of manipulation may lie in axoplasmic transport
events.

REFERENCES

ALBUQUERQUE, J. E., F. M. WARNICK, and O. SANSONE. The effects of
    vinblastine and colchicine on neural regulation of muscle.
    Ann. N. Y. Acad. Sci. 228:224-243, 1974.

ALLEN, R. D. Some new insights concerning cytoplasmic transport.
    Symp. Soc. Exptl. Biol. 8:15-26, 1974.

ALLEN, R. D., and N. KAMIYA, editors. *Primitive Motile Systems in
    Cell Biology.* New York: Academic Press, 1964.

BANKS, P., D. MAYOR, and P. MRAZ. Cytochalasin B and the intra-
    axonal movement of nonadrenaline storage vesicles. *Brain Res.*
    49:417-421, 1973.

BARONDES, S. H., and F. E. SAMSON. Axoplasmic transport. *Neurosci.
    Res. Prog. Bull.* 5:307-419, 1967.

BENSCH, K. G., and S. E. MALAWISTA. Microtubule crystals: A new
    biophysical phenomenon induced by vinca alkaloids. *J. Cell
    Biol.* 40:95-107, 1969.

BERL, S., S. PUSZKIN, and W. J. NICKLAS. Actomyosin-like protein
    in brain. *Science* 179:441-446, 1973.

BOEGMAN, R. J., P. L. WOOD, and L. PINAUD. Increased axoplasmic
    flow associated with pargyline under conditions which induce
    a myopathy. *Nature* 253:51-52, 1975.

BOESCH, J., P. MANKO, and M. CUÉNOD. Effect of colchicine on axonal transport of proteins in the pigeon visual pathways. *J. Neurobiol.* 2:123-132, 1972.

BRADLEY, W. G., and M. H. WILLIAMS. Axoplasmic flow in axonal neuropathies. *Brain* 96:235-246, 1973.

BRYAN, J. Biochemical properties of microtubules. *Fed. Proc.* 33:152-174, 1974.

BUNT, A. H., and R. D. LUND. Vinblastine induced blockage of orthograde and retrograde axonal transport of protein in retinal ganglion cells. *Exptl. Neurol.* 45:288-297, 1974.

BURTON, P. R., and H. L. FERNANDEZ. Delineation by lanthanum staining of filamentous elements associated with the surfaces of axonal microtubules. *J. Cell Sci.* 12:567-583, 1973.

BURTON, P. R., and R. E. HINKLEY. Further electron microscopic characterization of axoplasmic microtubules of the ventral nerve cord of the crayfish. *J. Submicr. Cytol.* 6:311-326, 1974.

CHOU, S. M., and H. A. HARTMANN. Axonal lesions and waltzing syndrome after IDPN administration in rats. *Acta Neuropathol.* 4:590-603, 1965.

COOPER, P. O., and R. S. SMITH. The movement of optically detectable organelles in myelinated axons of *Xenopus laevis.* *J. Physiol.* 242:77-97, 1974.

DAVISON, P., and B. WINSLOW. The protein subunit of calf brain neurofilament. *J. Neurobiol.* 5:119-133, 1974.

DROZ, B., and C. P. LeBLOND. Axonal migration of proteins in the central nervous system and peripheral nerves as shown by radioautography. *J. Comp. Neurol.* 121:325-345, 1963.

EDDS, K. Particle movements in artificial axopodia of *Echinosphaerium nucleofilum.* *J. Cell Biol.* 59:88a, 1973.

EDELMAN, G. Receptor interactions and mitogenesis in lymphoid cells. In: *Functional Linkage in Biomolecular Systems,* edited by F. O. Schmitt. New York: Raven Press, 1975, pp. 188-201.

ELAM, J. S., J. M. GOLDBERG, N. S. RADIN, and B. W. AGRANOFF. Rapid axonal transport of sulfated mucopolysaccharide proteins. *Science* 170:458-460, 1970.

FERNANDEZ, H. L., P. R. BURTON, and F. E. SAMSON. Axoplasmic
    transport in the crayfish nerve cord: The role of fibrillar
    constituents of neurons. *J. Cell Biol.* 51:176-192, 1971.

FERNANDEZ, H., and P. F. DAVISON. Axoplasmic transport in the
    crayfish nerve cord. *Proc. Natl. Acad. Sci. USA* 64:512-519,
    1969.

FERNANDEZ, H. F., and B. RAMIREZ. Muscle fibrillation induced by
    blockage of axoplasmic transport. *Brain Res.* 49:385-395,
    1974.

FINE , R. E. ,   A. L. BLITZ, S. E. HITCHCOCK, and B. KAMINER.
    Tropomyosin in brain and growing neurones. *Nature New Biol.*
    245:182-185, 1973.

FORMAN, D. S., A. L. PADJAN, and G. R. SIGGINS. Movements of
    organelles in frog axons studied by time-lapse cinematography
    and computer analysis. *Soc. Neurosci. Meeting,* Abs. 210, 1974.

GILLESPIE, E., R. J. LEVINE, and S. E. MALAWISTA. Histamine release
    from rat peritoneal mast cells: Inhibition by bolchicine and
    potentiation by deuterium oxide. *J. Pharmacol. Exptl. Ther.*
    164:158-165, 1968.

GRAFSTEIN, B. Axonal transport: Communication between soma and
    synapse. In: *Advances in Biochemical Psychology.* New York:
    Raven Press, 1969, pp. 11-25.

GRIFFIN, J. W., and D. L. PRICE. Axonal transport to and from the
    motor nerve ending. In: *Amyotrophic Lateral Sclerosis,*
    edited by J. M. Anders, R. T. Johnson, and M.A.B. Brazier.
    New York: Academic Press, 1976, pp. 33-67.

HENDRY, I. A., K. STOCKEL, H. THOENEN, and L. L. IVERSEN. The
    retrograde axonal transport of nerve growth factor. *Brain Res.*
    68:103-121, 1974.

HESLOP, J. P. Transport at the cellular level. *Symp. Soc. Exptl.*
    Biol. 28:209-227, 1974.

HINKLEY, R. E. Axonal microtubules and associated filaments
    stained by alcian blue. *J. Cell Sci.* 13:753-761, 1973.

HOKFELT, T., and A. DAHLSTROM. Electron microscopic observations
    on the distribution and transport of nonadrenaline storage
    particles after local treatment with mitosis inhibitors. *Acta*
    Physiol. Scand. Suppl. 357:10-11, 1971.

HOLMES, K. V., and P. W. CHOPPIN. Role of microtubules in movement
and alignment of nuclei in virus-induced syncytia. *J. Cell
Biol.* 39:526-543, 1968.

JAHN, T. L., and E. C. BOVEE. Protoplasmic movements within cells.
Physiol. Rev. 49:493-862, 1969.

JAMES, K.A.C., J. J. BRAY, I. G. MORGAN, and L. AUSTIN. Effect of
colchicine on the transport of axonal protein in the chicken.
Biochem. J. 117:767-771, 1970.

JASINSKI, A., A. GORBMAN, and T. J. HARA. Rate of movement and
redistribution of stainable neurosecretory granules in hypothalamic neurons. *Science* 154:776-778, 1966.

JOHNSON, G., R. S. SMITH, and G. S. LOCK. Accumulation of material
at severed ends of myelinated nerve fibers. *Am. J. Physiol.*
217:188-191, 1969.

KARLSSON, J. O., H. A. HANSSON, and J. SJÖSTRAND. Studies on
axonal transport of proteins in retinal ganglion cells of the
rabbit. *Z. Zellforsch. mikrosk. Anat.* 115:265-283, 1971.

KARLSSON, J., and J. SJÖSTRAND. Transport of labelled proteins in
the optic nerve and tract of the rabbit. *Brain Res.* 11:431-
439, 1968.

KEMPER, B., J. F. HABENER, A. RICH, and J. T. POTTS. Microtubules
and the intracellular conversion of proparathyroid hormone to
parathyroid hormone. *Endocrinology* 96:906-912, 1975.

KIRKPATRICK, J. B., J. J. BRAY, and S. M. PALMER. Visualization
of axoplasmic flow in vitro by nomanski microscopy. *Brain
Res.* 43:1-10, 1972.

KREUTZBERG, G. W. Neuronal dynamics and axonal flow. IV. Blockage
of intra-axonal enzyme transport by colchicine. *Proc. Natl.
Acad. Sci. USA* 62:722-728, 1969.

LABRIE, F., M. GAUTHIER, G. PELLETIER, P. BORGEAT, A. LEMAY, and
J.-J. GOUGE. Role of microtubules in basal and stimulated
release of growth hormone and prolactin in rat adenohypophysis
in vitro. *Endocrinology* 93:903-914, 1973.

LACY, P. E., S. L. HOWELL, D. A. YOUNG, and C. J. FINK. New
hypothesis of insulin secretion. *Nature* 219:1177-1179, 1968.

LASEK, R. J. Protein transport in neurons. *Int. Rev. Neurobiol.*
13:289-324, 1970.

LaVAIL, M. M., and J. H. LaVAIL.   Retrograde axonal transport in
    the central nervous system. *Brain Res.* 85:273-280, 1975.

LEVY, D. A., and J. A. CARLTON.   Influence of temperature on the
    inhibition by colchicine of allergic histamine release. *Proc.
    Soc. Exptl. Biol. Med.* 130:1333-1336, 1969.

LUBINSKA, L.   Axoplasmic streaming in regenerating and in normal
    nerve fibers. In: *Mechanisms of Neural Regeneration*
    (Progress in Brain Research), edited by M. Singer and J. P.
    Schade, Vol. 13. Amsterdam: Elsevier, 1964, pp. 1-66.

MALAWISTA, S. E.   Colchicine: A common mechanism for its anti-
    inflammatory and anti-miotic effects. *Arthritis Rheum.* 11:
    191-197, 1968.

MALAWISTA, S. E.   Colchicine-like effects of other antimitotic
    agents. *J. Cell Biol.* 49:848-855, 1971.

McCLURE, W. O.   The effect of drugs upon axoplasmic transport.
    Adv. Pharmacol. Chemother. 10:185-220, 1972.

McINTOSH, J. R.   An introduction to microtubules. *J. Supramolec.
    Struct.* 2:385-392, 1974.

OCHS, S.   Local supply of energy to the fast axoplasmic transport
    mechanism. *Proc. Natl. Acad. Sci. USA* 65:1279-1282, 1971a.

OCHS, S.   Dependence of fast axoplasmic transport in nerve on oxi-
    dative metabolism. *J. Neurochem.* 18:107-114, 1971b.

OCHS, S.   Fast axoplasmic transport in mammalian nerve in vitro
    after block of glycolysis with iodoacetic acid. *J. Neurochem.*
    18:833-843, 1971c.

OCHS, S.   Systems of material transport in nerve fibers. I.Axoplasmic
    transport related to nerve function and tropic control. *Ann.
    N. Y. Acad. Sci.* 228:202-223, 1974.

OLMSTEAD, J. B., and G. G. BORISY.   Characterization of MT assembly
    in porcine brain extracts by viscometry entry. *Annu. Rev.
    Biochem.* 42:507-540, 1973.

OOSAWA, F. *Polyelectrolytes.* New York: Marcel Dekker, Inc., 1971.

PALAY, S. L., and V. CHAM-PALAY.   The structural heterogeneity of
    central nervous tissue. In: *Metabolic Compartmentation in
    the Brain.* New York: MacMillan, 1972, pp. 187-207.

PLEASURE, D. E., K. C. MISHLER, and W. K. ENGEL. Axonal transport of proteins in experimental neuropathies. *Science* 166:524-525, 1969.

POISNER, A. M., and J. BERNSTEIN. A possible role of MTs in catecholamine release from the adrenal medulla. Effect of colchicine, vinca alkaloids and deuterium Oxide 2. *J. Pharmacol. Exptl. Ther.* 177:102-108, 1971.

POLLARD, T. O., and P. R. WEIKING. Actin and myosin and cell movement. *CRC Crit. Rev. Biochem.* 2:1-65, 1974.

PORTER, K. R. Cytoplasmic microtubules and their functions. In: *Principles of Biomolecular Organization*, CIBA Foundation Symp. London: J. and A. Churchill, 1966, pp. 308-345.

PRICE, D. L., and J. W. GRIFFIN. Neural transport of tetanus toxin. In: *Amyotrophic Lateral Sclerosis*, edited by J. M. Andrews, R. T. Johnson, and M.A.B. Brazier. New York: Academic Press, 1976, pp. 1-32.

PRICE, M. T. The effects of colchicine and lumicholchicine on the rapid phase of axonal transport in the rabbit visual system. *Brain Res.* 77:497-501, 1974.

SAMSON, F. E. Mechanism of axoplasmic transport. *J. Neurobiol.* 2:347-360, 1971.

SAMSON, F. E. Pharmacology of drugs that affect intracellular movement. *Annu. Rev. Pharmacol. Tox.* 16:143-159, 1976.

SCHMITT, F. O., and F. E. SAMSON. Neuronal fibrous protein. *Neurosci. Res. Prog. Bull.*, 1968.

SHELANSKI, M. L., and E. W. TAYLOR. Isolation of a protein subunit from microtubules. *J. Cell Biol.* 34:549-554, 1967.

SMITH, D. S., U. JARLFORS, and R. BERANEK. The organization of synaptic axoplasm in the lamprex (*Petromyzon marinus*) central nervous system. *J. Cell Biol.* 46:199-219, 1970.

SOIFER, D., Chairman, Conference on Biology of Cytoplasmic Microtubules. *Ann. N. Y. Acad. Sci.*, Vol. 253, 1975.

SYMPOSIA OF THE SOCIETY FOR EXPERIMENTAL BIOLOGY. Transport at the cellular level, No. 28. Cambridge: University Press, 1974.

TANI, E., and T. AMETANI. Substructure of microtubules in brain nerve cells as revealed by ruthenium red. *J. Cell Biol.* 46:159-165, 1970.

TAYLOR, E. W. The mechanism of colchicine inhibition of mitosis.
    I. Kinetics of inhibition and the binding of H^3-colchicine.
    J. Cell Biol. 25:145-160, 1965.

TEMPLE, R., and J. WOLFF. Stimulation of steroid secretion by
    antimicrotubular agents. *J. Biol. Chem.* 248:2691-2698, 1973.

THOA, N. G., G. F. WOOTEN, J. AXELROD, and I. J. KOPIN. Inhibition
    of release of dopamine β-hydroxylase and norepinephrine from
    sympathetic nerves by colchicine, vinblastine or cyto-
    chalasin-β. *Proc. Natl. Acad. Sci. USA* 69:520-522, 1972.

TRIFARO, J. M., B. COLLIER, A. LASTOWEKA, and D. STERN. Inhibition
    by colchicine and by vinblastine of acetylcholine-induced
    catecholamine release from the adrenal gland: An anticholi-
    nergic action, not an effect upon microtubules. *Molec. Phar-
    macol.* 8:264-267, 1972.

WEISENBERG, R. C., G. G. BORISY, and E. W. TAYLOR. The colchicine-
    binding protein of mammalian brain and its relation to micro-
    tubules. *Biochemistry* 7:4466-4479, 1968.

WEISS, P. Neuronal dynamics. *Neurosci. Res. Prog. Bull.* 5:371-
    400, 1967.

WEISS, P., and H. B. HISCOE. Experiments on the mechanism of nerve
    growth. *J. Exptl. Zool.* 107:315-395, 1948.

WILLIAMS, J. A., and J. WOLFF. Colchicine-binding proteins and the
    secretion of thyroid hormone. *J. Cell Biol.* 54:157-165, 1972.

WILSON, L., J. R. BAMBURG, S. B. MIZEL, L. M. GRISHAM, and K. M.
    CRESWELL. Interaction of drugs with microtubular proteins.
    Fed. Proc. 33:158-166, 1974.

WILSON, L., J. BRYAN, A. RUBY, and D. MAZIA. Precipitation of pro-
    teins by vinblastine and calcium ions. *Proc. Natl. Acad. Sci.
    USA* 66:807-814, 1970.

YIN, H., T. UKENA, and R. BERLIN. Effect of colchicine, colcemid,
    and vinblastine on the agglutination, by concanavalin A, of
    transformed cells. *Science* 178:867-868, 1972.

ZWEIG, M. H., and C. F. CHIGNELL. Interaction of some colchicine
    analogs, vinblastine and podophyllotoxin with rat brain micro-
    tubular protein. *J. Biochem. Pharmacol.* 22:2141-2150, 1973.

TRANSFER OF INFORMATION FROM EFFECTOR ORGANS TO INNERVATING

NEURONS BY RETROGRADE AXONAL TRANSPORT OF MACROMOLECULES

H. Thoenen, M. Schwab and Y.-A. Barde

Department of Pharmacology, Biocenter of the

University, Basel, Switzerland

INTRODUCTION

The functional capacity of integrated neuronal systems such as the human brain depends not only on the numerous synaptic contacts between their neurons, but also on the capability of these neurons to adapt their synaptic connectivity in response to changing functional requirements. This ability to undergo plastic adaptations represents a basic difference between the function of an integrated neuronal system and that of a computer. Thus, if a nerve impulse is transmitted from one neuron to the other by means of transmitter substances the response of the effector neuron is not confined to the short-term effects such as changes in the ionic permeability of the neuronal membrane. The response also involves changes in the macromolecular composition of the effector cell which may be reflected by covalent alterations of macromolecules, e.g., phosphorylation, or by changes in the rate of synthesis of macromolecules which directly or indirectly change the functional connection between neurons (cf. Cragg, 1970; Thoenen & Otten, 1976).

Although the impulse flow in axons is unidirectional, the trophic interaction is not confined to the orthograde direction. It is known that effector cells, neuronal or non-neuronal, have important influences on the innervating neurons. For instance, in his classical experiments with chick embryos Hamburger (1938) has shown that the volume of the peripheral organs determines the development of the corresponding sensory and motor systems in the spinal cord. Although these retrograde trophic effects have been evaluated under various experimental conditions the underlying mechanisms remained a matter of speculation. More recent experiments

311

in the peripheral sympathetic nervous system have opened up aspects
which seem to offer the opportunity to understand at least one possible mechanism by which effector cells influence innervating
neurons. Transplantation experiments have shown that the transplant and not the site of transplantation is essential for the
density and also qualitative composition of the re-innervating
fibers. For instance, if pieces of tissue of differing density
and composition of their autonomic innervation are transplanted
into the anterior eye chamber the original nerve fibers degenerate
and the transplant is re-innervated by nerve fibers originating
from the iris (Bjoerklund, Bjerre & Stenevi, 1974; Burnstock, 1974;
Olson & Malmfors, 1970). The density and pattern of re-innervation
occurs according to the autonomic innervation at the original site;
i.e., tissues with a dense adrenergic innervation are also densely
re-innervated and tissues with a cholinergic and/or adrenergic innervation become also qualitatively re-innervated according to
their original site (Burnstock, 1974; Olson & Malmfors, 1970).
Bjoerklund and collaborators (1974) made the important observation
that transplants pre-incubated in a medium containing nerve growth
factor (NGF) became more densely and more rapidly innervated by
adrenergic fibers than without pre-incubation. Furthermore, pre-
incubation of the transplants in a medium containing antibodies to
NGF markedly impaired the re-innervation of the transplant with
adrenergic nerve fibers. This together with other observations led
to the formulation of the hypothesis that NGF might act as a macromolecular messenger between effector organs and innervating neurons
(Hendry, 1976; Hendry & Iversen, 1973).

    In this chapter we will summarize and discuss the most impor-
tant requirements which should be fulfilled if NGF should act as a
macromolecular retrograde mediator of information between effector
organs and innervating neurons. We will also discuss more general
aspects of retrograde axonal transport related to the selectivity
of the transport of lectins and toxins which allow conclusions on
the composition of the cell membrane of the corresponding nerve
terminals, provide direct information on the site of action of
neuronal toxins and the use of (atoxic) fragments as carriers for
the transfer of viricide drugs in a highly selective manner.

                EVIDENCE FOR THE RETROGRADE AXONAL TRANSPORT
                     OF NGF IN ADRENERGIC NEURONS

    In addition to the stimulation of fiber outgrowth in explants
of sensory and adrenergic ganglia, one of the most characteristic
effects of NGF on adrenergic neurons is the selective induction of
tyrosine hydroxylase (TH) and dopamine β-hydroxylase (DBH) (Thoenen
et al., 1971). Although these enzymes exhibit the majority of their
activities in the adrenergic nerve terminals where more than 95% of

norepinephrine is produced, they are synthesized in the perikaryon and reach the nerve terminals by axoplasmic transport (Thoenen, Otten & Oesch, 1973). Thus, the regulation of their synthesis takes place in the perikaryon, and NGF as a regulator of their synthesis must act there. If NGF should function as a mediator between effector cells and innervating neurons a requirement would be that NGF is taken up by adrenergic nerve terminals and is transported to the perikaryon. Indeed, multiple evidence for such a transport has been provided. After unilateral injection of ^{125}I-NGF into the anterior eye chamber the radioactivity is preferentially accumulated in the superior cervical ganglia of the injected side (Figure 1) (Hendry et al., 1974). The difference between injected and contralateral sides only becomes apparent 6 h after injection. From this lag and the distance between the site of injection (vicinity of the nerve terminals) and the corresponding cell bodies in the superior cervical ganglion the transport rate can be calculated. This rate of transport amounts to about 2 to 3 mm/h and seems to be the same for both rats and mice (Hendry et al., 1974; Stoeckel, Schwab & Thoenen, 1975b), and is independent of age. The majority of the radioactivity accumulating in the superior cervical ganglion after retrograde transport is unchanged NGF in that more than 95% of the radioactivity extracted from the ganglia binds to solid phase monospecific anti-NGF antibodies and when subjected to SDS gel electrophoresis, migrates to the position of 2.5 S NGF (Figure 2) (Stoeckel et al., 1976; Stoeckel & Thoenen, 1975).

The preferential accumulation of radioactivity in the superior cervical ganglion of the injected side can be abolished by surgical interruption of the postganglionic axons. Moreover, the retrograde transport is sensitive to colchicine as is the rapid orthograde transport (Stoeckel, Schwab & Thoenen, 1975a, 1975b).

Most direct evidence for the retrograde axonal transport is provided by autoradiographic and histochemical studies. After unilateral injection of ^{125}-I-NGF, heavy labelling is restricted to a relatively small proportion of neurons, presumably the neurons which directly supply the injected organ (Iversen, Stoeckel & Thoenen, 1975; Schwab & Thoenen, 1977a). This selective labelling of single neurons by retrograde transport allows determination of the proportion of neurons supplying a specific organ and, additionally, whether the corresponding cell bodies have a particular topographical localization within the ganglion. Electron microscopic autoradiographic studies have shown that after intraocular injection of ^{125}-I-NGF the label is selectively located over the postganglionic adrenergic nerve fibers (Iversen, Stoeckel & Thoenen, 1975; Schwab & Thoenen, 1977a) (Figure 3). The most direct evidence was provided by ultra-histochemical procedures (Schwab, 1977), which showed that in peripheral adrenergic neurons of adult rats horseradish peroxidase is not transported to an appreciable extent if injected into the

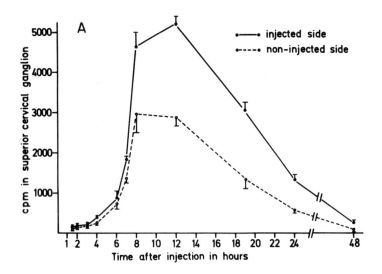

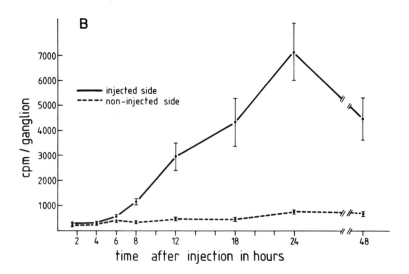

Figure 1. Time-course of accumulation of radioactivity in superior
cervical ganglia after unilateral injection of [125]-I-labelled NGF
(A) and DBH-antibodies (B). The larger accumulation of [125]-I-NGF
on the contralateral side as compared to [125]-I-DBH-antibodies results from the larger escape of NGF into the general circulation
due to its lower molecular weight (MW of NGF 26,500, DBH-antibodies
150,000) (Fillenz et al., 1976; Stoeckel & Thoenen, 1975).

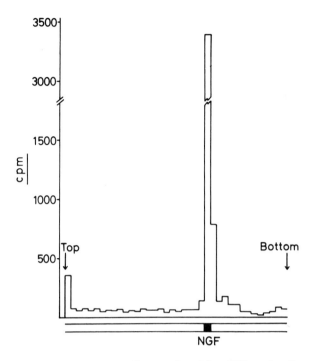

Figure 2.   Fifteen percent polyacrylamide SDS gel electrophoresis
of extracts of superior cervical ganglia 14 h after unilateral
intraocular injection of ^{125}I-NGF.   The position of the radioactivity is compared with that of native NGF (Stoeckel & Thoenen,
1975).

vicinity of the nerve terminals in similar concentrations as NGF.
However, horseradish peroxidase covalently coupled to NGF is transported in a similar manner as NGF, i.e., NGF acts as a carrier.
Since the enzymatic activity of horseradish peroxidase remains
intact after covalent binding it is possible to localize the complex NGF - horseradish peroxidase at the electron microscopic level
(Figure 4).   The advantage of this procedure over electron microscopic autoradiography is that the former provides a higher resolution: a localization of the label in a specific subcellular compartment is only possible by autoradiography after statistical
analysis.   There is, however, a perfect agreement between the
statistical analysis of the electron microscopic autoradiograms
(Figure 5) and the subcellular localization of the covalent coupling
product between NGF and horseradish peroxidase (Schwab, 1977;
Schwab & Thoenen, 1977a) (Figure 4).   In axons the reaction product
is virtually exclusively localized in vesicles and in cisternae of
smooth endoplasmic reticulum providing evidence that the retrograde

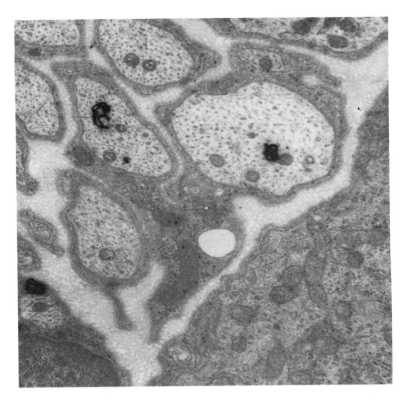

Figure 3. Electron microscopic autoradiogram of postganglionic adrenergic fibers in the rat superior cervical ganglion 14 h after injection of ^{125}I-NGF into the anterior eye chamber and the submandibular gland, two organs which receive a dense adrenergic innervation from the superior cervical ganglion. The autoradiographic silver grains clearly overlie axons. Magnification 25,000 X.

axonal transport is linked to similar subcellular structures as is the fast orthograde axonal transport. In the perikaryon not only is the reaction product localized in cisternae and vesicles of smooth endoplasmic reticulum but also in dense and multivesicular bodies, i.e., in lysosomal structures. It is noteworthy that neither in autoradiographic nor in ultrahistochemical studies could any evidence be found that NGF is accumulated in the cell nucleus of the adrenergic neuron, making it unlikely that the selective induction of TH and DBH by NGF is mediated by a direct template activation by NGF.

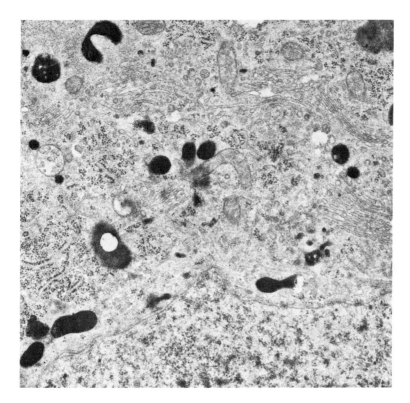

Figure 4. Perinuclear region of a sympathetic ganglion cell in the superior cervical ganglion 14 h after injection of an NGF-horseradish peroxidase coupling product into the anterior eye chamber and the submandibular gland. Reaction product (black precipitate) is localized in large lysosomal structures and in smaller, smooth vesicles. The nuclear membrane and the cell nucleus are free of label. Magnification 25,000 X.

SPECIFICITY OF RETROGRADE AXONAL TRANSPORT OF NGF

In order to obtain information as to whether the retrograde axonal transport of NGF depends on general, non-specific physico-chemical characteristics of this molecule such as molecular weight and net charge we labelled a series of macromolecules having a large range of molecular weights and isoelectric points (Stoeckel, Paravicini & Thoenen, 1974). These experiments showed that none of these molecules was transported retrogradely to a detectable extent in the peripheral adrenergic neurons (Figure 6). Of particular interest is the lack of retrograde transport of cytochrome C which has a molecular weight very similar to β-NGF (12,500 as compared to 13,260 of the monomer of β-NGF) and also a similar isoelectrical

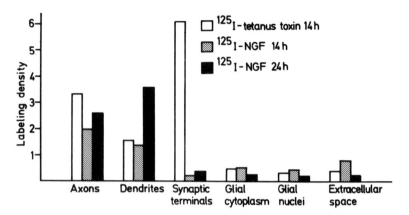

Figure 5. Density of silver grains over individual compartments in electron microscope autoradiograms of superior cervical ganglia 14 or 24 h after injection of ^{125}I-labelled NGF or tetanus toxin into the anterior eye chamber and the submandibular gland.

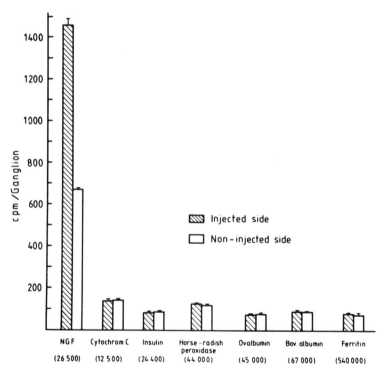

Figure 6. Accumulation of radioactivity in superior cervical ganglia 14 h after unilateral injection of ^{125}I-NGF and various other ^{125}I-labelled proteins (Stoeckel, Paravicini & Thoenen, 1974).

point (9.8 as compared to 9.3 of β-NGF). Thus, these data indicate that highly specific criteria must be fulfilled as a prerequisite for retrograde axonal transport. This aspect will be discussed in more detail below.

The selectivity and specificity refer not only to the molecules to be transported but also to the type of neuron. For instance, retrograde axonal transport of NGF is confined to adrenergic and sensory neurons, the two types of neurons which are responsive to NGF. The adrenergic neurons are responsive throughout the whole life span, the sensory neurons only during a restricted period of ontogenesis. In contrast, no retrograde axonal transport of NGF was detectable in motor neurons under experimental conditions under which the retrograde axonal transport of tetanus toxin could clearly be demonstrated (Stoeckel, Schwab & Thoenen, 1975b).

FUNCTIONAL IMPORTANCE OF RETROGRADE AXONAL TRANSPORT OF NGF

As already mentioned above, one of the characteristic effects of NGF on adrenergic neurons is the selective induction of TH and DBH. After unilateral injection of NGF into the anterior eye chamber and submaxillary gland the TH induction on the injected side was significantly higher than on the contralateral side (Figure 7) (Paravicini, Stoeckel & Thoenen, 1975). This difference becomes even more impressive if one takes into account that the experimental procedure (anaesthesia and unilateral injection) itself leads to a stress-mediated neuronal TH induction of about 20%. This non-NGF-mediated induction must be subtracted from both sides - unilateral injection of cytochrome C which served as a control for NGF led to a bilateral identical neuronally-mediated TH induction of about 20% - resulting in an increase of the ratio between injected and non-injected side. Moreover, it should be borne in mind that by injection of NGF into the anterior eye chamber and the submaxillary gland only about 15 to 20% of all the adrenergic nerve terminals originating from the superior cervical ganglia have been exposed to these high concentrations. If all the nerve terminals would have been exposed unilaterally to the same high NGF concentrations as in the anterior eye chamber and the submaxillary gland a ratio of the TH induction between injected and non-injected side of about 20:1 might be expected. Moreover, there is also good evidence that a major part of the NGF escaping from the site of injection into the general circulation reaches the perikaryon of all adrenergic neurons by retrograde axonal transport (Otten et al., 1977; Stoeckel et al., 1976).

By far the weakest link in the chain of arguments favoring the role of NGF as a messenger between effector cells and innervating neurons is the demonstration of the NGF supply by the target organ.

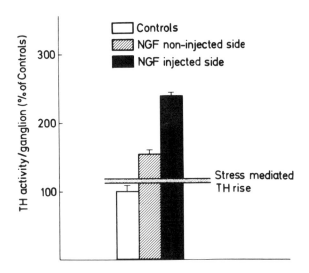

Figure 7. Effect of unilateral injection of 2.5 S NGF into the
anterior eye chamber on TH activity in the superior cervical
ganglion determined 48 h after injection. The "stress-mediated"
increase in TH activity was evaluated by unilateral injection of
cytochrome C, a molecule which has a molecular weight and isoelectrical point very similar to 2.5 S NGF (Paravicini, Stoeckel &
Thoenen, 1975).

This supply could result from the de novo synthesis, activation
from a precursor or storage of NGF (synthesized in remote parts of
the body) in the corresponding effector organs. There are multiple
reasons for the lack of reliable information on this important
aspect. The determination of NGF in effector organs requires very
sensitive assays. Several radioimmunoassays have been developed
(Hendry, 1972; Johnson, Gorden & Kopin, 1971; Murphy et al., 1975)
and subsequently NGF has been reported to be present in almost
every sample tested. However, the interpretation of these data
raises some important problems. First, the range of the published
values not only for tissues but also for serum is impressively
large, ranging in mouse serum from 2 to more than 1000 ng/ml
(Hendry, 1972; Johnson, Gorden & Kopin, 1971). Second, the predicted values do not correlate with those obtained by bioassay,
which are invariably much lower.

These discrepancies may be explained in two ways. First, it
has been shown that the antigen preparation used to raise antibodies is, in some cases, not pure enough in that it contains, in
addition to NGF, mouse γ-globulins which act as very good antigens
(Carstairs et al., 1977). When the serum of the immunized animal

is subsequently used to perform radioimmunoassays, it is therefore possible that the protein actually measured might be something other than NGF, for instance, γ-globulins. Second, it has been known for a long time that NGF is a very "sticky" molecule, i.e., it tends to adsorb to other molecules (Hogue-Angeletti, 1969). Indeed, the proteins contained in tissue homogenate and mammalian serum do adsorb NGF. This can be shown by gel filtration, using iodinated NGF. In the presence of serum protein, for instance, the radioactivity is eluted at molecular weights much higher than that of NGF. A consequence of such an adsorption would be that in single-site radioimmunoassays, where the competition between a given amount of labelled NGF and possible cross-reacting substance is measured, any macromolecule adsorbing labelled NGF would appear as NGF in the sample being assayed. This can be shown in experiments containing detergents, which by reducing unspecific adsorption also reduce the apparent level of NGF (Barde, Suda & Thoenen, unpublished observations).

Finally, the bioassay itself, a very sensitive way to determine NGF levels semi-quantitatively, is subject to pitfalls. For instance, it is known that radial emigration of non-neuronal cells from the dorsal root ganglia can mimic fiber outgrowth (Herrup, Stickgold & Shooter, 1974). In addition, it is possible that agents other than NGF may induce real fiber outgrowth although the features of these fibers are generally different from those induced by NGF (Frazier et al., 1973). Therefore, in the bioassay, as in the radioimmunoassay, very strict criteria have to be employed, the most important here being the blockade of fiber outgrowth by monospecific anti-NGF antibodies.

A further complicating factor in evaluating the production of NGF by effector organs is the fact that the uptake by nerve terminals and the subsequent retrograde axonal transport represents a very efficient mechanism of removal. Thus, the determination of the level of NGF in an effector organ, even if it should be possible in a reliable manner, will provide neither definitive information on the rate of de novo synthesis of NGF, nor information concerning possible formation from a precursor.

Although there is no direct evidence for the physiological role of locally released NGF for the development and maintenance of function of the innervating adrenergic neurons, there is strong indirect evidence for such an action. The treatment of newborn animals with 6-hydroxydopamine or antibodies to NGF results in a destruction of major parts of the peripheral sympathetic nervous system (Levi-Montalcini et al., 1975; Levi-Montalcini & Angeletti, 1968). The former amine has the ability to destroy adrenergic nerve terminals in adult and newborn animals (Levi-Montalcini et al., 1975). However, in newborn animals the destruction of nerve

terminals is followed by degeneration of the corresponding adrenergic cell bodies. Since degeneration of the adrenergic cell bodies
could be prevented by treatment with NGF without preventing the destruction of the nerve terminals, it was suggested that the deleterious effect of 6-hydroxydopamine on adrenergic neurons in newborn animals results from the interruption of the normal supply of
NGF from the periphery by retrograde axonal transport   (Levi-
Montalcini et al., 1975).

     This interpretation is in full agreement with the experiments
of Hendry who showed that axotomy in the early postnatal period also
led to a degeneration of the corresponding cell bodies which could
be prevented by treatment with NGF during the first three postnatal
weeks (Hendry, 1975; Hendry & Campbell, 1976). With increasing age
the irreversible damage of axotomy became gradually smaller and
disappeared about three weeks after birth. This decrease with age
of the irreversible damage due to axotomy is in good agreement with
the decremental effect of NGF antibodies: both axotomy and NGF-
antibodies have only a transient effect in adult animals (Otten,
Goedert & Thoenen, 1977). Interestingly, some important effects of
axotomy can also be largely prevented in adult animals by the administration of NGF. For instance, in guinea pig superior cervical
ganglia, axotomy or local application of colchicine results in an
impairment of ganglionic transmission after preganglionic electrical
stimulation (Purves, 1975, 1976). This impaired transmission is reflected by the morphologically detectable detachment and retraction
of the preganglionic nerve terminals from their postsynaptic counterparts.   Both the morphological and electrophysiological consequences of axotomy can be prevented to a large extent by administra-
tration of NGF (Purves & Nja, 1976) supporting the concept that in
adults as in the neonate, changes in the adrenergic cell body after
axotomy mainly reflect the interruption of the normal supply of NGF
from the periphery.

                GENERAL ASPECTS OF RETROGRADE AXONAL AND
                TRANSSYNAPTIC TRANSPORT OF MACROMOLECULES

           (a) Retrograde Axonal Transport as a Tool to Obtain
           Information on the Composition of the Nerve Terminal
                 Membrane of the Transporting Neurons

     Two groups of macromolecules can be distinguished according to
the efficiency of their retrograde axonal transport. As already
discussed above, for the majority of macromolecules, e.g., horseradish peroxidase, albumin, ferritin, etc., a retrograde axonal
transport can be demonstrated only if they are injected into the
vicinity of nerve terminals in extremely large amounts. It is possible that this non-specific retrograde axonal transport of virtually all macromolecules which reach the synaptic cleft reflects

a "trapping" of these macromolecules during the process of transmitter liberation by exocytosis. In contrast, a few macromolecules
are taken up by nerve terminals and are transported retrogradely if
injected at much lower concentrations. So far, such a selective,
highly specific transport has been found for NGF (MW 26,500), tetanus
toxin (MW 160,000), a non-toxic fragment of the tetanus toxin (MW
46,000), cholera toxin (MW 84,000), the lectins - wheat germ agglutinin (MW 35,000), ricin (MW 60,000), and phytohaemagglutinin (MW
110,000), and for antibodies against DBH (MW 150,000) (Bizzini,
Stoeckel & Schwab, 1977; Fillenz et al., 1976; Hendry et al., 1974;
Stoeckel, Paravicini & Thoenen, 1974; Stoeckel, Schwab & Thoenen,
1975b, 1977; Ziegler, Thomas & Jacobowitz, 1976).

The selectivity of the retrograde axonal transport of these
macromolecules seems to be due to the presence of specific binding
sites for these molecules at the nerve terminal membrane and their
high affinity binding initiating their internalization by a so-
far-unknown mechanism (Schwab & Thoenen, 1977b; Stoeckel, Schwab &
Thoenen, 1977; Dumas et al., in preparation). The causal relationship between the high affinity binding of the ligands to surface
receptors and retrograde transport is also supported by the fact
that the highly efficient retrograde axonal transport of cholera
and tetanus toxin, which occurs in all peripheral neurons studied,
is blocked by the simultaneous injection of gangliosides to which
these two toxins are known to have a high affinity, choleratoxin to
the monosialoganglioside GM_1 and tetanus toxin to the di- and tri-
sialogangliosides GD_{1b} and GT_1 (van Heyningen, 1974; Stoeckel,
Schwab & Thoenen, 1977).

On the other hand, the selective retrograde axonal transport
of NGF is confined to peripheral adrenergic and sensory neurons,
but does not occur in motoneurons (Stoeckel, Schwab & Thoenen,
1975b). This agrees with the fact that high affinity surface receptors for NGF are present only on adrenergic and sensory ganglia
(Banerjee, Cuatrecasas & Snyder, 1976; Herrup, Stickgold & Shooter,
1974). Moreover, oxidation of the tryptophan residues of the NGF
molecule causes a gradual loss of its biological activity as determined in the chick dorsal root assay concomitant with a gradually
decreasing affinity to the binding sites and the disappearance of
retrograde axonal transport (Stoeckel, Paravicini & Thoenen, 1974).
The retrograde axonal transport of DBH-antibodies is confined to
the adrenergic neurons in which DBH is present in the amine storage
vesicles in a soluble and membrane-bound form (Fillenz et al.,
1976). The retrograde axonal transport of DBH supports the suggestion that the vesicular membrane, in consequence of transmitter
liberation by exocytosis, is at least temporarily incorporated into
the cell membrane of the nerve terminal and that DBH becomes accessible to DBH-antibodies as an integral membrane constituent.

The binding concept as a prerequisite for initiation of uptake by nerve terminals and subsequent retrograde axonal transport is also demonstrated by the fact that horseradish peroxidase, a molecule which is not transported in measurable quantities if injected in low concentrations, is transported in relatively high amounts if coupled to biologically active NGF (Schwab, 1977).

The most direct evidence for the importance of high affinity binding to nerve terminals evolves from recent morphological studies in the rat iris. These studies have shown that colloidal gold particles (acting as an electron-dense tracer) coated with tetanus toxin become clearly associated with the neuronal membrane of the nerve terminals followed by internalization and subsequent retrograde axonal transport. In contrast, albumin-coated gold particles were neither associated with neuronal membranes nor taken up by nerve terminals (Schwab & Thoenen, 1977b).

All these data speak strongly in favor of the concept that a high affinity binding is a prerequisite for uptake and retrograde axonal transport. Moreover, since, for many molecules which are transported, their affinity for specific sugars of cell surface membrane glycoproteins or glycolipids is well documented, this offers a unique opportunity to obtain information on the composition of the membrane of the nerve terminals of single species of neurons. It is extremely unlikely that such information could be obtained using contemporary biochemical techniques.

(b)   Transsynaptic Transport of Macromolecules

Electron microscopic autoradiography of rat sympathetic ganglia has shown that after retrograde axonal transport of tetanus toxin to the cell bodies, the statistical distribution of the silver grains over the various subcellular compartments was the same as after retrograde axonal transport of NGF (Figure 5) (Schwab & Thoenen, 1977a). However, in addition in the former case, radioactivity could also be detected inside presynaptic terminals forming contacts with the dendrites and cell bodies of the neurons labelled by retrograde axonal transport. Similar labelled terminals synapsing with labelled motoneurons were found after retrograde transport of ^{125}I-tetanus toxin to the spinal cord (Schwab & Thoenen, 1976). Since the labelling density over the glia was very low in comparison to the extremely high labelling of the presynaptic terminals and since it has been shown that the blood-brain barrier precludes the other routes by which tetanus toxin could reach the cell bodies of the motor cells in the spinal cord, this labelling of the presynaptic terminals suggests a retrograde transsynaptic transfer of tetanus toxin. Surprisingly, this retrograde transsynaptic migration was confined to tetanus toxin and did not occur after retrograde axonal transport of NGF or various lectins in the sympathetic ganglion (Schwab & Thoenen, 1977a; unpublished results). The mechanism of this selective transfer of a macromolecule from post-synaptic to presynaptic structures is still unclear.

So far evidence for a biological significance of the retro-grade axonal transport has been provided for NGF only. However, it seems to be reasonable to assume that the pathway of retrograde axonal transport eventually followed by transsynaptic transfer could have more general implications as a manner of communication between individual neurons and between neurons and non-neuronal cells. Endogenous molecules could carry specific signals from the target cell to the main centers of macromolecular synthesis in the perikaryon of the innervating neuron and even further, transsynap-tically to second order neurons. It is well known from in vivo and tissue culture experiments that general "trophic" influences as well as specific signals are produced by target organs and act on innervating neurons. This aspect has been discussed in more detail in connection with the mechanism and site of action of NGF. How-ever, these retrograde phenomena are not confined to cells sensitive to NGF. Many lines of evidence suggest that the signal for chro-matolysis, i.e., the complex response of the cell body to lesion of its axon, is propagated by retrograde transport (Cragg, 1970).

(c) Pathophysiological and Possible Therapeutic Aspects

The transsynaptic transfer of tetanus toxin following its retrograde axonal transport answers the question how the toxin, which cannot reach the spinal cord across the blood-brain barrier, reaches its site of action, namely the inhibitory nerve terminals ending on spinal cord motoneurons. Electrophysiological and bio-chemical studies have shown earlier that tetanus toxin acts by selectively blocking the release of the inhibitory transmitters glycine and γ-aminobutyric acid (Curtis & DeGroat, 1968; Curtis et al., 1973; Osborne & Bradford, 1973). In addition to tetanus toxin a series of neutrotropic viruses have been shown to reach their targets by retrograde axonal transport (herpes, rabies, pseudo-rabies, possibly poliomyelitis) (Blinzinger & Anzil, 1974; Kristens-son, Gehtti & Wisniewski, 1974; Murphy et al., 1973; Price, Katz & Notkins, 1975; Walz, Price & Notkins, 1974). Both toxins and viruses can reach the central nervous system or peripheral autonomic ganglia from local sites of production or by general distribution via the blood stream by binding to peripheral nerve terminals and subsequent retrograde transport. For the understanding of the mechanism of viral infection and possible specific therapeutic ap-proaches to neurotropic viral disorders it is essential to learn more about the manner of their interaction with the nerve cell mem-brane as a prerequisite of their internalization for subsequent retrograde axonal transport.

In the course of studies with tetanus toxin, a non-toxic fragment of 46,000 has been prepared by Bizzini and coworkers at the Institut Pasteur in Paris (Bizzini, Stoeckel & Schwab, 1977). In spite of the loss of toxicity, the ability to bind to di- and tri-sialogangliosides was fully preserved as was its retrograde axonal transport. Such molecules could be used as carriers for drug molecules which are, per se, active against a specific virus for example but do not reach the site of action in the body. The enrichment of specific binding sites for tetanus toxin in neuronal membranes additionally provides the base for the preparation of a specific neurotropic carrier. Moreover, since carrier-drug complexes will most probably use the same intracellular compartment for retrograde axonal transport as the target virus, this represents a further mechanism of subcellular enrichment with respect to the site of action.

REFERENCES

BANERJEE, S. P., P. CUATRECASAS, and S. H. SNYDER. Solubilization of nerve growth factor receptors of rabbit superior cervical ganglia. *J. Biol. Chem.* 251:5680-5685, 1976.

BIZZINI, B., K. STOECKEL, and M. E. SCHWAB. An antigenic polypeptide fragment isolated from tetanus toxin: Chemical characterization, binding to gangliosides and retrograde axonal transport in various neuron systems. *J. Neurochem.* 28:529-542, 1977.

BJOERKLUND, A., B. BJERRE, and U. STENEVI. Has nerve growth factor a role in the regeneration of central and peripheral catecholamine neurons? In: *Dynamics of Degeneration and Growth in Neurons*, edited by K. Fuxe, L. Olson, and Y. Zotterman. New York: Pergamon Press, 1974, pp. 389-409.

BLINZINGER, K., and A. P. ANZIL. Neuronal route of infection in viral diseases of the central nervous system. *Lancet* 7: 1374-1377, 1974.

BURNSTOCK, G. Degeneration and orientation of growth of autonomic nerves in relation to smooth muscle in joint tissue cultures and anterior eye chamber transplants. In: *Dynamics of Degeneration and Growth in Neurons,* edited by K. Fuxe, L. Olson, and Y. Zotterman. New York: Pergamon Press, 1974, pp. 509-520.

CARSTAIRS, J. R., R. C. EDWARDS, F. L. PEARCE, C. A. VERNON, and S. J. WALTER. Immunogenic contaminants in mouse nerve growth factor. *Eur. J. Biochem.* 77:311-317, 1977.

CRAGG, B. G. What is the signal for chromatolysis? *Brain Res.* 23:1-21, 1970.

CURTIS, D. R., and W. C. DeGROAT. Tetanus toxin and spinal inhibition. *Brain Res.* 10:208-212, 1968.

CURTIS, D. R., D. FELIX, C.J.A. GAME, and R. M. McCULLOCH. Tetanus toxin and the synaptic release of GABA. *Brain Res.* 51:358-362, 1973.

FILLENZ, M., C. GAGNON, K. STOECKEL, and H. THOENEN. Selective uptake and retrograde axonal transport of dopamine β-hydroxylase antibodies in peripheral adrenergic neurons. *Brain Res.* 114:293-303, 1976.

FRAZIER, W. A., C. E. OHLENDORF, L. F. BOYD, L. ALOE, E. M. JOHNSON, J. A. FERRENDELL, and R. A. BRADSHAW. Mechanism of action of nerve growth factor and cyclic AMP on neurite outgrowth in embryonic chick sensory ganglia: Demonstration of independent pathways of stimulation. *Proc. Natl. Acad. Sci. US* 70:2448-2452, 1973.

HAMBURGER, V. The effects of wing bud extirpation on the development of the central nervous system in chick embryos. *J. Exptl. Biol.* 68:449-494, 1938.

HENDRY, I. A. Developmental changes in tissue and plasma concentrations of the biologically active species of nerve growth factor in the mouse by using a two-site radioimmunoassay. *Biochem. J.* 128:1265-1272, 1972.

HENDRY, I. A. The response of adrenergic neurons to axotomy and nerve growth factor. *Brain Res.* 94:87-97, 1975.

HENDRY, I. A. Control in the development of the vertebrate sympathetic nervous system. In: *Reviews of Neuroscience.* New York: Raven Press, 1976, vol. 2, pp. 149-194.

HENDRY, I. A., and J. CAMPBELL. Morphometric analysis of rat superior cervical ganglion after axotomy and nerve growth factor treatment. *J. Neurocytol.* 5:351-360, 1976.

HENDRY, I. A., and L. L. IVERSEN. Reduction in the concentration of nerve growth factor in mice after sialectomy and castration. *Nature* 243:500-504, 1973.

HENDRY, I. A., K. STOECKEL, H. THOENEN, and L. L. IVERSEN. The retrograde axonal transport of nerve growth factor. *Brain Res.* 68:103-121, 1974.

HERRUP, K., R. STICKGOLD, and E. M. SHOOTER. The role of the nerve
  growth factor in the development of sensory and sympathetic
  ganglion. *Ann. N. Y. Acad. Sci.* 228:381-392, 1974.

HEYNINGEN, W. E. VAN. Gangliosides as membrane receptors for
  tetanus toxin, cholera toxin and serotonin. *Nature* 249:
  415-417, 1974.

HOGUE-ANGELETTI, R. Nerve growth factor (NGF) from snake venom and
  mouse submaxillary gland: Interaction with serum proteins.
  Brain Res. 12:234-247, 1969.

IVERSEN, L. L., K. STOECKEL, and H. THOENEN. Autoradiographic
  studies of the retrograde axonal transport of nerve growth
  factor in mouse sympathetic neurons. *Brain Res.* 88:37-43,
  1975.

JOHNSON, R. G., R. GORDEN, and I. J. KOPIN. A sensitive radioimmunoassay for 7S nerve growth factor antigens in serum and
  tissues. *J. Neurochem.* 18:2355-2362, 1971.

KRISTENSSON, K., B. GEHTTI, and H. M. WISNIEWSKI. Study of the
  propagation of herpes simplex virus (type 2) into the brain
  after intraocular injection. *Brain Res.* 69:189-202, 1974.

LEVI-MONTALCINI, R., L. ALOE, E. MUGNAINI, F. OESCH, and H.
  THOENEN. Nerve growth factor induces volume increase and
  enhances tyrosine hydroxylase synthesis in chemically axoto-
  mized sympathetic ganglia of newborn rats. *Proc. Natl. Acad.
  Sci. US* 72:595-599, 1975.

LEVI-MONTALCINI, R., and P. U. ANGELETTI. Nerve growth factor.
  Physiol. Rev. 48:534-569, 1968.

MURPHY, F. A., S. P. BAUER, A. K. HARRISON, and W. C. WINN, Jr.
  Comparative pathogenesis of rabies and rabies-like viruses.
  Viral infection and transit from inoculation site to the
  central nervous system. *Lab. Invest.* 28:361-376, 1973.

MURPHY, R. A., N. Z. PANTAZIS, B.G.W. ARNASON, and M. YOUNG.
  Secretion of a nerve growth factor by mouse neuroblastoma
  cells in culture. *Proc. Natl. Acad. Sci. US* 72:1895-1898,
  1975.

OLSON, L., and T. MALMFORS. Growth characteristics of adrenergic
  nerves in the adult rat. *Acta Physiol. Scand. Suppl.* 348:
  1-112, 1970.

OSBORNE, R. H., and H. F. BRADFORD. Tetanus toxin inhibits amino
  acid release from nerve endings in vitro. *Nature New Biol.*
  244:157-158, 1973.

OTTEN, U., M. GOEDERT, and H. THOENEN. Role of nerve growth factor
    for development and maintenance of function of sympathetic
    neurons and adrenal medullary cells. In: *Proc. Satellite
    Symp. Inter. Soc. Neurochem., Saint-Vincent, Italy*. Basel:
    Karger S. A., 1977, in press.

OTTEN, U., M. SCHWAB, C. GAGNON, and H. THOENEN. Selective induc-
    tion of tyrosine hydroxylase and dopamine β-hydroxylase by
    nerve growth factor: Comparison between adrenal medulla and
    sympathetic ganglia of adult and newborn rats. *Brain Res*.
    133:291-303, 1977.

PARAVICINI, U., K. STOECKEL, and H. THOENEN. Biological importance
    of retrograde axonal transport of nerve growth factor in
    adrenergic neurons. *Brain Res*. 84:279-291, 1975.

PRICE, R. W., B. J. KATZ, and A. L. NOTKINS. Latent infection of
    the peripheral ANS with herpes simplex virus. *Nature* 257:
    686-688, 1975.

PURVES, D. Functional and structural changes in mammalian sympa-
    thetic neurones following interruption of their axons. *J.
    Physiol*. 252:429-463, 1975.

PURVES, D. Functional and structural changes in mammalian sympa-
    thetic neurones following colchicine application to post-
    ganglionic nerves. *J. Physiol*. 259:159-175, 1976.

PURVES, D., and A. NJA. Effect of nerve growth factor on synaptic
    depression after axotomy. *Nature* 260:535-536, 1976.

SCHWAB, M. E. Ultrastructural localization of a nerve growth fac-
    tor - horseradish peroxidase (NGF-HRP) coupling product after
    retrograde axonal transport in adrenergic neurons. *Brain Res*.
    130:190-196, 1977.

SCHWAB, M. E., and H. THOENEN. Electron microscopic evidence for a
    transsynaptic migration of tetanus toxin in spinal cord moto-
    neurons: An autoradiographic and morphometric study. *Brain
    Res*. 105:213-227, 1976.

SCHWAB, M. E., and H. THOENEN. Selective transsynaptic migration
    of tetanus toxin after retrograde axonal transport in periph-
    eral sympathetic nerves: A comparison with nerve growth factor.
    Brain Res. 122:459-474, 1977a.

SCHWAB, M. E., and H. THOENEN. Selective binding, uptake and retro-
    grade transport of tetanus toxin by nerve terminals in the rat
    iris. *J. Cell Biol*. 1977b, in press.

STOECKEL, K., G. GUROFF, M. SCHWAB, and H. THOENEN. The significance of retrograde axonal transport for the accumulation of systemically administered nerve growth factor (NGF) in the rat superior cervical ganglion. *Brain Res.* 109:271-284, 1976.

STOECKEL, K., U. PARAVICINI, and H. THOENEN. Specificity of the retrograde axonal transport of nerve growth factor. *Brain Res.* 76:413-421, 1974.

STOECKEL, K., M. SCHWAB, and H. THOENEN. Specificity of retrograde transport of nerve growth factor (NGF) in sensory neurons: A biochemical and morphological study. *Brain Res.* 89:1-14, 1975a.

STOECKEL, K., M. SCHWAB, and H. THOENEN. Comparison between the retrograde axonal transport of nerve growth factor and tetanus toxin in motor, sensory and adrenergic neurons. *Brain Res.* 99:1-16, 1975b.

STOECKEL, K., M. E. SCHWAB, and H. THOENEN. Role of gangliosides in the uptake and retrograde axonal transport of cholera and tetanus toxin as compared to nerve growth factor and wheat germ agglutinin. *Brain Res.* 132:273-285, 1977.

STOECKEL, K., and H. THOENEN. Specificity and biological importance of retrograde axonal transport of nerve growth factor. In: *Proc. Sixth Inter. Congr. Pharm., Helsinki, Finland,* edited by J. Tuomisto and M. K. Paasonen. New York: Pergamon Press, 1975, vol. II, pp. 285-296.

THOENEN, H., P. U. ANGELETTI, R. LEVI-MONTALCINI, and R. KETTLER. Selective induction of tyrosine hydroxylase and dopamine β-hydroxylase in the rat superior cervical ganglia by nerve growth factor. *Proc. Natl. Acad. Sci. US* 68:1598-1602, 1971.

THOENEN, H., and U. OTTEN. Molecular events in transsynaptic regulation of the synthesis of macromolecules. In: *Essays in Neurochemistry and Neuropharmacology,* edited by M.B.H. Youdim, W. Lovenberg, D. F. Sharman, and J. R. Lagnado. New York: J. Wiley & Sons Ltd., 1976, vol. 1, pp. 73-101.

THOENEN, H., U. OTTEN, and F. OESCH. Axoplasmic transport of enzymes involved in the synthesis of noradrenaline: Relationship between the rate of the transport and subcellular distribution. *Brain Res.* 62:471-475, 1973.

WALZ, M. A., R. W. PRICE, and A. L. NOTKINS. Latent ganglionic
    infection with herpes simplex virus types 1 and 2: Viral
    reactivation in vivo after neurectomy. *Science* 184:1185-
    1187, 1974.

ZIEGLER, M. G., J. A. THOMAS, and D. M. JACOBOWITZ. Retrograde
    axonal transport of antibody to dopamine β-hydroxylase.
    Brain Res. 104:390-395, 1976.

DISCUSSION AND SHORT REPORTS ON AXONAL TRANSPORT

Johan Sjöstrand, Initiator of Discussion

DR. JOHAN SJÖSTRAND: Before presenting my report, I would
like to ask for questions and comments concerning anterograde and
retrograde transport.

DR. KORR: A question for Dr. Samson. In that beautiful film
on axoplasmic transport, all the movement of the organelles seems
to be retrograde. They are returning, presumably, from the endings. Why don't we see the motion that brought them there in the
first place?

DR. SAMSON: I think you have to remember that you are looking through a special window in both instances, with the radioactive labeling of proteins, and now the visual viewing of objects
under the microscope. The visual microscope will show only certain
large particles, and when you use this window, most of the traffic
is going retrograde. However, the comment is made in the film that
probably there was more anterograde traffic, but it was not visible
to them. Now, the origin of that retrograde traffic is probably
mixed: things that may be returning in larger aggregate than came
down anterograde; things that may have actually been generated out
at the terminals; and then, thirdly, the kind of materials that may
be taken up into lysosome-like structures that Dr. Thoenen referred
to, that might now be a little more visible than the original structure would be, going downstream.

DR. KORR: But then the implication is that the mitochondria,
for example, are assembled in the endings.

DR. SAMSON: I think you have to remember that you are looking
at a very small spatial feature, and that it would be hard to know
what the net direction of mitochondria would be under these kinds
of observations.

DR. COOTE: I would like to ask Dr. Samson or Dr. Thoenen whether activity of the neurons influences axoplasmic flow of material at all, in either direction?

DR. SAMSON: I think that Dr. Worth is going to have some data on that, so why don't we save that question.

DR. OTTO APPENZELLER: There is some clinical evidence that in tetanus there is an excessive discharge of autonomic neurons. Johnson and Spalding published in the *Lancet* some years ago a paper showing that there are bursts of hypertension and bursts of sweating that cannot be related to anything else except to an excessive unrestrained discharge of autonomic neurons.   I think your work, showing that tetanus toxin is also taken up by sympathetic neurons and goes across the synaptic cleft in those structures, is pertinent to this clinical observation, which heretofore had been difficult to explain.

DR. THOENEN: Yes, I absolutely agree.   I think that tetanus toxin is transported so far in any single neuron we have investigated--not only the periphery, but also in the central nervous system.   And, just to mention an interesting little story.   We thought it would be nice to study the transport of tetanus toxin in the in vitro system.   We set up a frog system, and it didn't work at all.   When we went back to the literature, we found that frogs are not susceptible to tetanus toxin, and that solved the mystery.

DR. STEPHEN BRIMIJOIN: I wonder if Dr. Thoenen has identified any fragments of the tetanus toxin molecule which are taken up by the neurons and carried back to the cell body but not transferred across the next synapse, into the presynaptic nerve terminal.   Have you identified any fragments that behave in that way?   You mentioned a nontoxic fragment that was taken up.   I wonder if you have been able to separate not just the toxicity but this special property of being able to jump synapses.

DR. THOENEN: The fragment we have isolated also goes across the synapse.   But these are not "natural" fragments; you have to split them off proteolytically.   Certainly, we cannot trace every single molecule, but more than 95% of the radioactivity travels with the original tetanus toxin.   So we know that the presynaptic terminals are reached by intact tetanus toxin.

DR. BRIMIJOIN: I raise this question because one of the nicest demonstrations where retrograde transport and transsynaptic transfer are involved in the toxicity of tetanus would be to identify a subfragment which is toxic when applied to the spinal cord, but which is nontoxic when confined to the periphery, because it isn't able to make this jump to the receptors.

DR. THOENEN: Well, this dissociation is not possible so far.

DR. SJÖSTRAND: I would like to ask a question before we start discussion of the impairment of axonal transport. In one of your slides, Dr. Thoenen, you indicated that the transport was within the smooth axoplasmic reticulum, whereas in the anterograde transport system, many people have argued that it is associated with the microtubules. Do you have any indication that different transport mechanisms are involved and, therefore, that some trauma or some pathophysiological factor could affect the two systems differently?

DR. THOENEN: I would say "no" because from the experiments of Bernard Droz, the retrograde system, as far as you can trace it, is associated with endoplasmic reticulum. To my mind, there is no direct association with the microtubules--maybe Sidney Ochs will tell us more about it--but you need an intact microtubule system for both anterograde and retrograde transport. The question is, what is the connection between the microtubules and the sacs of endoplasmic reticulum which obviously contain the molecules? There must be some kind of association of the transported molecules with the membrane, because, if you imagine the affinity constants of an antibody to an antigen, you have an affinity constant of 10 at least, or 11, or even more. So I think there is little chance that they are only swimming around in this sac. As for the microtubules, I think they provide the railroad track for the anterograde and the retrograde transport, and that the endoplasmic reticulum sacs are the carriers. I think that Sidney's research will provide us very soon the machine which is moving the whole thing. Would you agree that this view is reasonable?

DR. SIDNEY OCHS: I am very happy to agree with that point.

DR. SJÖSTRAND: I think we have time for one final question, before we start out with the impairment section, and then we can return to these papers.

DR. LYNNE WEAVER: I am not sure to whom to address my question, so I'll just pose it generally. Is there a reported action of prostaglandins on the rate of axoplasmic transport? The reason I am asking is because there is some recent work, as yet unpublished, regarding water reabsorption in the collecting duct of the kidney, which is beginning to show that an action of prostaglandins mediated through calcium influences microfilament aggregation, which then ultimately leads to differences in permeability between cells. And it would be an interesting corollary if there were some action of prostaglandins on microfilaments in neurons, which had something to do with the reported ability of prostaglandins to modulate neural activities and neural transmissions.

DR. SJÖSTRAND: Dr. Thoenen, would you answer?

DR. THOENEN: I think you know more about it. One has to be very careful to distinguish between the rate of transport and the amount of material transported. And several reports have shown that lowering the calcium concentration affects not the rate of anterograde transport, but the quantity. So that calcium could be involved in the linking of the molecules which are transported to the carrier, but the linear rate is a different thing. I can speak only for the retrograde transport in a given neuron and I have to answer, first, that prostaglandins might in this manner indirectly affect the amount which is transported. I don't know about the rate.

On the other hand, this is something that I have to emphasize: For a given neuron, the rate of transport of all the molecules is always the same. But it is different from one neuron to the other. For instance, in the rat, for the adrenergic neurons it is about 2 to 3 mm/h, in the sensory neurons it is 12 to 15 mm/h and in the motor neurons, it is about 7 mm/h. We have the impression that it is high-affinity, specific binding sites on the surface which are the requirements for internalization, but this is still under in-vestigation. We don't know whether or what kind of cross-linkage is involved. But then, all the molecules are handed over, obvi-ously, to a common carrier, because as I have shown you, the nerve growth factors linked to horseradish peroxidase, toluidine to tetanus toxin, and as in the simpler and more elegant method with coated gold particles -- are also transported at the same rate.

IMPAIRMENT OF INTRANEURAL MICROCIRCULATION, BLOOD-NERVE BARRIER AND AXONAL TRANSPORT IN EXPERIMENTAL NERVE ISCHEMIA AND COMPRESSION

J. Sjöstrand[1,3], B. Rydevik[2], G. Lundborg[2,4], and

W. G. McLean[5]

Studies on experimental ischemia and compression of peripheral nerves are reviewed. It is concluded that any trauma to a nerve trunk may induce microvascular injury in the nerve. A slight trauma may cause epineurial micro-bleedings, oedema, etc. Severe trauma, e.g., prolonged experimental tourniquet ischemia or compression, involves injury to endoneurial capillaries (blood-nerve barrier) leading to intrafascicular oedema. The establishment of post-ischemic or post-traumatic interfascicular oedema coincides in time with severe disturbances in nerve function.

In other studies graded compression was applied directly to exposed nerve trunks by means of a "mini-cuff". It was found that 2 h of compression with 200 to 400 mm Hg induced break-down of the blood-nerve barrier. Local nerve compression with pressures of 50 to 400 mm Hg acutely blocked anterograde axonal transport in sensory vagal fibers. Reversal of transport blockade generally occurred within a day after compression at 50 mm Hg; with higher pressures recovery occurred in most cases within one week. The duration of the transport blocks was related to the magnitude of the pressures applied.

---

[1]Institute of Neurobiology, Fack, S-400 33 Göteborg 33, Sweden.
[2]Laboratory of Experimental Biology, Department of Anatomy.
[3]Department of Ophthalmology.
[4]Division of Hand Surgery, Department of Orthopaedic Surgery I
[5]University of Göteborg, Göteborg, Sweden.
Department of Pharmacology, School of Pharmacy, Liverpool Polytechnic, Liverpool, England.

INTRODUCTION

The peripheral nerve is a complex structure composed of nerve
fibers as well as supporting connective tissue elements constituted
by the epi-, peri- and endoneurium. Consequently, trauma to a
nerve not only affects the nerve fibers, but also the cell and vascular components of the intraneural connective tissue. The intraneural microvessels respond readily to trauma by increasing their
permeability, and oedema formation in the epineurium may be an
early indication of nerve injury.

Interference with intraneural blood flow may have varying consequences for nerve function, depending on the degree of ischemia
induced. Proper nerve function requires a continuous supply of
oxygen by the endoneurial capillaries, and total ischemia is followed by deterioration of impulse transmission within 30 to 90 min
(Gerard, 1930; Lehmann, 1937; Lundborg, 1970). However, if the
intraneural blood flow is then re-established, recovery of nerve
function follows the restoration of the blood flow (Lundborg, 1970).

A slight trauma, e.g., moderate compression, might induce
microvascular injury, limited to the superficial layers of the
nerve, as indicated by microbleedings and oedema formation in the
epineurium. The fascicles are embedded in loose epineurial connective tissue and their contents are protected by the strong
perineurial membrane which acts as a diffusion barrier to macromolecules such as proteins (Martin, 1964; Olsson et al., 1971;
Shanta, 1968). Thus, an epineurial oedema cannot penetrate an intact perineurium and reach the endoneurial space, but if such an
oedema becomes long-standing it might be transferred into epineurial scar tissue with secondary constrictive effects on the
fascicles.

A severe trauma may involve injury also to the intrafascicular
capillaries. The endothelium of these vessels normally constitutes
a blood-nerve barrier in correspondence to the blood-brain barrier
of the central nervous system (Olsson et al., 1971; Waksman, 1961).
The local environment of the endoneurial space is normally controlled by the joint action of this blood-nerve barrier and the
perineurial barrier, and derangement of one or both of these barriers, as observed after experimental mechanical, ischemic and
chemical trauma (Lundborg, 1970; Mellick & Cavanagh, 1967; Olsson,
1966; Olsson et al., 1971; Olsson & Kristensson, 1973; Rydevik et
al., 1976; Rydevik & Lundborg, 1977) might have serious consequences
also for the nerve function.

Within the axons there is a continuous transport of macromolecules and organelles both from the cell body to the synaptic
terminals and in a retrograde direction (for review, see Lubińska,
1975; Ochs, 1975). Recent studies have demonstrated that axonal

transport is partially or completely blocked by local ischemia or compression (Andersson & Hendrickson, 1974; Levy, 1974; Minckler et al., 1976; Ochs, 1974; Quigley & Anderson, 1976); a local supply of energy is needed to support the axonal transport.

Thus, interference with intraneural microvascular flow might compromise the excitability of nerve fibers, as well as the axonal transport. As compression of a nerve trunk might involve oblitera-tion of intraneural vessels and mechanical deformation of nerve fibers, it might be difficult or impossible to separate the vascu-lar and mechanical factors respectively in various compression lesions of peripheral nerves. While the mechanical deformation of nerve fibers has been put forward as a principal factor in severe compression lesions, induced under pneumatic cuffs around extremi-ties (Fowler et al., 1972), the vascular factor was stressed in the etiology of the carpal tunnel syndrome by Sunderland (1976).

The aim of this presentation is to give some current aspects on how the peripheral nerve might respond to experimental trauma, and to present some data from our own experiments on the effects of ischemia and local graded compression on intraneural microcircula-tion, blood-nerve barrier and axonal transport.

METHODS

Rabbits of both sexes were used. The animals were anesthetized by intravenous injection of 25 to 30 mg/kg body weight of sodium pentobarbital (Nembutal[R]) into a marginal ear vein. Additional doses of the anesthetic were given, when necessary, to maintain sufficient depth of anesthesia.

The tibial nerve was used for the study of intraneural micro-circulation and nerve barriers (Lundborg & Brånemark, 1968; Lund-borg, 1970; Lundborg & Rydevik, 1973; Rydevik & Lundborg, 1977). This nerve contains both sensory and motor fibers, it is multi-fascicular and can easily be exposed 2 cm proximal to the ankle. The cervical vagus nerve was used for axonal transport analyses (McLean et al., 1976; Rydevik et al., 1977).

Ischemia was induced in the hind limb of rabbits by applying a small pneumatic tourniquet around the thigh; the cuff was inflated with air, so that the blood flow to the distal parts of the limb was totally arrested (Lundborg, 1970). After various periods up to 10 h, the tourniquet was removed and the recovery of intraneural microcirculation, permeability of intraneural microvessels and perineurial sheath and nerve function were analysed.

In other experiments local, graded compression was applied to
the tibial and vagus nerves with a specially designed chamber made
of Plexiglas and rubber membranes (Rydevik & Lundborg, 1977;
Rydevik et al., 1977). This chamber was placed around the nerve
and connected to a pressure system. By varying the pressure in the
chamber (50-200-400 mm Hg) and the time of application, the nerves
could be subjected to graded, controlled compression injuries. Following release of the compression, permeability of the microvessels
and perineurium as well as axonal transport were analysed up to
14 days after the injury.

Intraneural Microcirculation

The tibial nerve was transilluminated by a quartz glass rod
and the intraneural circulation in various experimental situations
was analysed in a modified Leitz intravital microscope (Lundborg,
1970; Lundborg & Brånemark, 1968) (Figure 1). Low voltage xenon
lamps provided the source of light. Heat absorbing filters were
used to minimize any increase in local tissue temperature. In addition, the studies were performed in the green part of the
spectrum at about 5000 Å.

Permeability of Intraneural Blood Microvessels
and Perineurial Sheath

The permeability of intraneural microvessels was analysed by
fluorescent microscopic tracing of intravenously injected albumin
labelled with Evans blue, according to Steinwall and Klatzo (1965)

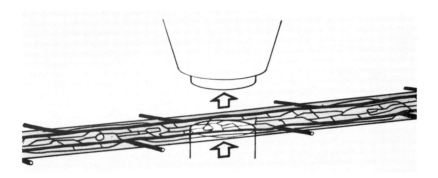

Figure 1. Schematic representation of vital microscopic observation
of intraneural microcirculation. Here the regional vascular supply
of the nerve has been excluded. (From Lundborg, 1970, by kind permission of the editor of *Scand. J. Plast. Reconstr. Surg.*)

and Olsson (1968).   The solution was prepared by mixing 5% bovine
albumin with 1% Evans blue.   The standard dose of the solution here
called EBA, was 1 ml/100 g body weight.   The EBA conjugate was slowly
injected into an ear vein.   Thirty minutes later, the animals were
sacrificed by an overdose of anesthetic.   Specimens from the nerve
were removed and fixed in 4% buffered formaldehyde for 24 h.   Frozen
longitudinal sections were mounted in 50% aqueous glycerine and immediately examined in a Leitz fluorescence microscope equipped with
an Osram HBO 200 high-pressure mercury lamp (Figure 2a).   The filters
used were BG 12/3 mm as excitation filter and K 510 as barrier filter.
Under these conditions the EBA complex can easily be traced by its
red fluorescence.   Photographic recordings were made with a Leitz
Orthomat microscope camera and Kodak Ektachrome high-speed film.

The barrier function of the perineurial sheath after the various experimental procedures was investigated by applying the Evans
blue-albumin conjugate locally around the nerve in situ.   After 2 h
of contact between the nerve and the conjugate, the animals were
sacrificed and specimens were removed from the test segment of the
nerve.   Fluorescent microscopic tracing of the distribution of the
EBA complex was performed by the method described above.

Nerve Function

Impulse conduction capacities after ischemia and compression
were tested with neurophysiological techniques.   The tibial nerve
was stimulated distally with two electrodes carefully placed
around the nerve trunk.   The recording electrodes were placed
proximally at various levels of the nerve trunk depending on the
experimental procedure (Lundborg, 1970; Rydevik et al., 1976).
Compound action potentials were recorded by a differential pre-
amplifier connected to a cathode ray oscilloscope (Tektronix 502).

Axonal Transport

The nodose ganglion of the vagus nerve was gently exposed and
20 µl (100 µCi) of ^{3}H-leucine in 0.9% NaCl (L-4.5 ^{3}H-leucine,
58 Ci/mmol, Radiochemical Centre, Amersham, England) was injected
sub-epineurially into the nodose ganglion through a 30-gauge stain-
less steel needle.   The fast axonal transport of ^{3}H-labelled proteins
along the cervical vagus nerve was measured as described previously
(McLean et al., 1976) and the effect of local compression (see above)
was studied.   In acute experiments (i.e., without recovery from
compression) vagus nerves were compressed 2 h after labelling with
^{3}H-leucine; in others, recovery from compression of up to 14 days
was allowed before the ganglia were labelled.

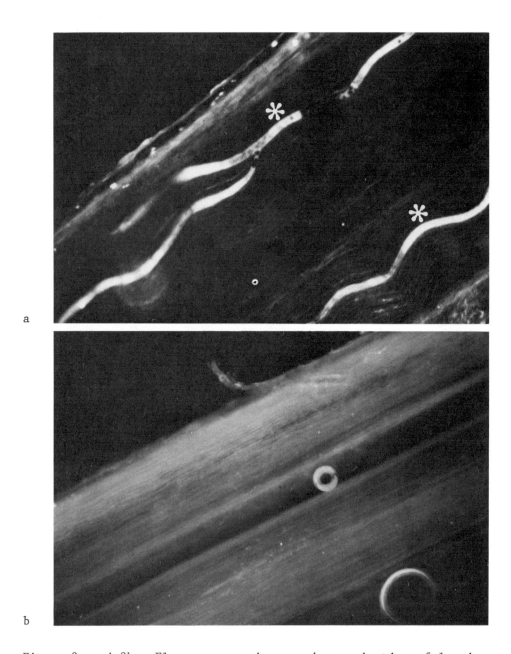

Figure 2a and 2b. Fluorescence microscopic examination of longitudinal sections of rabbit tibial nerve. Evans-Blue-albumin (EBA)
has been injected 30 min prior to removal of specimens. a: Control
nerve. Two fascicles are shown. The red-fluorescent EBA-complex

(Legend continued to next page.)

In all experiments, the animals were killed 4 h after injection of isotope. The nodose ganglion and the cervical vagus nerve were rapidly dissected out and placed on ice. The nerve was then cut into 2.5 mm pieces and these were transferred individually to 2 ml 10% trichloracetic acid (TCA) for 24 h at 4°C. The nerve pieces were washed once in cold TCA, dissolved in Soluene[R] (Packard) and measured in Permablend[R] (Packard) scintillation fluid in a Packard Tricarb liquid scintillation spectrometer with automatic quenching (for details, see McLean et al., 1976).

RESULTS AND DISCUSSION

Vascularization of Peripheral Nerves

Most studies on the vascularization of peripheral nerves have been performed with injection techniques. In these studies the vascular system has been perfused with various dyes, plastics, silicone rubber or contrast media (Adams, 1942; Blunt, 1957; Edshage, 1964; Lundborg, 1970; Smith, 1966a). These methods often give a good picture of the architecture of the intraneural microvascular bed (Figure 3), but they do not give a true picture of the hemodynamics and intraneural microvascular flow patterns. However, recently Lundborg et al. have used vital microscopic technique in order to analyse intraneural microvascular flow patterns in vivo under various experimental conditions (Figure 1) (Lundborg, 1970; Lundborg & Brånemark, 1968; Lundborg & Rydevik, 1973).

In these studies the existence of two integrated but functionally independent microvascular systems, the extrinsic and intrinsic systems, has been verified. The extrinsic system consists of vessels approaching the nerve trunk segmentally along its course, usually in a "mesoneurium". These vessels originate from adjacent arteries and veins, and they usually have a coiled appearance with great reserve in length, thus allowing considerable changes in position of the nerve before the vessels become stretched and the blood flow impaired. When these local nutrient vessels reach the

---

(here: white) has perfused endoneurial capillaries x). The dye is strictly confined to the lumina of these vessels which contrast distinctly to the green nerve tissue (here: greyish-black). b: Tibial nerve after 8 h ischemia followed by EBA-injection. The ischemia has induced increased permeability of the endoneurial capillaries leading to the formation of intrafascicular oedema. This is indicated by the diffuse orange-red fluorescence (here: white) in the endoneurial space.

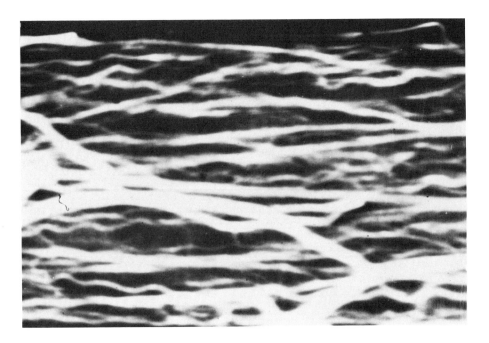

Figure 3. Microangiographic appearance of a segment of rabbit's tibial nerve. The vascular system of the nerve has been perfused with X-ray contrast medium (for details see Lundborg, 1970),

epineurium, they divide into ascending and descending branches, thereby contributing to the intrinsic system.

The vessels in the epineurium, predominantly of venular type, frequently communicate with those in the perineurium and the endo-neurium. The endoneurial vascular bed consists mainly of capillaries running parallel with the long axis of the nerve. The intrafascicular vessels communicate with those located extrafascicularly by numerous anastomoses, which often pierce the perineurial membrane obliquely.

Effects of Mobilization, Transsection and Stretching on Intraneural Microcirculation

If a nerve trunk is mobilized and its regional, extrinsic vessels thereby excluded, the quality of the intraneural microcirculation depends on the capacity of the intrinsic longitudinal collateral vessels. The significance of these collaterals has been

discussed extensively in the literature and some authors have claimed
that nerves can be mobilized over long distances with no or only
minimal interference with their function (Adams, 1943; Bentley &
Schlapp, 1943a; Denny-Brown & Brenner, 1944; Kline et al., 1972),
while others have stressed the importance of the extrinsic vessels
(Causey & Stratman, 1953; Okada, 1905; Smith, 1966b).

In our vital microscopic experiments it was found very difficult
to impair the intraneural microcirculation by excluding the extrinsic
vascular supply; the whole tibial-sciatic nerve (width 1.5 mm and
length 15 cm) could be mobilized without any visible disturbances of
its microvascular flow in the middle of the nerve (Lundborg, 1970)
(Figure 1).

Severance of the tibial nerve did not seem to affect the intraneural microcirculation, not even most terminally in the cut end
where a mainly normal capillary circulation could be observed
(Lundborg, 1970).

However, when stretching was applied to the cut nerve, its
microcirculation was impaired over a long distance at a relatively
moderate degree of tension (Figure 4). With increasing tension the
intraneural microcirculation was gradually compromised. The first
signs of circulatory disturbances appeared at 8% elongation and at
15% there was a total standstill of blood flow in all intraneural

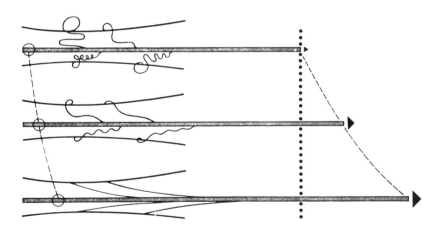

Figure 4. Various degrees of tension applied to a nerve trunk.
With increasing tension the extrinsic vessels are stretched and
finally strangulated. (From Lundborg, 1970, by kind permission of
the editor of *Scand J. Plast. Reconstr. Surg.*)

microvessels (Lundborg & Rydevik, 1973). However, if the tension
was then released the intraneural circulation rapidly recovered.

Effects of Ischemia and Compression on Intraneural
Microcirculation and Blood-Nerve Barrier

Ischemia of peripheral nerve tissue can be seen in various
clinical situations. Severe trauma to a limb, for example, may disrupt major blood vessels, which may render all the tissues in the
extremity ischemic for a long period until the blood flow is restored. Surgery in extremities is routinely performed in a blood-
free field, achieved by arresting the blood flow to the limb by a
pneumatic tourniquet. This procedure facilitates the surgical
dissections, but it can, under certain circumstances, be harmful
to the nerve and muscle structures in the limb (Dahlback, 1970;
Lundborg, 1972; Moldaver, 1954; Rudge, 1974; Solonen and Hjelt,
1968). The relative importance of ischemia and compression from
the cuff, respectively, for the occurrence of nerve lesion after
tourniquet application has been extensively discussed (Bentley &
Schlapp, 1943b; Denny-Brown & Brenner, 1944; Fowler et al., 1972;
Lundborg, 1970, 1972, 1975). Critical limits for time of ischemia
and degree of pressure in the cuff are, however, still open to
discussion.

In addition to these acute compression lesions, peripheral
nerves may also be subjected to more long-standing compression in
association with various entrapment syndromes. The role of ischemia and compression, respectively, in the carpal tunnel syndrome
has recently been extensively discussed by Sunderland (1976). Also
nerve roots can be expected to suffer from chronic compression in
association with certain degenerative conditions in the cervical
and lumbar spine, as reactive changes in the vertebrae could
diminish the diameter of the intervertebral foramina. Herniations
of intervertebral discs may, among other effects, also mechanically
compress the nerve root in question.

The Ischemic Factor. The effects of ischemia, induced in
rabbit's hind limb by a pneumatic cuff, were analysed by Lundborg
(1970, 1975) with special reference to intraneural microcirculation,
oedema formation and nerve function. The nerves investigated were
the tibial nerve (situated distal to the cuff and subjected to
ischemia only) and the sciatic nerve (subjected also to compression
of the cuff). The findings in the tibial nerve illustrate the
ischemic factor in the development of nerve injury after prolonged
circulatory arrest. Two, four and six hours of ischemia was followed by a rapid restoration of intraneural microvascular blood
flow. Even after eight and ten hours of ischemia there was an
immediate recovery of blood flow in the major part of the microvessels in the nerve.

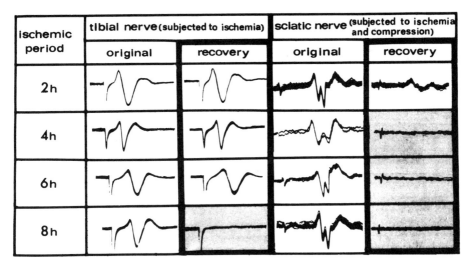

ischemic period	tibial nerve (subjected to ischemia)		sciatic nerve (subjected to ischemia and compression)	
	original	recovery	original	recovery
2h				
4h				
6h				
8h				

Figure 5. Diagram on effects of ischemia and compression on nerve function in experiments with a tourniquet. In the tibial nerve (situated distal to the cuff) nerve function did not recover after 8 h ischemia, while there was no return of function after as little as 4 h in the sciatic nerve (situated at the level of the cuff). The occurrence of persistent loss of nerve function corresponded well to the establishment of endoneurial oedema, which is indicated by grey colour in the diagram. (From Lundborg, 1970, by kind permission of the editor of *Scand. J. Plast. Reconstr. Surg.*)

The analysis of the permeability of the endoneurial micro-vessels revealed that not even 6 h ischemia gave an ischemic injury to the walls of these vessels, prominent enough to give leakage of albumin. However, following restoration of flow after 8 to 10 h ischemia there was a marked oedema in the endoneurial space as a result of anoxic injury to the vascular endothelium (Figure 2b).

After 6 h ischemia there was a rapid restoration of the conduction capacity of the tibial nerve, while there was no return of nerve function after 8 to 10 h of ischemia (Figure 5). Thus, the establishment of a post-ischemic endoneurial oedema corresponded well to a persistent loss of nerve function.

An intrafascicular oedema alters the local environment of the axons by deranging the ionic balance. The oedema may also, because of the unyielding properties of the perineurial membrane, increase the intrafascicular pressure, leading to further impairment of the intrafascicular microcirculation. Moreover, a long-standing oedema might be invaded by fibroblasts and transferred to an endoneurial fibrotic scar.

The Compression Factor. In the study by Lundborg (1970, 1975), the sciatic nerve was subjected not only to ischemia, but also to compression from the cuff. In this nerve also there was a relationship between endoneurial oedema and occurrence of severe nerve injury, but this injury was present in the sciatic nerve already after 4 h of cuff compression as compared to 8 to 10 h of ischemia in the tibial nerve. Thus, apparently the compression of the cuff played a major role in the development of nerve injury in this situation, and the ischemia per se, induced distally in the limb, was of subordinate importance. The mechanical factor in tourniquet compression was stressed also by Fowler et al. (1972) who demonstrated displacement of the nodes of Ranvier and local demyelination beneath the edges of cuffs, inflated around the lower limb of baboons.

We have found that the intraneural microvascular damage may also be considerable in corresponding situations. In recent experimental investigations (Rydevik & Lundborg, 1977), the mechanisms behind oedema formation in peripheral nerves following local, graded compression trauma utilizing the previously mentioned "compression-chamber" have been analysed. Preliminary results indicate that compression by 200 to 400 mm Hg for 2 h may induce a breakdown of the blood-nerve barrier leading to intrafascicular oedema, located at the edges of the compressed nerve segment. The barrier function of the perineurial sheath, however, seems to be unaffected by a compression trauma of this magnitude. This means that the oedema cannot escape through the perineurium, but is restricted to the intrafascicular space until it may be absorbed by endoneurial vessels. The reversibility of post-traumatic intraneural oedema is presently the subject for further investigation.

Effect of Ischemia and Compression on Axonal Transport

Both rapid (415 mm/day) and slow (24 mm/day) rates of axonal transport of proteins have been demonstrated in sensory fibres of rabbit vagus nerve after injection of ^{3}H-leucine into the nodose ganglion (McLean et al., 1976). These two phases of axonal transport found in the sensory axons are identical in rates to those found in the vagal motor fibres (Sjöstrand, 1969).

We have studied the effect of local compression on the rapid axonal transport in sensory vagal fibres (Rydevik et al., 1977). In these experiments 4 h were allowed for the synthesis of protein in the cell body, transport along the cervical vagus nerve and time for radioactive proteins to accumulate in the case of transport block caused by the local compression. Previous studies by Sjöstrand (1969) have shown that nerve ligature performed 2 h after isotope injection results in a subsequent accumulation of

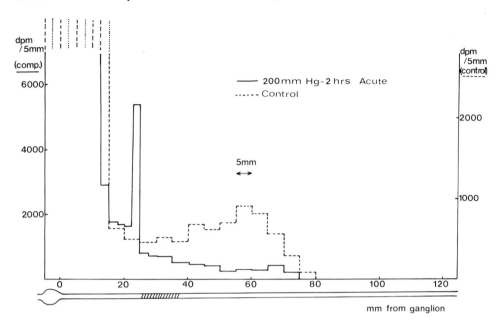

Figure 6.   The effect of nerve compression on fast axonal transport of ^{3}H-labelled proteins in rabbit vagus nerves. The profiles demonstrate the distribution of ^{3}H-labelled material along the vagus nerves 4 h after injection of ^{3}H-leucine into the nodose ganglia in an untreated nerve (interrupted line) and a nerve subjected to a pressure of 200 mm Hg for 2 h (solid line) within the indicated zone. A total block of axonal transport can be seen in the compressed nerve.

protein-bound radioactivity just proximal to the ligation. Therefore, in the acute compression experiments the local compression was applied 2 h following isotope injection, and the animals were killed at the end of a 2 h compression period.

The profile of the distribution of labelled proteins in the vagus nerve 4 h after the injection into the nodose ganglion is illustrated in Figure 6. In untreated nerves a wave front of labelled proteins was seen in agreement with previous studies (McLean et al., 1976). That this wave front was due to axonal transport of proteins labelled in the nodose ganglion is confirmed by the fact that the contralateral nerve which was exposed to a similar amount of blood-borne ^{3}H-leucine did not show the same radioactivity, and also by the fact that only a small percentage of the radioactivity was TCA soluble.

In nerves which had been subjected to local compression, an acute accumulation of labelled proteins was found in the region of compression (Figure 6). When compression was applied for 2 h even such low pressure as 50 mm Hg caused blockage of the rapid axonal transport which was, however, reversible within one day. The higher pressures tested, i.e., 200 mm Hg and 400 mm Hg, applied for 2 h induced a corresponding block (Figure 6), which was more pronounced in these nerves. Reversal of transport blockade occurred in most cases within 3 days after compression at 200 mm Hg for 2 h and within 7 days after compression at 400 mm Hg for 2 h (Rydevik et al., 1977). Time required for recovery of normal transport was correlated with the magnitude of the pressure applied and recovered transport was mostly found within the first week after compression.

Some effects of elevated pressure on axonal transport have been reported previously. In the optic nerves of monkeys, both fast (Andersson & Hendrickson, 1974; Quigley & Anderson, 1976) and slow (Levy, 1974) axonal transport are blocked by elevated intraocular pressure. A recovery of fast transport to normal levels as early as 4 h after restoration of pressure to normal levels was reported by Quigley and Andersson (1976).

In peripheral nerves, Ochs (1974) has demonstrated that application of a thigh cuff inflated to 300 mm Hg results in a blockade of fast axonal transport in the sciatic nerve of the cat and that transport recovered from such compression if the pressure levels were maintained not longer than 4 h.

There are also examples of the recovery of axonal transport from the effects of drugs, or from blockade by cooling. Rapid recovery of fast transport from the inhibiting effect of cooling has been observed in sympathetic nerves (Banks et al., 1975; Brimijoin & Helland, 1976), while the inhibition of fast axonal transport in the pigeon optic nerve is not reversed until 42 days after colchicine application (Cuénod et al., 1972). It is clear that axonal transport can recover from blockade without nerve regeneration, and it has been calculated that neuronal degeneration need not occur even after six weeks of axonal transport block by colchicine (Cuénod et al., 1972).

The mechanism by which nerve compression may block axonal transport is still unclear. Local ischemia, whether by interruption of the endoneurial microcirculation or by prevention of the diffusion of oxygen from tissues surrounding the nerve trunk can lead to local blockage of axonal transport (Levy & Adams, 1975; Ochs, 1971). Recovery of axonal transport was observed after ischemia for up to 1 h produced by local application of petroleum jelly to the sciatic nerve trunk or up to 4 h if the ischemia was caused by an inflated cuff on the limb (Ochs, 1974). In those studies, only immediate recovery from anoxia was investigated. In the work presented here, the rather slow reversal of the transport block seems inconsistent with a recovery of the axons from local ischemia. Intra-axonal changes caused by compression have not yet been examined. Displacement of axoplasm at the site of compression would be expected to lead to a block of transport by disruption of, for example, the cytoplasmic microtubules, known to be involved in the transport process. Equally, disruption of the axonal membrane, or a change in its ionic environment as may be caused by endoneurial oedema, could alter the ionic balance of the axoplasm. Fast axonal transport is known to be influenced by alterations in ion concentration (Edström, 1975).

ACKNOWLEDGEMENTS

This review is based on studies supported by grants from The Swedish Medical Research Council (projects Nr 2226 and 3513); Trygg-Hansas fond för personskadeforskning; Riksföreningen för Trafik-och Polioskadade; Faculty of Medicine, University of Göteborg; the Göteborg Medical Society and European Molecular Biology Organization.

REFERENCES

ADAMS, W. E. The blood supply of nerves. I. Historical review. *J. Anat.* 76:223-241, 1942.

ADAMS, W. E. The blood supply of nerves. II. The effects of exclusion of its regional sources of supply on the sciatic nerve of the rabbit. *J. Anat.* 77:243-250, 1943.

ANDERSSON, D. R., and A. HENDRICKSON. Effect of intraocular pressure on rapid axoplasmic transport in monkey optic nerve. *Invest. Ophthalmol.* 13:771-783, 1974.

BANKS, P., D. MAYOR, and T. OWEN. Effects of low temperature on microtubules in the non-myelinated axons of post-ganglionic sympathetic nerves. *Brain Res.* 83:277-292, 1975.

BENTLEY, F. H., and W. SCHLAPP. Experiments on the blood supply of nerves. *J. Physiol.* 102:62-71, 1943a.

BENTLEY, F. H., and W. SCHLAPP. The effects of pressure on the conduction in peripheral nerve. *J. Physiol.* 102:72-82, 1943b.

BLUNT, M. J. Functional and clinical implications of the vascular
    anatomy of nerves. *Postgrad. Med. J.* 33:68-72, 1957.

BRIMIJOIN, S., and L. HELLAND. Rapid retrograde transport of
    dopamine-β-hydroxylase as examined by the the stop-flow tech-
    nique. *Brain Res.* 102:217-228, 1976.

CAUSEY, G., and C. J. STRATMAN. The relative importance of the
    blood supply and the continuity of the axon in recovery after
    prolonged stimulation of mammalian nerve. *J. Physiol.* 120:
    173-182, 1953.

CUÉNOD, M., J. BOESCH, P. MARKO, M. PERISIC, C. SANDVI, and J.
    SCHONBACH. Contributions of axoplasmic transport to synaptic
    structures and functions. *Intern. J. Neurosci.* 4:77-87, 1972.

DAHLBÄCK, L.-O. Effects of temporary ischemia on striated muscle
    fibers and motor end-plates. *Scand. J. Plast. Reconstr. Surg.*
    Suppl. 7, 1970.

DENNY-BROWN, D., and C. BRENNER. Paralysis of nerve induced by
    direct pressure and by tourniquet. *Arch. Neurol. Psychiat.*
    51:1-26, 1944.

EDSHAGE, S. Peripheral nerve suture. A technique for improved
    intraneural topography. Evaluation of some suture materials.
    Acta Chir. Scand. Suppl. 331, 1964.

EDSTRÖM, A. Ionic requirements for rapid axonal transport in vitro
    in frog sciatic nerves. *Acta Physiol. Scand.* 93:104-111,
    1975.

FOWLER, R. J., G. DANTA, and R. W. GILLIAT. Recovery of nerve
    conduction after a pneumatic tourniquet: Observations on the
    hind-limb of the baboon. *J. Neurol. Neurosurg. Psychiat.*
    35:638-647, 1972.

GERARD, R. W. The response of nerve to oxygen lack. *Am. J.
    Physiol.* 92:498-541, 1930.

KLINE, D. G., E. R. HACKETT, G. D. DAVIS, and M. B. MYERS. Effects
    of mobilization and the blood supply and regeneration of in-
    jured nerves. *J. Surg. Res.* 12:254-266, 1972.

LEHMANN, J. E. The effects of asphyxia on mammalian nerve fibres.
    Am. J. Physiol. 119:111-120, 1937.

LEVY, N. S. The effects of elevated intraocular pressure on slow
    axonal protein flow. *Invest. Ophthalmol.* 13:691-695, 1974.

LEVY, N. S., and C. K. ADAMS. Slow axonal protein transport and visual function following retinal and optic nerve ischaemia. *Invest. Ophthalmol.* 14:91-97, 1975.

LUBIŃSKA, L. On axoplasmic flow. *Int. Rev. Neurobiol.* 17:241-296, 1975.

LUNDBORG, G. Ischemic nerve injury. Experimental studies on intraneural microvascular pathophysiology and nerve function in a limb subjected to temporary circulatory arrest. *Scand. J. Plast. Reconstr. Surg.* Suppl., 6, 1970.

LUNDBORG, G. Limb ischemia and nerve injury. *Arch. Surg.* 104:631-632, 1972.

LUNDBORG, G. Structure and function of the intraneural microvessels as related to trauma, edema formation and nerve function. *J. Bone Jt. Surg.* 57A:938-948, 1975.

LUNDBORG, G., and P.-I. BRÅNEMARK. Microvascular structure and function of peripheral nerves. Vital microscopic studies of the tibial nerve in the rabbit. *Adv. Microcirc.* 1:66-88, 1968.

LUNDBORG, G., and B. RYDEVIK. Effects of stretching the tibial nerve of the rabbit. A preliminary study of the intraneural circulation and the barrier function of the perineurium. *J. Bone Jt. Surg.* 55B:390-401, 1973.

MARTIN, K. H. Untersuchungen über die perineurale Diffusionsbarriäre an gefriertrockneten Nerven. *Zeitschr. f. Zellforsch. Mikr. Anat.* 64:404-428, 1964.

McLEAN, W. G., M. FRIZELL, and J. SJÖSTRAND. Slow axonal transport of proteins in sensory fibres of rabbit vagus nerve. *J. Neurochem.* 26:1213-1216, 1976.

MELLICK, R., and J. B. CAVANAGH. Longitudinal movement of radioiodinated albumin within extravascular space in peripheral nerves following three systems of experimental trauma. *J. Neurol. Neurosurg. Psychiat.* 30:458-463, 1967.

MINCKLER, D. S., M.O.M. TSO, and L. E. ZIMMERMAN. A light microscopic autoradiographic study of axoplasmic transport in the optic nerve head during ocular hypotony, increased intraocular pressure, and papilledema. *Am. J. Ophthalmol.* 82:741-757, 1976.

MOLDAVER, J. Tourniquet paralysis syndrome. *Arch. Surg.* 68:136-
    144, 1954.

OCHS, S. Local supply of energy to the fast axoplasmic transport
    mechanism. *Proc. Natl. Acad. Sci. US* 68:1279-1282, 1971.

OCHS. S. Energy metabolism and supply of ~p to the fast axoplasmic
    transport mechanism in nerve. *Fed. Proc.* 33:1049-1058, 1974.

OCHS, S. Axoplasmic transport. In: *The Nervous System,* edited by
    D. B. Tower. New York: Raven Press, vol. 1, 1975, p. 137-146.

OKADA, E. Experimentelle Untersuchungen über die vasculäre Trophik
    des peripheren Nerven. *Arb. Neurol. Inst. Univ. Wien* 12:
    59-108, 1905.

OLSSON, Y. Studies on vascular permeability in peripheral nerves.
    I. Distribution of circulating fluorescent serum albumin in
    normal, crushed and sectioned rat sciatic nerve. *Acta Neuro-
    path.* 7:1-15, 1966.

OLSSON, Y. Studies on vascular permeability in peripheral nerves.
    III. Permeability changes of vasa nervorum and scudation of
    serum albumin in INH-induced neuropathy of the rat. *Acta
    Neuropath.* 11:103-112, 1968.

OLSSON, Y., and K. KRISTENSSON. The perineurium as a diffusion
    barrier to protein tracers following trauma to nerves. *Acta
    Neuropath.* 23:105-111, 1973.

OLSSON, Y., K. KRISTENSSON, and I. KLATZO. Permeability of blood
    vessels and connective tissue sheaths in the peripheral nervous
    system to exogenous proteins. *Acta Neuropath.* Suppl. V:61-
    69, 1971.

QUIGLEY, H. A., and D. R. ANDERSON. The dynamics and location of
    axonal transport blockade by acute intraocular pressure eleva-
    tion in primate optic nerve. *Invest. Ophthalmol.* 15:606-616,
    1976.

ROBERTS, J. T. The effects of occlusive arterial diseases of the
    extremities on the blood supply of nerves. Experimental and
    clinical studies on the role of vasa nervorum. *Am. Heart J.*
    35:369-392, 1948.

RUDGE, P. Tourniquet paralysis with prolonged conduction block;
    an electrophysiological study. *J. Bone Jt. Surg.* 56B:716-
    720, 1974.

RYDEVIK, B., P.-I. BRÅNEMARK, C. NORDBORG, W. G. McLEAN, J.
    SJÖSTRAND, and M. FOGELBERG. Effects of chymopapain on nerve
    tissue. An experimental study on the structure and function
    of peripheral nerve tissue in rabbits after local application
    of chymopapain. *Spine* 1:137-148, 1976.

RYDEVIK, B., and G. LUNDBORG. Permeability of intraneural micro-
    vessels and perineurium in acute, graded experimental nerve
    compression. *Scand. J. Plast. Reconstr. Surg.* In press.

RYDEVIK, B., W. G. McLEAN, J. SJÖSTRAND, and G. LUNDBORG. Blockage
    of axonal transport induced by acute, graded compression of
    the rabbit vagus nerve. In preparation (1977).

SHANTA, T. R., and G. H. BOURNE. The perineurial epithelium - A
    new concept. In: *Structure and Function of Nervous Tissue,*
    vol. 1, Structure, edited by G. H. Bourne. London: Academic
    Press, 1968, p. 379-459.

SJÖSTRAND, J. Rapid axoplasmic transport of labelled proteins in
    the vagus and hypoglossal nerves of the rabbit. *Exp. Brain
    Res.* 8:105-112, 1969.

SMITH, J. W. Factors influencing nerve repair. I. Blood supply
    of peripheral nerves. *Arch. Surg.* 93:335-341, 1966a.

SMITH, J. W. Factors influencing nerve repair. II. Collateral
    circulation of peripheral nerves. *Arch. Surg.* 93:433-437,
    1966b.

SOLONEN, K. A., and L. HJELT. Morphological changes in striated
    muscle during ischemia. A clinical and histological study in
    man. *Acta Orthop. Scand.* 39:13-19, 1968.

STEINWALL, O., and I. KLATZO. Double tracer methods in studies on
    blood-brain barrier dysfunction and brain edema. *Acta
    Neurol. Scand.* 41, Suppl. 13:591-595, 1965.

SUNDERLAND, S. The nerve lesion in the carpal tunnel syndrome. *J.
    Neurol. Neurosurg. Psych.* 39:615-626, 1976.

WAKSMAN, B. H. Experimental study of diphtheritic polyneuritis in
    the rabbit and guinea pig. III. The blood-nerve barrier in
    the rabbit. *J. Neuropath. Exp. Neurol.* 20:35-77, 1961.

DISCUSSION

DR. KORR: If I may, then, draw my own summary from your paper, you have made it clear that, in research as well as in practice, we need to keep in mind that at least three factors may be affected by nerve compression, stretching or other nerve trauma, and that they may differ in their susceptibilities, namely, conduction, axonal transport and blood-nerve barrier. Is that right?

DR. SJÖSTRAND: Yes, but I would add two things. One, that conduction block, transport impairment and intraneural oedema may also differ in their reversibility; and, two, that anterograde and retrograde transport may also be differentially affected. Dr. Thoenen has shown us that impairment of the retrograde would primarily affect the nerve cell body. Anterograde would most likely be reflected in the target cells, as well as in the axon and its terminals.

We need experimental models that can examine all these factors together so that we can eventually tell, in a clinical situation, how each has been affected. I know that later on in the discussion, Dr. McComas will comment on that in the clinical perspective. But first, I will call on Dr. Ochs and ask him to comment about factors in transport mechanisms that could be affected in the pathological condition.

DR. SIDNEY OCHS: Thank you very much. I would like to comment on the reversibility of axoplasmic transport from a period of anoxia which my colleague, Dr. Leone, and I had worked on (Leone & Ochs, 1973, 1978).

A cuff placed high on the hind limb of cats was used to produce a period of anoxia by anemic compression. There is a difference in using this technique compared to a tourniquet in that the edge effect is not as prominent when using the wide cuff. Pressures of 300 mm Hg were applied, but the true pressure is lower in the tissue at the nerve. We had earlier shown that this level of ap-

357

plied pressure was adequate to acutely block axoplasmic transport
(Ochs, 1975). We then went on to study different periods of compression for reversibility of conduction of the nerve action
potential and axoplasmic transport through those regions. Transport was followed by injecting the precursor ^{3}H-leucine into the
cat L7 dorsal root ganglion by our usual technique and looking for
transport over times long enough so that labeled proteins are
carried through the region which had been blocked.

In brief, we could maintain cuff compressions for up to about
6 to 7 hr and still get reversibility of function. However, the
time required for recovery from anoxia was greater the longer the
period of compression. Such studies were done at 38°C. If a lower
temperature was used, even longer times of compression could be
endured before irreversible block took place. Presumably, this is
due to the high Q_{10} of nerve. Beyond 7 hr, failure of function and
Wallerian degeneration will occur.

An interesting phenomenon found was the later return of axoplasmic transport after recovery of conduction of the action potential. This dissociation of recovery of action potential
conduction and axoplasmic transport is still under study.

REFERENCES

LEONE, J., and S. OCHS. Reversibility of fast axoplasmic trans-
    port following different durations of anoxic block in vitro
    and in vivo. *Abstr. Soc. Neurosci.* 3:147, 1973.

LEONE, J., and S. OCHS. Anoxic block and recovery of axoplasmic
    transport and electrical excitability of nerve. (Submitted
    for publication)

OCHS, S. Axoplasmic transport - A basis for neural pathology. In:
    Peripheral Neuropathy, edited by J. P. Dyck, P. K. Thomas, and
    E. H. Lambert, vol. 1, chap. 12. Philadelphia: Saunders,
    1975, pp. 213-230.

DR. SJÖSTRAND: Thank you, Dr. Ochs, for these very interesting observations. Please tell us now about your study on calcium
in relation to axonal transport.

CALCIUM AND THE MECHANISM OF AXOPLASMIC TRANSPORT

S. Ochs, S.-Y. Chan, and R. Worth

Departments of Physiology and Medical Biophysics

Indiana University School of Medicine, Indianapolis

It is a truism that clinical problems will be solved through a deeper knowledge of the basic mechanisms of the body. With respect to the nervous system, our understanding has been advanced in recent years through the uncovering of a new basic aspect of nerve function, namely, the movement of materials from their site of synthesis in the nerve cell bodies outward in the fibers (Ochs, 1975). This process, termed axoplasmic transport, carries materials in the anterograde direction within nerve fibers of all sizes at a constant rate of close to 410 mm/day in all mammalian species so far examined (Ochs, 1972a). In our studies, a labeled precursor, ^{3}H-leucine, is injected into the L7 dorsal root ganglia or into the spinal cord supplying the sciatic nerve and at later times, a crest of labeled incorporated proteins and polypeptides is seen to move down the nerve. Biochemical analysis shows that a wide range of labeled materials are moved down the fibers. Some of these materials and the later downflow behind the crest supply the axon and terminal processes with essential components required to maintain their function. Various aspects of transport, including retrograde transport and slow transport, have been touched on by the other speakers of this workshop.

Here we describe a new aspect of the mechanism underlying the fast axoplasmic transport process, its requirement for Ca^{2+} (Ochs, Worth & Chen, 1977a, 1977b). This was of special interest to us in that in the transport filament model we had proposed to account for fast axoplasmic transport Ca^{2+} was considered to play a role (Ochs, 1971). In the model shown in Figure 1, materials synthesized in the cell are considered to be bound to transport filaments which

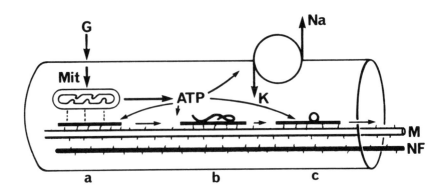

Figure 1. Transport filament hypothesis. Glucose (G) enters the
fiber and after glycolysis, oxidative phosphorylation in the mitochondrion (Mit) gives rise to ATP. The $\sim$P of ATP supplies energy
to the sodium pump controlling the level of Na^+ and K^+ in the fiber
and also to the cross-bridges activating the transport filaments.
These are shown as black bars to which the various components
transported are bound and so carried down the fiber by cross-
bridge activity. The components transported include the mitochondria (a) attaching temporarily as indicated by dashed lines
to the transport filament thus giving rise to either fast forward
or retrograde movement (though with a slow net forward movement),
soluble protein (b) shown as a folded or globular configuration,
polypeptides and small particulates (c). Simpler molecules are
also bound to the transport filaments. Thus, a wide range of components are transported at the same fast rate. The cross-bridges
between the transport filament and the microtubules presumably act
in similar fashion to the sliding filament theory of muscle and
the MgCa ATPase found in nerve utilizes ATP as the source of energy.
M - microtubules; NF - neurofilaments.

are then moved down along microtubules by cross-arms in analogy
to the sliding filament mechanism of muscle contraction.

We had shown in in vitro studies that transport can be maintained as long as oxidative metabolism continues to supply the ATP
needed to maintain axoplasmic transport (Ochs, 1974). The ATP
energy could be utilized by the $Mg^{2+}-Ca^{2+}$ ATPase present in
peripheral nerve (Khan & Ochs, 1974). Thus, we might expect that
transport depends on the presence of one or other of these di-
valent cations. However, using the in vitro technique we and
others had previously failed to find evidence for a dependence of
transport on Ca^{2+} (Edström, 1974; Hammerschlag, Dravid & Chiu, 1975).

Transport in vitro continued at the usual rate and with normal crest shape with the nerves placed in media free of either Ca^{2+} or Mg^{2+} and with or without EGTA added.

The perineurial sheath is known to act as an effective permeability barrier in nerve (Krnjević, 1955) and we considered that this could account for the apparent insensitivity of transport in vitro to a deficiency of Ca^{2+} in the medium. A desheathed nerve preparation was developed to test this point. It was essential that a long enough length of nerve be desheathed so as to allow time for a changed concentration of Ca^{2+} in the medium to have its effects, within an incubation period of some 4 h. For this purpose, the peroneal branch of the cat sciatic nerve was found suitable. This preparation also gave us an additional bonus in that the tibial branch which remains sheathed, served as a control.

The L7 dorsal root ganglia were injected with 10μ Ci of ^3H-leucine according to our usual procedure. The precursor is rapidly taken up by the cell bodies and incorporated into protein and polypeptides within some 10 to 20 min. Usually 2 or sometimes 3 h were allowed for the labeled polypeptides to move down into the fibers of the tibial and peroneal nerve branches of the sciatic nerves. The nerves were removed from the animals, the peroneal branch desheathed and the nerves put into flasks containing 10 to 20 ml of the desired solution and incubated for 3 to 5 h at $38^{\circ}C$ while they were vigorously oxygenated with 95% O_2 + 5% CO_2. Afterwards, the outflow patterns in the peroneal and tibial branches of the nerve were determined in the usual fashion by cutting each into 5 mm portions and counting their radioactivity to assess the pattern of outflow of labeled materials.

With the lactated Ringer solution as the in vitro medium, the outflow in both the desheathed peroneal and sheathed tibial branches was similar, each branch showing the usual outflow crest and rate of transport at close to 410 mm/day. Again, the usual outflow was seen when 3 to 5 mM Ca^{2+} was added to an isotonic NaCl medium (Figure 2). When lower concentrations of Ca^{2+} down to 1.5 mM were used, an addition of 4 mM K^+ to the medium was needed to prevent some decrement of the crest seen at these lower concentrations of Ca^{2+}.

When the nerve preparation was placed in Ca^{2+}-free medium, e.g., isotonic NaCl, axoplasmic transport was blocked in the desheathed peroneal nerves after an average time of 2.6 h (Figure 3). A similar block time was found when EGTA was added to a lactated Ringer solution. This was taken as further evidence that Ca^{2+} is a key factor in the maintenance of axoplasmic transport.

A series of experiments were conducted using Mg^{2+} instead of Ca^{2+} in the incubation medium. We found that full transport was

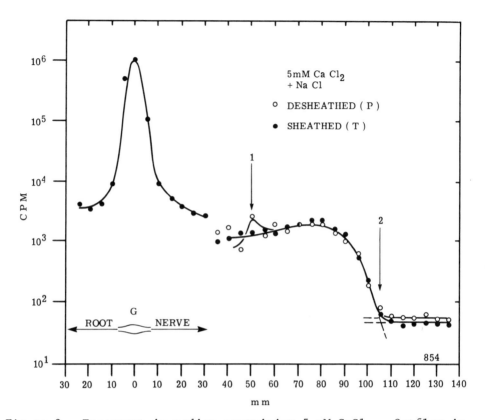

Figure 2.   Transport in medium containing 5 mM CaCl$_2$.   Outflow in
the desheathed peroneal branch (o) and the sheathed tibial branch
(●) is shown.   After 2 h of downflow in vivo, the peroneal nerve
was desheathed and the nerve placed in an in vitro medium of 5 mM
CaCl$_2$ and 140 mM NaCl for an additional 4 h.   The points represent
labeled materials present in 5 mm segments cut from the dorsal
root, L7 ganglion (G) and nerve.   Each branch, the tibial (T) and
peroneal (P), are taken separately from a point 30 mm below the
ganglion.   A small degree of damming of activity is seen in the
peroneal branch where desheathing begins (arrow 1).   The fronts of
activity move to the same position (arrow 2) indicating similar
rates.   Activity in counts per minute (c.p.m.) is given on the
ordinate on a logarithmic scale.   The position of sections is
shown in mm from zero taken at the peak of activity in the ganglion.

not maintained with Mg^{2+} as it was with Ca^{2+}, indicating that Ca^{2+}
may be specifically required for the maintenance of axoplasmic
transport.   However, the block time found when using 5 mM Mg^{2+}
was 3.5 h, an hour longer than the block time in a Ca^{2+}-free

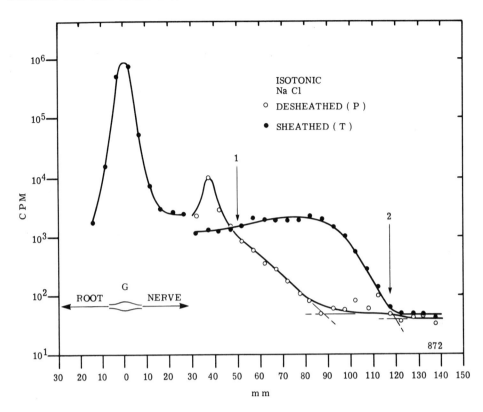

Figure 3.   Transport in Ca-free medium.   Outflow in a sciatic nerve in vitro and its desheathed peroneal branch (o) and sheathed tibial branch (●) under conditions similar to Figure 2.   A peak of dammed activity is seen above arrow 1, approximately where the peroneal nerve is desheathed.   This is followed by a steep descent to baseline at about 85 mm.   The sheathed tibial nerve shows axoplasmic transport is unaffected, with the front at the expected distance (arrow 2).

medium.   This might suggest that Mg^{2+} can partially substitute for Ca^{2+}, directly or perhaps in a nonspecific fashion.   This point is under further study.

In those experiments where a block of transport was seen in the desheathed peroneal branch in a Ca^{2+}-free medium, apparently normal transport continued in the sheathed tibial branch.   That finding is consistent with all our previous observations showing a lack of effect on Ca^{2+} depletion on axoplasmic transport in sciatic nerves in vitro where the sheath is intact.

In addition to the block found in Ca^{2+}-free media in the desheathed nerve, another phenomenon was observed, a block of axoplasmic transport when higher than normal concentrations of Ca^{2+}
were present in the medium. A progressively earlier block time
was seen with the higher levels of Ca^{2+} over the range of 25 to
100 mM. At the highest Ca^{2+} concentrations (95 to 100 mM), transport was blocked within less than 2 h of incubation. Again, it is
of interest that the sheathed tibial nerves were not affected by
these high concentrations of Ca^{2+}, normal transport proceeded as
usual.

Our findings with Ca^{2+}-free media and high Ca^{2+} concentrations
suggest that Ca^{2+} is normally regulated in the fibers within some
limited range to maintain normal transport. The actual amount of
Ca^{2+} entering the fibers when an excess of Ca^{2+} is present in the
medium or the amount of Ca^{2+} leaving the fibers when Ca^{2+} has been
removed from the medium is at present unknown. Also unknown are
the resulting concentration changes of Ca^{2+} in the axoplasm.
Studies now in progress in our laboratory may help assess these
points.

We may attempt to account for the block of axoplasmic transport
we have seen with a deficiency or an excess of Ca^{2+} in the medium
on the basis of what is known concerning Ca^{2+} in other cells. A
particularly favorable preparation for such studies is the cephalo-
pod giant axon which was found to have a free Ca^{2+} concentration of
approximately 10^{-7} M (Baker, 1972; Blaustein, 1974). This low
level of Ca^{2+} is maintained in the face of the relatively high
level of Ca^{2+} present in the extraneural compartment which causes
Ca^{2+} to move into the cell. Several mechanisms are responsible for
the low level of Ca^{2+} in the axoplasm; a Ca^{2+} exchange carrier in
the membrane (Brinley, Spangler & Mullins, 1975), the carrier possibly dependent on ATP (Di Polo, 1976), a sequestration of Ca^{2+}
within the mitochondrion (Carafoli & Crompton, 1976), and likely
as well in the endoplasmic reticulum, and a Ca-binding protein
(CaBP) recently found in the cat sciatic nerve which is moved down
by the fast transport mechanism (Iqbal & Ochs, 1976).

A removal of Ca^{2+} from the medium in which the desheathed
nerve preparation is incubated likely lowers the level of free Ca^{2+}
normally present in the fibers below that required to maintain
transport. We do not, however, know the concentration of free Ca^{2+}
in the axoplasm of mammalian nerve fibers although we suspect it is
probably similar to that measured in other cells.

One other possibility, however, can be excluded as the basis
of the block, namely, the effect of Ca^{2+} removal from the medium
to cause a lowering of the level of ATP and creatine phosphate ($\sim$P)
in the desheathed nerve. We found a fall of $\sim$P of approximately

22% in 3 h. This reduction of $\sim$P was not in itself responsible for the block of axoplasmic transport. We found that desheathed nerves exposed to the Ca^{2+}-free medium were able to sustain action potentials for at least 2 h after the onset of the block of axoplasmic transport. The level of $\sim$P remaining in the fibers thus is sufficient to supply the Na-pump required to maintain excitability and presumably as well to supply energy to the transport mechanism. This conclusion is based on our earlier findings that a block of axoplasmic transport and action potentials occurs some 15 min after initiation of anoxia, at a time when the $\sim$P level falls by 50% (Ochs, 1974).

It is of interest that a similar reduction of $\sim$P had been observed in nerves exposed to high concentrations of oxalate, a Ca^{2+}-chelating agent which causes a block of transport we had presumed to be due to the reduction in free Ca^{2+} inside the nerve fibers (Ochs, 1972b).

The block of transport caused by high concentrations of Ca^{2+} in the medium might come about by an interference with ATP production in the mitochondrion, or the utilization of ATP by the Mg^{2+}-Ca^{2+} ATPase in accord with the transport filament model. Another possibility is that higher levels of Ca^{2+} entering the fibers may bring about a disassembly of microtubules. In preliminary electron microscopic studies we found a marked depletion of microtubules in nerve fibers exposed to high levels of Ca^{2+}. However, further studies are required to establish if this is in fact a causal relation.

In any case, we have seen that Ca^{2+} is fundamentally involved in axoplasmic transport. We may expect that a disturbance of Ca^{2+} regulation brought about by toxic agents, by genetic diseases, by trauma or other causes, can block transport and in turn bring about neural defects. Some agents may change the permeability of the perineurial sheaths and cause a disturbance of the Ca^{2+} present in the endoneurial compartment thus bringing about a defect of axoplasmic transport on that account. These possibilities warrant further investigation in our search for explanations of neuropathological processes.

Acknowledgment

Debbie Jadhav and Larry Smith helped in the course of these experiments and we wish to thank them and the Illustration Department for the figures. This work was supported by grant No. R01 NS 8706-07 from the National Institutes of Health and by grant No. BNS 75-03868-A03 from the National Science Foundation.

REFERENCES

BAKER, P. F. Transport and metabolism of calcium ions in nerve. *Progr. Biophys. Mol. Biol.* 24:177-223, 1972.

BLAUSTEIN, M. P. The interrelationship between sodium and calcium fluxes across cell membranes. *Rev. Physiol. Biochem. Pharmacol.* 70:33-82, 1974.

BRINLEY, F. J., Jr., S. G. SPANGLER, and L. J. MULLINS. Calcium and EDTA fluxes in dialyzed squid axons. *J. Gen. Physiol.* 66:223-250, 1975.

CARAFOLI, E., and M. CROMPTON. Calcium ions and mitochondria. In: *Calcium in Biological Systems (Symp. Soc. Exptl. Biol.)*, vol. 30, edited by C. J. Duncan. London: Cambridge University Press, 1976, pp. 89-115.

DI POLO, R. The influence of nucleotides on calcium fluxes. *Fed. Proc.* 35:2579-2582, 1976.

EDSTRÖM, A. Effects of Ca^{2+} and Mg^{2+} on rapid axonal transport of proteins in vitro in frog sciatic nerves. *J. Cell Biol.* 61: 812-818, 1974.

HAMMERSCHLAG, R., A. R. DRAVID, and A. Y. CHIU. Mechanism of axonal transport. A proposed role for calcium ions. *Science* 188:273-275, 1975.

IQBAL, Z., and S. OCHS. Calcium binding protein in brain synaptosomes. *Soc. Neurosci. Abstr.* 2(1):47, 1976.

KHAN, M. A., and S. OCHS. Magnesium or calcium activated ATPase in mammalian nerve. *Brain Res.* 81:413-426, 1974.

KRNJEVIĆ, K. The distribution of Na and K in cat nerves. *J. Physiol.* 128:473-488, 1955.

OCHS, S. Characteristics and a model for fast axoplasmic transport in nerve. *J. Neurobiol.* 2:331-345, 1971.

OCHS, S. Rate of fast axoplasmic transport in mammalian nerve fibers. *J. Physiol.* 227:627-645, 1972a.

OCHS, S. Fast transport of materials in mammalian nerve fibers. *Science* 176:252-260, 1972b.

OCHS, S. Energy metabolism and supply of ~P to the fast axoplasmic transport mechanism in nerve. *Fed. Proc.* 33:1049-1058, 1974.

OCHS, S.   Axoplasmic transport.   In: *The Nervous System (The Basic Neurosciences)*, vol. 1, edited by D. B. Tower.   New York: Raven Press, 1975, pp. 137-146.

OCHS, S., R. WORTH, and S.-Y. CHAN.   Dependence of axoplasmic transport on calcium shown in the desheathed peroneal nerve. *Soc. Neurosci. Abstr.*   3:31, 1977a.

OCHS, S., R. M. WORTH, and S.-Y. CHAN.   Calcium requirement for axoplasmic transport in mammalian nerve.   *Nature*   270:748-750, 1977b.

DISCUSSION

DR. JOHAN SJÖSTRAND: Thank you, Dr. Ochs. I think your study brings up the very important question about the perineurial barrier in the clinical situation. When we carried our compression traumas up to the highest pressure level of 600 mm Hg for 4 h, we never had a breakdown of the perineurial barrier, so it seems to be extremely resistant, at least, to compression trauma. I think clinical evidence indicates that we can have blocked nerve conduction for considerable times and still have a survival of axons. I would like to ask Dr. McComas to comment on the pathophysiology of the different nerve traumas.

DR. ALAN J. McCOMAS: I would like to tell you of some observations on man which may have their explanation in terms either of abnormal axoplasmic flow or of preservation of axoplasmic flow at the time when impulse conduction is impaired. I would like to begin by reminding you that underlying this discussion of axoplasmic transport is the big question, to what extent is axoplasmic transport responsible for the trophic action of nerve on tissue, or tissue on nerve, or nerve on other nerve cells. As most of you know, there is a big debate going on at the moment between those who say that axoplasmic transport is very important in trophic mechanisms, and others who say that it isn't so important and that the main influence is an impulse-mediated one. Until recently, the advocates of the impulse-mediated hypothesis appeared to be winning. For example, if you subjected a muscle to disuse, either by blocking impulse conduction with tetrodotoxin or by applying tubocurarine to the neuromuscular junction, you could produce within a few hours the beginnings of denervation phenomena in the muscle fibers.

There is a corollary to that. If surgically denervated muscle is stimulated electrically, denervation phenomena are prevented from taking place. The laboratory which has been most active in this field is that of Lømo and his collaborators in Norway.

369

Now, for those very reasons, an impulse-based mechanism, at least a _purely_ impulse-based mechanism, seems rather unlikely, at any rate for man. The reason for that is that most of us are relatively inactive. There are few periods during an ordinary week when we make maximum use of our muscles, and that means that some of our motor units are simply not discharging at all, perhaps for 99% of the time.

Over and beyond that, there is another type of thinking based on the phenomenon of the neurapraxic lesion. A neurapraxic lesion is the clinical counterpart of the nerve compression which we have been hearing about from Dr. Ochs and Dr. Sjöstrand. If a nerve is crushed or otherwise damaged, a block of impulse conduction through the damaged region is possible, and yet the same fibers are excitable further down the nerve. Patients who have neurapraxic lesions seldom have any significant atrophy in the muscle fibers. Furthermore, if you put a recording needle electrode in the muscle belly of the paralyzed muscle, you do not find fibrillation activity, which is ordinarily a sign of denervation. So, one could argue backwards, and say that maintenance of muscle fiber size and prevention of fibrillation activity do not depend on the continued receipt of impulses by the muscle fiber. This is our own observation, but, in point of fact, it had been made much earlier in cats by Denny-Brown and Brenner. More recently, Westgaard has made neurapraxic lesions in baboons, and has shown that, conversely, a neurapraxic disuse model produces very little denervation in the muscle fibers. What I am saying is that it is probable in the higher primates, including man, that something other than impulse-mediated activity is important in subserving trophic mechanisms. The inference, of course, is that this is axoplasmic transport.

We have been puzzled by some patients who have nerve injuries, who do not show denervation phenomena, and yet, when the nerve fibers are stimulated beyond the lesion, there is no response from the muscle. Now, we know from other situations that if a nerve is cut, or if there is a severe neuropathy from any cause such that the axon degenerates, then of course the full panoply of denervation phenomena, including atrophy and fibrillation, occur.

We are forced to postulate that there is something in between the classical neurapraxic lesion and axonal degeneration. It seems as if one may have some sort of compressive lesion of an axon which will turn off excitability in the motor nerve terminals, and yet, will still permit a trophic influence to be exerted by the nerve fiber on the muscle fiber. Sometimes these patients have quite a dramatic recovery of excitability in the muscle, although it is unlikely from its shape and latency measurements that there could have been either regeneration or remyelination of the nerve fiber. I think it is something much more subtle, a switching on of excitability in the nerve terminals.

Remember that not only is the neuron soma responsible for maintaining the integrity of the target tissue to which it has a synaptic connection, but of course it is also maintaining itself. And
we wonder whether an abnormality in axoplasmic flow may be responsible for a clinical phenomenon which Dr. Adrian Upton and I described a few years ago--the double crush syndrome. We had
observed that perhaps the majority of patients in whom one could
electrophysiologically demonstrate a peripheral entrapment neuropathy (we were using particularly the carpal tunnel syndrome) had
not only clinical but electrophysiological evidence of an associated
abnormality in the more proximal paths of the nerve fibers. We
wondered whether some impairment of axoplasmic flow at a proximal
point in the nerve might make the nerve unusually susceptible to
compression lower down, and we are probably all subjecting our
median nerves to stress in the carpal tunnel. What I am saying is
that if there is something else wrong with the axon at another
point then you may get a frank entrapment of neuropathy.

The last clinical observation I would make, again related to
the work of Dr. Sjöstrand and of Dr. Thoenen, is that it is possible in man to get electrophysiological evidence of transsynaptic
degeneration, not just of muscle, but also inside the central
nervous system. One can imagine the sort of amplifying action
which can go on in a patient due to this destruction of a population of axons or nerve cells at one given point.

May I conclude with some other observations? Recently, we
have been looking at patients with amputations of their hands,
some as long as 30 years ago. We have been stimulating the nerve
stump, and recording such things as the compound action potential
in the nerve, the contralateral somatosensory root response, and a
rather complex reflex in the triceps muscle. First of all, the
compound action potential is very much smaller on the side of the
amputation, which suggests that many of the axons undergo frank
degeneration when they are no longer connected to periphery. Second, though later components in the somatosensory response are
quite well preserved, the earliest part, which is dependent on the
dorsal column system, is very small indeed. Third, rather surprisingly, the reflex effects that we test are quite strong.

DR. SJÖSTRAND: Dr. Worth, would you now respond to the question about the relationship between electrical activity and axonal
transport?

DR. ROBERT M. WORTH: We have been interested for some time
in the relationship between membrane phenomena and axoplasmic
transport. There are a number of studies in the literature using
widely varying rates of stimulation to try to assess this problem.
We used the experimental system that Dr. Ochs has just described

to study the effect of rapid stimulation on axoplasmic transport.
The L7 dorsal root ganglion of the cat was injected with ^{3}H-leucine,
and the sciatic nerve was removed and placed in a temperature- and
humidity-controlled oxygenated chamber from which one could stimulate and monitor the action potential. We selected a rate of 350
pulses per second--knowing that this was a rate much higher than
the average physiological rate of conduction in the nerve--so that
we could be sure of getting a maximal response on transport. This
was the highest rate that could be used and still avoid trouble in
some nerves with refractory periods and the alternation phenomenon.

Figure 1 shows the results in a control nerve (shown by open
circles) and a nerve stimulated for about 2 h (shown by closed
circles). I think you can see there is a discrepancy in the downflow distance of the labeled substances; the material in the stimulated nerve does not go as far as that in the control nerve.

We used the formula, $\left[\dfrac{d - 18.5\, t_o}{t_i}\right] \div \left[\text{antilog } .03(T - 38)\right]$,

to calculate the transport rate while the nerve was actually in
the chamber being stimulated. Basically we took the parameter d
(the total downflow distance of the labeled material), subtracted
a correction factor for the time that the nerve spent in the cat
prior to its insertion in the chamber, then divided it by the time
that the nerve was in the chamber and being stimulated. The results were then corrected to allow us to compare the rates at 38°C,
the normal body temperature of the cat.

The question then arose as to whether the discrepancy in downflow distance was caused by a change in rate or the transported material just reached a certain point and then stopped altogether.
This problem was approached by looking at the results from experiments of different durations. We took the parameter of the difference in downflow distance--this is not rate but the difference in
absolute downflow distance between the stimulated and controlled
nerves--expressed as Δd and plotted it as a function of the stimulation duration in hours. The regression line was determined. The
regression coefficient, 2.7, is significantly different from zero.
This demonstrates that the discrepancy in downflow distance is dependent on time. Thus, the phenomenon is one of an alteration in
rate, rather than an absolute cessation of transport.

For a series of 29 experiments, the rate was 416 mm/24 h in
the control nerves; in the stimulated nerve it was 337 mm/24 h. It
will be noted that the control value is quite close to the 410 mm/
day which has previously been reported from our laboratory. This
indicates that the downflow rate in these experiments, prior to
insertion of the nerves in the chamber, was 18.5 mm/h (hence, the
selection of this value for use in the formula noted above). This
rate is within the range of 17 ± 2 mm/h derived from many prior

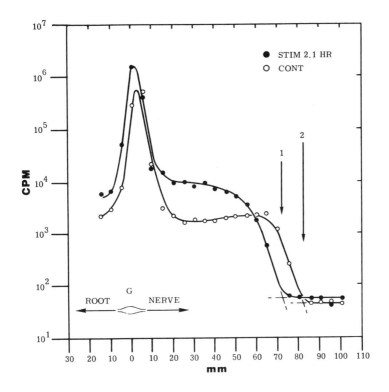

Figure 1. Axoplasmic transport pattern in stimulated (●) vs
control (o) nerves. Dorsal root ganglion of both nerves injected
with ^{3}H-leucine. Stimulation carried out for 2.1 h at 350 pps.
Ordinate: counts per minute, log scale. Abscissa: distance from
injection site in mm. Arrow 1: distance label transported in
stimulated nerve. Arrow 2: transport distance in control nerve.

experiments. The difference in rate between stimulated and control
nerves is significant at the $p \ll 0.001$ level. In the course of
assessing the etiology of this rate alteration we have looked at
high-energy phosphate levels and found that they are not significantly different between the stimulated and control nerves.

DR. FRED SAMSON: I regret that there has not been more time
for questions and comments on this topic, but there will be further
opportunity in the concluding session tomorrow. I now call on
Dr. Michael A. Nigro for his presentation.

TROPHIC CHANGES IN AFFLICTIONS OF THE MOTOR UNIT

Michael A. Nigro

Glendale Neurological Associates, P.C., Osteopathic

Birmingham, Michigan

The motor unit includes the anterior horn cell, nerve fiber, motor end plate and muscle fiber. Varying pathology of any or all parts of the motor unit may produce significant, albeit clinically indistinguishable, trophic changes in the skin, muscle, joints and long bones. In some instances, early changes suggest particular clinical disorders, for example, spinal muscle atrophy and Duchenne's muscular dystrophy. Quite often the distinguishing features are transitory or not at all present. The onset may occur in infancy, childhood or adulthood and progression may be slow, rapid, stuttering or quickly arrested, and these factors modify the extent of pathology and subsequent trophic changes. Muscles may become flaccid, firm or knotty on palpation.

Atrophy is common but, alternatively, hypertrophy may be seen in selective muscles. Strength is usually impaired whether involvement is proximal, distal, patchy or global. Joints may be unusually lax or severely deformed with limited range of motion as a result of contracture. Lumbar lordosis may be exaggerated upon ambulation and dorsal kyphoscoliosis may be so advanced that it results in impaired pulmonary function. Dry brittle skin may ulcerate and become infected and subcutaneous calcification may complicate inflammatory myopathies, and periarticular calcification may accompany joint contracture in immobile limbs.

In the following discussion, I would like to present several diverse disorders that affect the motor unit, the resultant effects on trophic function and related neuropathology and pathogenesis. This will be an attempt to highlight how vulnerable the motor unit is and how limited or extensive the resultant trophic effect may be.

Progressive neuromuscular disease with absence of sensory involvement is typical in virtually all of the muscular dystrophies,
and these are fairly common in clinical practice. Duchenne's
pseudohypertrophic muscular dystrophy can be considered the prototype and other dystrophies are usually less severe in progression
and often of later onset. Limb girdle and Duchenne's dystrophies
usually affect proximal limb muscles and shoulder and pelvic girdle.
In facioscapulohumeral dystrophy, facial weakness is quite prominent, with later atrophy of biceps, abdominal wall weakness and
shoulder weakness.

In most instances the diagnosis of muscular dystrophy can be
made by clinical presentation, pedigree analysis, electromyography,
enzyme elevation and confirmation by muscle biopsy.

Controversy has always marked attempts to explain the pathogenesis of the muscular dystrophies (Appenzeller & Ogin, 1975;
Eulenburg, 1877; McComas, Sica & Upton, 1974; Rowland, 1976).
Today it is suggested that alteration of surface membranes in
either physiologic activity or structure may explain the pathogenesis of muscular dystrophy (Rowland, 1976). Recent studies
have revealed abnormal responses of erythrocyte ATPase and adenyl
cyclase to epinephrine. Similar results in dystrophic muscle preparations suggest a genetic defect in membranes of dystrophy patients (Mawatari, Schonberg & Olarte, 1976). The neurogenic and
vascular theories have been extensively studied and subjected to
considerable controversy. The dispute of the "sick motor neurone"
and muscular dystrophy persists. In studying intramuscular innervation, Coërs and Tellerman-Tappet (1977) found no increase in
collateral ramifications of subterminal axons. This indicated
that primary axonal disease played no role in pathogenesis of muscular dystrophy. The dystrophies are alike in producing weakness,
having a hereditable etiologic basis and having similar abnormalities on muscle biopsy. This makes classification easier but despite these similarities the pathogenesis of the dystrophies may
ultimately require several different explanations with perhaps a
link between membrane defect, vascular and neurogenic pathways.

Typically, altered biomechanics, with lumbar lordosis and
dorsal kyphoscoliosis, result from progressive and asymmetric
muscle atrophy and weakness (Figures 1 and 2). Restricted range
of motion with joint contracture and resultant painful arthropathies is quite common. The limbs become cool, especially the
dependent lower extremities. Skin turgor is reduced. Initially
tone is reduced in affected muscles and later atrophy and fibrosis
result, with muscle bulk replaced by firm woody mass.

The first description of pseudohypertrophic muscular dystrophy is generally attributed to Duchenne who wrote in 1861 of
"paraplegic hypertrophique de l'enfance de cause cerebrale". By

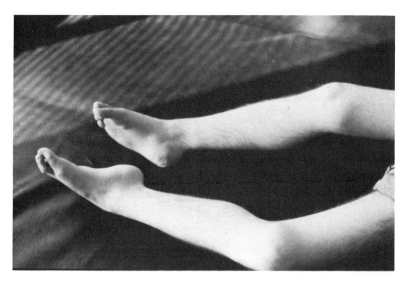

Figure 1. Flexion contracture at knee with pes equinovarus deformity of the foot in child with Duchenne's muscular dystrophy.

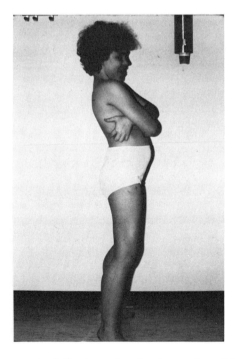

Figure 2. Exaggerated lumbar lordosis and calf hypertrophy.

1877, 110 cases were accumulated (Eulenburg, 1877). Included, however, were a disproportionate number of females and males with onset in second and third decades. The clinical description has not changed significantly:

> "By degrees it grows harder to stand without support, the gait becomes waddling . . . depresses the point of the toe and raises the inner edge of the foot. As the process extends to the thighs, sitting down and rising from the sitting posture become extremely difficult . . . in the latter he seeks to assist himself by bracing his hands firmly on the thigh . . . lying on his back the legs are usually spread apart, especially at the knees while the feet are nearer each other; . . . position of pes varo-equinus . . . peculiar changes in the carriage of the body are developed, namely a considerable lordosis of the lumbar spine and a compensatory kyphotic curve in the thoracic spine . . ."

In Duchenne's x-linked recessive progressive muscular dys-trophy, typical changes on muscle biopsy include phagocytosis of muscle fiber, internalization of nuclei, random fiber hypertrophy and regenerating fibers (Dubowitz & Brooke, 1973) (Figure 3). Without concomitant sensory impairment, arthropathies become a significant feature of the incapacitating nonambulatory state. Unfortunately, obesity due to sedentary confinement and over-eating add to the prominence of these symptoms. Duchenne's dys-trophy often requires surgical intervention either to prevent or ultimately to treat the deformities that result.

In myotonia dystrophica multiple organ systems are involved. Cardiac conduction defects may lead to complete heart block. Af-fective disturbances, smooth-muscle esophageal weakness, cataracts, frontal baldness, testicular atrophy and impaired hormonal metabo-lism may be seen in this autosomal dominantly heritable disease. Atrophy and weakness are distal and the sternocleidomastoideus is prominently affected. Persistent contraction of muscle is accom-panied by repetitive electrical activity that persists after ces-sation of stimulus or voluntary effort. An unusual feature of myotonia is the appearance of profound hypotonia and weakness that can be seen when the neonate is affected, in which case the myo-tonic phenomenon is little expressed. In either manner of pre-sentation, weakness and atrophy may be so severe that ambulation is limited and wheelchair confinement may rarely occur. In adult forms of myotonia, the muscle biopsy reveals typical myopathic changes, i.e., changes in fiber size, degeneration and regenera-tion, fibrosis, and, in addition, increased numbers of ring fibers, multiple internal nuclei and angular fibers (Dubowitz & Brooke, 1973) (Figure 4). In contrast, neonatal myopathic dystrophy is

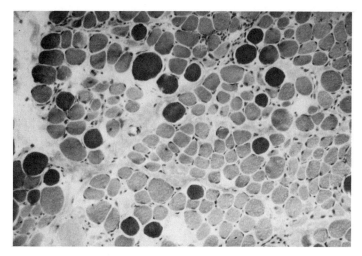

Figure 3.   Hematoxylin and eosin stain, cross section.   Internalization of nuclei, random fiber hypertrophy, phagocytosis of muscle
fibers.   Duchenne's muscular dystrophy.

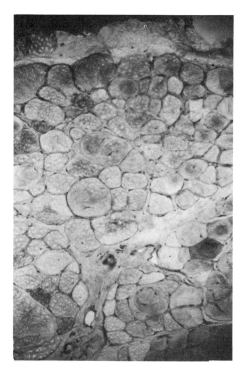

Figure 4.   PAS stain, frozen section, cross section.   Angular
fibers, Ringbiden fibers and several degenerating fibers.

characterized by indistinguishable fiber types, small round muscle
fibers and large vesicular internal nuclei but lacking degeneration
(Sarnat & Selbert, 1976).

    Spinal muscle atrophy of the juvenile or adult onset is a motor
neuron disease without significant sensory impairment. These familial disorders were first described and separated from the muscular
dystrophies by Kugelberg and Welander (1956). Many subgroups have
subsequently been defined (Hausmanowa-Petrusewicz et al., 1968) with
consideration that they represent variations of a single disorder.
Muscle stretch reflexes are absent from infancy or early childhood,
and tone is uniformly reduced and generalized weakness is prominent.
Electromyographic changes typically reveal reduced interference pattern, increased recruitment of large motor units of long duration
with fibrillations and fasciculations seen at rest. Biopsy of
muscle reveals group atrophy involving Type I and II fibers with
hypertrophy (reinnervated fibers) often of Type II fibers with
fibrous connective tissue interspersed (Dubowitz & Brooke, 1973)
(Figure 5). Reduction of spinal anterior horn cells, with reduced
volume of axis cylinders in peripheral nerves, is also noted.

    There is distal joint derangement with uncomfortable vertebral
deformities (Figure 6). Chronic joint pathology is a result of
altered biomechanics due to muscular atrophy with loss of suppor-
tive structure. Initially hypermobile joints are evident but later
severe and painful joint deformity results. Prophylactic bracing,
active and passive exercises and orthopedic surgery may offer
significant relief of pain.

    Hereditary disorders of central and peripheral nervous system
myelin are rather rare. In Krabbe's globoid leukodystrophy and
metachromatic leukodystrophy (MLD) progressive central nervous
system deterioration (dementia, spasticity, impaired consciousness)
with accompanying peripheral neuropathy is characteristic. "Neuralgic pain" is a common symptom and is often difficult to manage
(Stanbury, Wyngaarden & Fredrickson, 1972).

    Infantile, juvenile and adult forms of MLD are recognized.
Autosomal recessive inheritance pattern is documented and a defect
in arylsulfatase A activity has been defined (Stanbury, Wyngaarden
& Fredrickson, 1973). A result of this deficiency of active arylsulfatase A is an accumulation of sulfatides and a decrease in
total lipids in myelin (Stanbury, Wyngaarden & Fredrickson, 1973).
Lysosomal storage of undegraded cerebroside sulfate results in defective lysosomal activity in myelin and this may be further complicated by the mechanical-electrochemical effects of the sulfate
accumulation (Dyck, Thomas & Lambert, 1975). The following case is
representative of the disorder: A four-year-old girl presented
with limp of the left lower extremity and was found to have

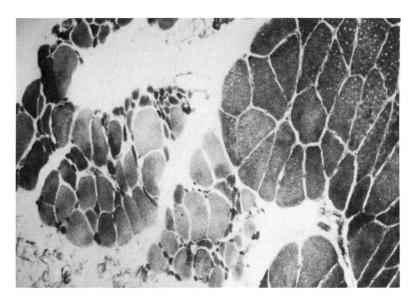

Figure 5.   DPNH - TR stain 400X cross section.   Group atrophy
Type I and II fibers.   Predominant Type II fiber hypertrophy.

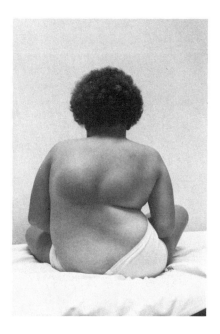

Figure 6.   Kyphoscoliosis in a child with juvenile onset spinal
muscle atrophy.

eversion of that limb on orthopedic examination. She experienced
a gradual deterioration in memory, social skills and became more
irritable. Within six months of diagnosis, she was aphasic and
could not comprehend even the simplest commands, exhibited tonic
extension of the lower extremities, was crying constantly and
appeared in pain. Weight loss and uniform muscle atrophy developed.
Initial laboratory studies included: elevated CSF protein of
60 mg% and prolonged motor nerve conduction velocities of 14 meters
per second at the peroneal and 24 meters per second at the ulnar
nerve. The urine sediment was positive for metachromatic staining
of renal epithelial cells utilizing cresyl-violet stain. Peripheral
nerve biopsy revealed a diagnostic abnormality of brown metachrom-
asia staining with crystal violet and toluidine blue (Figure 7).
Fibroblast arylsulfatase A activity of the proband was markedly reduced (1.48 n mal/min; control is greater than 10), and for the
parents 6.9 and 4.7. Urine arylsulfatase A was 0.99 µg/ml (greater
than 1.3). Computed tomography initially was normal but within six
months of diagnosis, suggested patchy area of periventricular demyelination of periventricular regions (Figure 8).

Krabbe's disease, globoid cell leukodystrophy (GCL), is due
to a decreased activity of cerebroside β-galactosidase. Lactosylceramide activity is also markedly reduced. There is a marked
reduction in cholesterol esters and long-chain fatty acids (Dyck,
Thomas & Lambert, 1975). In peripheral nerves inclusions are seen
in approximately half of the myelinated and unmyelinated fibers
with "membrane-bound cytoplasmic inclusions . . . moderate to
marked dilatation of the endoplasmic reticulum" (Dyck, Thomas &
Lambert, 1975). Onset is in early infancy with progressive deterioration and death by three to four years of age. Regression of
early milestones, spasticity, marked irritability with spontaneous
crying and seeming neuralgic pain are also noted with progression
to coma. Peripheral neuropathy is typical and usually not easily
identified unless electrodiagnostic studies are done. A patient
with Krabbe's disease is described below.

At six months of age, A. J. presented with regression of milestones, no longer being able to sit and less responsive to all
forms of external stimuli. Her condition deteriorated gradually
and was characterized by irritability, crying and increasing muscle
tone and a marked startle response. Pertinent laboratory data included elevated CSF protein (55 mg%), slow motor nerve conduction
velocity of 30 meters per second. The lactosylceramide level of
proband fibroblast was 1.8 n mal/hr/mg. Autopsy revealed
generalized cortical atrophy with extensive loss of myelin with
proliferation of histiocytes and twisted tubules or crystals within
paravascular macrophages, pathognomonic of cerebroside deposition
(Figures 9 and 10). Early in the disease no remarkable peripheral
nerve myelin abnormality was found on biopsy.

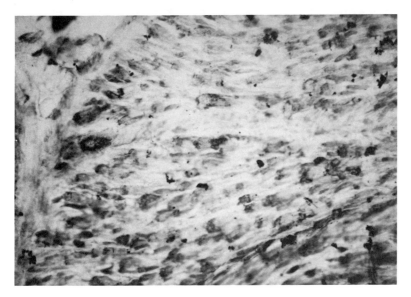

Figure 7. Cresyl-violet stain of peripheral nerve. Clumps of metachromatic staining "smudged" accumulations.

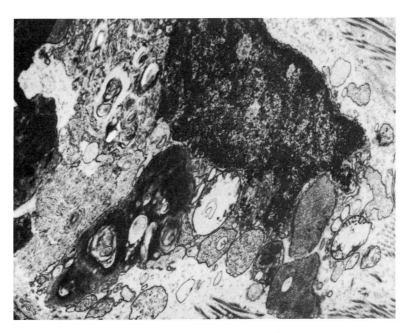

Figure 8. Electron micrograph of peripheral nerve. Large dense collection of metachromatic inclusion in myelin.

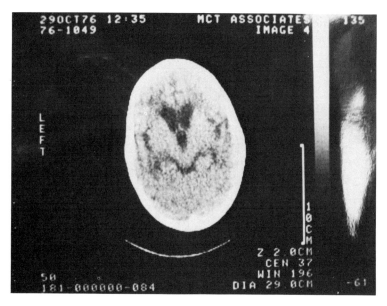

Figure 9. Computed tomogram of brain revealing ventricular dilatation and periventricular diminished densities, an indication of
affected white matter in metachromatic leukodystrophy.

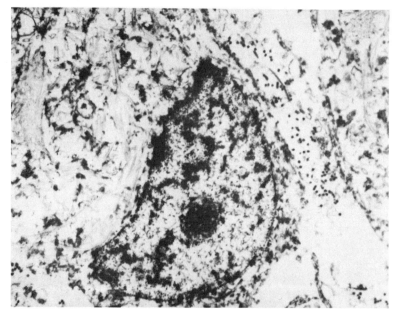

Figure 10. Krabbe's disease revealing twisted tubules.

In both of these hereditary leukodystrophies, defective myelin formation and accumulation of undegraded lipid results in neuralgic pain as an uncomfortable symptom. This is overshadowed by progressive deterioration, spasticity and coma that ultimately result. The continuous spasticity and uniform atrophy of muscles is prominent (Figure 11). Deformity of the limbs is a result of altered muscle tone and opisthotonous is not uncommon. With the sedentary life, accompanying demineralization of bone is frequent. Therapy for these disorders remains a considerable problem.

Chronic hypertrophic interstitial neuritis (HMSN Type III or Déjérine-Sottas) is an uncommon hereditary neuropathy with onset in early childhood (Déjérine & Sottas, 1893). The pattern of inheritance is autosomal recessive. The patient described below exhibited typical features of this disorder.

He was the product of a first-cousin union. He was not walking by 20 months of age and subsequently with ambulation he exhibited clumsiness, frequent falling and he never was able to run well. On examination at age seven, he had no muscle stretch reflexes in the extremities and muscle tone was uniformly reduced with moderate distal weakness. Vibration and position sense were

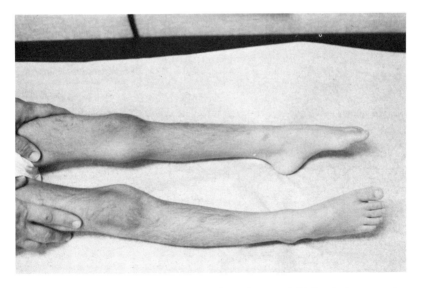

Figure 11. Tonic extensor spasticity in a child with metachromatic leukodystrophy.

mildly impaired with touch and pinprick preserved. Nerve conduction studies revealed the following: Peroneal nerve-18 meters per second, ulnar nerve-20 meters per second, and sural nerve-6 milliseconds. The CSF protein was elevated at 80 mg% and sural nerve biopsy indicated a marked decrease in the thickness of the myelin with reduplication of Schwann cell cytoplasm. There was increased connective tissue separating the nerve fibers. These changes were consistent with hypertrophic neuropathy. Electromyogram did not reveal any active denervation. Over the past year, the child has not shown any progressive involvement. He has not had any pain occurring in relationship to this neuropathy and there has been no joint contracture or spinal abnormality to date.

Axonal flow abnormalities have been described (Brimijoin, Capek & Dyck, 1973) and studies suggest impaired cerebroside formation in peripheral myelin and liver.

Typically in HMSN III there is no altered pain perception in earlier years. Sensory impairment is limited to kinesthesia, touch and pressure. Altered biomechanics with increased lumbar lordosis, dorsal kyphoscoliosis, and joint contracture (club feet) are the only sources for pain in this disorder and are not seen early. No remarkable changes in skin turgor are noted.

In another hereditary neuropathy, hereditary sensory neuropathy (HSN Type II), the unusual feature of marked joint deformity and destructive arthropathy with self-mutilation without pain perception is noted. It is characterized by autosomal recessive inheritance and typically the onset is in early infancy. This is in sharp contrast to HSMN III since motor nerve function is much less affected. There is another disorder, HSMN I, which is autosomal dominant in inheritance, but does not make its appearance until much later in life and similar destructive arthropathies are noted (Dyck, Thomas & Lambert, 1975).

The diagnosis is suggested when self-mutilation presents in infancy and other causes such as Lesch-Nyhan, congenital indifference to pain and Riley-Day dysautonomia are ruled out.

Studies have indicated minimal slowing of motor nerve velocities with failure to elicit sural evoked potentials (Ohta et al., 1973). Dyck pointed out the reduced number of unmyelinated fibers distally with virtual absence of myelinated fibers. They indicated this was a progressive disorder because of axis cylinder changes, more distal involvement, and denervation in muscle biopsy (Ohta et al., 1973). Our experience with this disorder supports this finding, as described in case study which follows.

At seven months of age, C. C. was brought because her parents noted repeated self-mutilation. The infant had bitten off the distal one-quarter of her tongue and was constantly biting and chewing on her fingers. There was no consanguinity. The past history was unremarkable and social and motor development appeared normal to the parents. On examination, she exhibited reduced and delayed responses to pinprick stimulation and deep pain in all extremities, trunk and face. The tongue was partially amputated (Figure 12) and healing wounds of the fingers were present. The muscle stretch reflexes were only trace in all limbs, and muscle tone was minimally, but uniformly, reduced. Development was not affected. Chemistries including cerebrospinal fluid analysis, lactic acid of blood and CSF, urine and serum uric acid, lipoprotein electrophoresis and amino acid analysis were all normal. The sural latency was prolonged at 7 milliseconds. Peroneal nerve motor velocity was 44 meters per second. The peripheral nerve biopsy revealed an increase in the interstitial element including the Schwann cell processes and collagen fibers around small nerve fibers (Figure 13).

In this instance, acropathy, self-mutilation and amputation will occur without an appreciation of pain. The protective function of pain is evident, since without this annoying sensation, serious progressive and destructive joint injury will occur. The patient can do little to prevent it, since the onset is so early in infancy and the parents are often at a total loss to deal with the problem, except for providing mechanical restrictions to prevent further mutilation or having the child's teeth extracted.

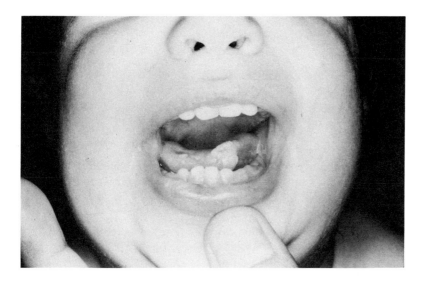

Figure 12. Self-mutilation of tongue in infant with HSN Type II.

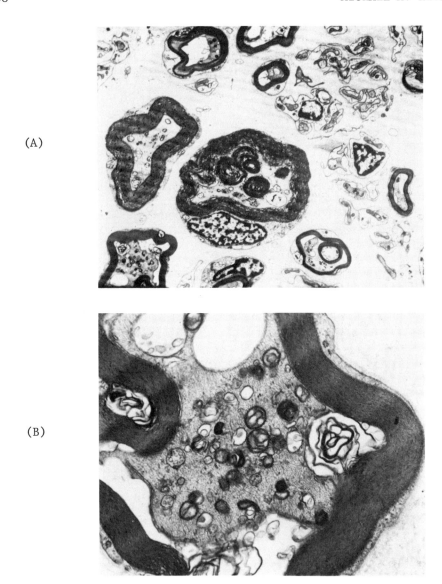

(A)

(B)

Figure 13. Electron microscopy in patient with HSN Type II.
(A) Increase in interstitial elements; (B) Axonal inclusions.

     Dermatomyositis is a nonfamilial inflammatory myopathy affect-
ing children and adults. Diagnosis may be simple or elusive depending on the abundance or lack of clinical signs and confirmatory
laboratory studies. Muscle weakness may be restricted or global,
skin lesions clinically appear as heliotrope of eyelids and linear

striations of fingernails or phalanges. Muscles can be tender to
palpation or ache with slight movement. In most instances, the
disease is self-limited or may respond to corticosteroids with
little trophic effect aside from temporary weakness and reversible
atrophy. Especially in the childhood form the course may be un-
remitting, unresponsive to immunosuppressive drugs and ultimately

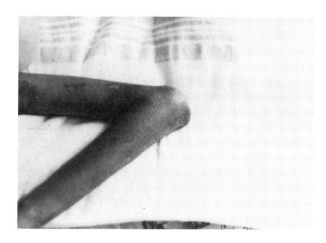

Figure 14. Trophic changes in dermatomyositis.

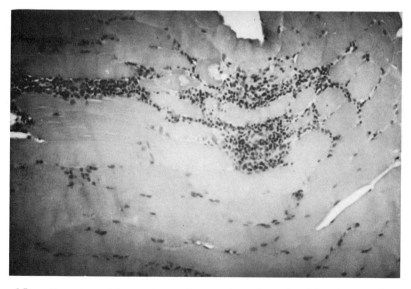

Figure 15. Hematoxylin and eosin stain, longitudinal section.
Infiltrates of inflammatory cells with areas of fiber phagocytosis.

resulting in the most severe contracture deformities of joints, secondary calcinosis universalis and total muscle atrophy with replacement by unyielding firm fibrous tissue (Figure 14). Ulceration of skin with chronic cutaneous infection is a major problem.

In the most typical case, creatine phosphokinase is elevated, sedimentation rate is raised, the electromyogram reveals myopathic potentials and denervation. The muscle biopsy reveals inflammatory myopathy with degeneration and regeneration of muscle fibers, infiltrates of chronic inflammatory cells, active phagocytosis and interstitial fibrosis (Pierson & Currie, 1974) (Figure 15).

In all of the described disorders involving the motor unit, trophic changes of variable degree are present. Demineralization of bone is a long-term effect of chronic weakness and impaired ambulation. As a result, fracture may occur more easily and healing may be prolonged. An interesting corollary to this is the worsening of symptoms that occurs in patients with neuromuscular disease following prolonged bedrest associated with fractures.

Hereditary, mutant and acquired diseases have specific effects on the motor unit. As a result, trophic changes are seen to a variable degree and at different stages of active and inactive disease.

REFERENCES

APPENZELLER, O., and G. OGIN. Pathogenesis of muscular dystrophies: Sympathetic neurovascular components. *Arch. Neurol.* 32:2-4, 1975.

BRIMIJOIN, S., P. CAPEK, and P. J. DYCK. Axonal transport of dopamine β-hydroxylase by human sural nerves in vitro. *Science* 180:1295-1297, 1973.

COËRS, C., and N. TELLERMAN-TAPPET. Morphological changes of motor units in Duchenne's muscular dystrophy. *Arch. Neurol.* 34: 396-402, 1977.

DÉJÉRINE, J., and J. SOTTAS. Sur la nevrité: Interstitielle, hypertrophique et progressive de l'enfance. *C. R. Soc. Biol., Paris* 45:63-70, 1893.

DUBOWITZ, V., and M. H. BROOKE. *Muscle Biopsy: A Modern Approach.* London: W. B. Saunders, 1973, p. 154-158.

DYCK, P. J., P. K. THOMAS, and E. H. LAMBERT. *Peripheral Neuropathy,* vol. 2. Philadelphia: W. B. Saunders Co., 1975, p. 794-804.

EULENBURG, A. Diseases of the nervous system. In: *Cyclopedia of the Practice of Medicine,* vol. 14, edited by R. A. Ziemssen. (Publisher unknown) 1877, p. 153-179.

HAUSMANOWA-PETRUSEWICZ, I., W. ASKANAS, B. BADURSKA, B. EMERYK, A. FIDZIAŃSKA, W. GARBALIŃSKA, L. HETNARSKA, H. JEDRZEJOWSKA, Z. KAMIENIECKA, I. NIEBRÓJ-DOBOSZ, J. PROT, and E. SAWICKA. Infantile and juvenile spinal muscular atrophy. *J. Neurol. Sci.* 6:269-287, 1968.

KUGELBURG, E., and L. WELANDER. Hereditofamilial juvenile muscular atrophy simulating muscular dystrophy. *Arch. Neurol. Psychiat.* 75:500-505, 1956.

MAWATARI, S., M. SCHONBERG, and M. OLARTE. Biochemical abnormalities of erythrocyte membranes in Duchenne's dystrophy. *Arch. Neurol.* 33:489-494, 1976.

McCOMAS, A. J., R.E.P. SICA, and A.R.M. UPTON. Multiple muscle analysis of motor units in muscular dystrophy. *Arch. Neurol.* 30:249-251, 1974.

OHTA, M., R. D. ELLEFSON, E. H. LAMBERT, and P. J. DYCK. Hereditary sensory neuropathy, Type III. *Arch. Neurol.* 29:23-37, 1973.

PIERSON, C. M., and S. CURRIE. *Disorders of Voluntary Muscle,* edited by John Walton. London: Churchill Livingston, 1974, p. 627-634.

ROWLAND, L. P. Pathogenesis of muscular dystrophies. *Arch. Neurol.* 33:315-321, 1976.

SARNAT, H. B., and S. W. SELBERT. Maturational arrest of fetal muscle in neonatal myotonic dystrophy. *Arch. Neurol.* 33: 466-474, 1976.

STANBURY, J. B., J. B. WYNGAARDEN, and D. S. FREDRICKSON. *The Metabolic Basis of Inherited Disease,* 3rd ed. New York: McGraw-Hill, 1972.

WING FLAPPING AND OTHER MOVING TOPICS: A DEVELOPMENTAL PERSPECTIVE

Martin Balaban

Department of Zoology

Michigan State University, East Lansing, Michigan

G. E. Coghill (1929) attempted to describe the sequence of steps involved in the differentiation of the central nervous system of ambystoma following his careful observations upon the development of their walking and swimming behaviors. The central premise of his work was that the development and elaboration of behavior patterns was the manifestation of an orderly sequence of steps of differentiation in the embryonic nervous system (Hamburger, 1963).

Indeed, many other neuroembryologists have used behavioral measures in their studies of neuronal development. Hamburger et al. (1965, 1966), following observations upon the development of chick embryo motility cycles, asked questions concerning the role played by sensory feedback upon the maturation of the spinal cord. Székely (1963), Detwiler (1936), Weiss (1955), Narayanan and Hamburger (1971), and Straznicky (1963) were all concerned with the development of regional specificities within the spinal cords of amphibians and chick embryos. Their assays following surgical manipulations were behavioral assays. These included observations upon both the coordination of limb movement (e.g., walking in amphibians) and qualitative differences in motor patterns of limbs (e.g., wing flapping vs. alternating leg movements in the bird). Sperry (1951) was interested in the central neural structures involved in the representation of the sensory world of animals. He studied both the visual and tactual systems. His observations consisted of recording amphibian orientations to visually and tactually presented stimuli. Finally, Sperry (1965) and Weiss (1955) were concerned with the plasticity of neural control circuits, once they had developed. Again, assays of the results of their manipulations consisted of either animal locomotory or orientation behaviors.

393

The reader should refer to Hamburger (1976), Keating (1976), Meyer
and Sperry (1976), Landmesser (1976), Székely (1976), and Fambrough
(1976) for the most recent reviews in this area of developmental
neurobiology.

Rather than a further pursuit of the developmental behavior
literature from the point of view of the light that it can shed
upon the general principles of nervous system development, it will
be the purpose of this review to extract from the developmental
neurobiological literature that information pertinent to identifying both the location of and properties of the different neuronal
circuits underlying organized motor output. In particular we shall
be concerned with those neural mechanisms related to motility
cycles, the muscular coordination involved in single limb movements,
and the qualitative differences in motor patterns of limbs (e.g.,
wing flapping vs. alternating leg stepping movements) in the bird.

Hamburger (1976) described the inception and development of
chick motility as follows: "It begins around 3½ days (of incubation)
with a slight nodding of the head and in subsequent days extends to
the whole body . . . . the amount of motility increases to reach a
peak around 13 to 14 days (total time to hatching around 21 days).
Until then movements are performed periodically, activity phases
alternating with inactivity phases . . .". Hamburger (1963) further
reported that responses to tactile stimulation cannot be observed
until 7 to 7½ days of incubation, that is, until 3½ to 4 days following the inception of motility. Earlier, Windle and Orr (1934)
claimed that though many sensory neurons have already sent
processes from the spinal ganglia, both peripherally into a limb
and centrally to form the dorsal funiculus prior to day 7, collaterals are not yet sent into the grey matter. During day 7, collaterals from afferent fibers in the dorsal funiculus were observed to
contact commissural and association interneurons. Windle and Orr
(1934) reported that both spinal commissural and associational
interneurons make contact with motoneuron dendrites during day 4
of development. Indeed, Foelix and Oppenheim (1973) and Oppenheim
et al. (1975) reported the first axodendritic synapses in the
lumbosacral cord at day 5 in the chick. These synapses are presumably between motoneurons and either commissural or association
interneurons.

Since the initiation of motility occurs at least 4 days prior
to the first observed contact between afferent fiber collaterals
and either commissural or association interneurons, it can be concluded that the central neural circuitry necessary for the control
of motility cycles in chick embryos occurs independently of sensory
influence.

Hamburger et al. (1966) decided to test directly the hypothesis that sensory input was not necessary for the maintenance and

development of motility patterns in the chick embryo. The dorsal
halves of the lumbosacral cords of 2 day embryos (prior to motility
performance) were extirpated. This included the neural crest, which
is the precursor of the spinal ganglia. To eliminate input from
rostral parts of the nervous system (e.g., brain), several segments
of the thoracic spinal cord were also removed, thus effectively
isolating the ventral lumbosacral cord. Experimental and control
embryos showed no difference in motility qualitatively for up to
15 to 17 days of observation. In short, the embryos in which both
exteroceptive and proprioceptive input had been eliminated, with the
removal of the spinal ganglia, still performed qualitatively normal
motility cycles. The legs, of course, showed no response to tactile
stimulation.

Bekoff et al. (1975) have presented electromyographic evidence
from two pairs of ankle muscles in chick embryos that the activity
of muscles within a single limb is coordinated at day 7 (shortly
after the inception of limb movement). The synergists (peroneus
and gastrocnemius) were coactivated; the antagonists (tibialis and
gastrocnemius) recordings showed a phase delay between onset of
activity in each during an activity cycle. While such recordings
were not made upon embryos whose spinal ganglia had been removed,
if we accept the observations of Hamburger et al. (1966), that movements of the operated embryos were qualitatively like that of controls, we come to the conclusion that chick embryos, at least up to
the age of 15 to 17 days, can perform coordinated muscular movements
without the benefit of proprioceptive feedback.

We conclude from all of the above that both the first movements
and continued activity cycles appear to be entirely of spinal origin, with neither sensory nor descending supraspinal inputs being
necessary.

Secondly, that control of these motility cycles resides either
in the ventral horns or within the commissural and association interneurons of the local segments of the spinal cord that innervates the
limb under observation. Hamburger (1976) further postulated that
the motility observed was the result of autonomously generated
electrophysiological activity of neurons in the ventral spinal cord
(see Provine 1973, for review). The actual structure of such a
local control mechanism has yet to be demonstrated.

We cannot conclude, however, that sensory input and feedback
(proprioceptive) never has an effect upon the quality of motility
cycle performance. Hamburger (1976) described the quality of
motility as, "The most prominent features of motility are abrupt,
convulsive-type, jerky movements and the apparent lack of coordination. Movements of different parts of the body, such as head,
trunk, wings, legs, tail, occur independently of each other in

unpredictable, random combinations. There is little change in this unorganized performance, except that the amount of motility increases to reach a peak around 13 to 14 days." Later on, towards the end of the chick embryonic phase, around day 19, this uncoordinated picture changes. One aspect of this change is the appearance of coordination of movement between the two legs. The legs begin to move alternately, that is, in a stepping fashion. Nikundiwe (1972) has reported that following the early removal of the sensory ganglia the legs later lose this alternating, stepping, coordinated activity. The role of sensory feedback in the later stages of chick motor development needs to be further studied.

Limbs transplanted to the thoracic body wall and innervated by thoracic segments of the spinal cord in urodeles do not exhibit coordinated stepping movements (Detwiler, 1920). If, however, a supernumerary limb is transplanted near to the normal limb and receives innervation from the brachial plexus, coordinated stepping movements develop in the transplanted limb (Detwiler and Carpenter, 1929; Weiss, 1937). Findings such as these point to functional differences between limb and non-limb segments of the spinal cord.

The only difference observed between limb innervating (brachial and lumbosacral) segments of the spinal cord and the non-limb innervating segments (thoracic) appears to be that limb innervating segments have more cells present. Hamburger (1958), Harris (1965), and Levi-Montalcini (1950) all present evidence indicating that the enlarged ventral horns (brachial and lumbosacral) develop from a continuous motor column as a result of cell proliferation and degeneration during growth. The cells in the limb segments of the cord have a lower rate of cell death than in other segments.

Further evidence implicating regional functional differences between limb innervating and non-limb innervating segments of the spinal cord is shown in the following.

Székely and Szentágothai (1962) and Székely and Czéh (1971) transplanted pieces of spinal cord (minus sensory ganglia) and limbs into the dorsal fin of salamander larvae. Neural connections developed between the transplanted limbs and cord. The fin is composed of gelatinous connective tissue with a rich blood supply. It serves as an excellent culture chamber for the survival and further differentiation of transplanted tissues. Since the fin does not normally contain muscle tissue or motoneuronal fibers, all movements in these experiments reflect those of the transplanted tissues. Regular stepping movements of the limb graft were observed when the spinal transplant was from the brachial region of the donor larva. Electromyographic recordings from these limbs showed normal muscle activity patterns. Limb movements were described as irregular twitches when the spinal cord transplants were taken from the thoracic region. The movements of the grafted limbs remained unaltered even when the host's spinal cord was destroyed.

Székely (1963) transplanted brachial or lumbosacral spinal cord segments into the place of thoracic segments and implanted either hind or fore supernumerary limbs at the same level in urodele embryos. After these limbs had become innervated by the grafted cords, limb movements in larvae and in metamorphosed animals were observed. The supernumerary limbs of these animals showed regular coordinated stepping movements, in which the rhythm of movement was determined by the origin of the grafted spinal cord segments. If the extra limbs were innervated by grafted brachial segments, they moved in synchrony with the normal forelimbs. If innervated by grafted lumbosacral segments, they moved in synchrony with the normal hindlimbs, regardless of whether fore- or hindlimbs were transplanted.

An important aspect of the observations was the reported quality of movement of the transplanted supernumerary limbs. During locomotion, in the intact animal, there is a considerably large excursion, greater than 90°, in the elbow joint and only a limited movement in the knee. When a forelimb pair is innervated by transplanted lumbosacral segments, the elbow moves only to a limited extent. This probably corresponds to the small excursion observed in the normal knee joint. A forelimb with lumbosacral innervation therefore assumes a hindlimb movement pattern.

Similar quality differences in motor performances have been observed in chickens. After replacing brachial segments of spinal cords with lumbosacral segments during the third day of incubation of chicken embryos, Straznicky (1963) observed the characteristics of wing movements after the chickens had hatched. The wings did not perform wing-like flutter movements. Instead, there was only an elevation and abduction of moderate excursion in the shoulder, and a very slight elbow extension. These movements occurred at the same time as stepping movements of the leg.

When Straznicky (1963) replaced the wing with a leg primordium in an otherwise normal chick embryo, the knee and ankle joints remained in an extended position after hatching. A movement similar to fluttering occurred in the hip joint of the transplanted leg at the same time as the movement of the normal wing on the other side was observed. Therefore, Straznicky was able to demonstrate a wing that produced leg type of movements and a leg that fluttered like a wing depending upon the identity of the cord segment innervating the limb.

Narayanan and Hamburger (1971) both substantiated Straznicky's findings and extended his results. They transplanted brachial spinal cord segments in place of lumbosacral cord in chick embryos and observed leg movements following hatching. The legs, rather than performing alternating stepping movements, were ab- and adducted synchronously and in parallel, as in wing flapping.

These results indicate that not only the rhythm but also the character of movement (fore- or hindlimb type, leg or wing type) is predetermined in the limb innervating spinal cord segments. We also infer that the brachial segments and lumbosacral segments generate different activity output patterns for the movement of forelimbs and hindlimbs, or of wings and legs, respectively.

Straznicky (1963) and Narayanan and Hamburger (1971) both demonstrated that the specificity of behavioral quality of both the brachial and lumbosacral cord segments is fixed very early in development (stages 15-16) in chick embryos. Székely (1963) showed with urodeles that the functional specificities of both the brachial and lumbosacral segments of the spinal cord were already determined immediately after the closure of the medullary tube. However, Detwiler (1923) has shown that thoracic segments in amphibians, if transferred in early embryonic stages, do replace the function of brachial segments. Early thoracic segments may be considered as "neutral" spinal cord.

Is there anything for us to learn about the neural mechanisms underlying limb behavior from a study of the ability of early thoracic segments to assume brachial segment functions? Székely (1976) reports that normal limb movements develop in amphibians if transplantation of thoracic cord segments in place of brachial cord segments occurs early in development. Transplantations made at increasingly older stages fail to develop movements; first in the shoulder, then in the elbow, and finally at later stages, the limb remains motionless. In effect, with increasing age of transplantation, the original thoracic cord segments fail to assume brachial regional function in a proximo-distal direction with respect to the anatomical positions of the limb musculature. Székely (1976) presented electromyographic evidence that muscle groups of both motionless joints and moving joints were active. There is, in fact, evidence that stronger activity occurred in some muscles of motionless joints than in their counterparts in moving limb joints. Differences, however, were recorded between the timing pattern of different muscle activities in limbs that did move and those that did not move. Székely feels that the central neural mechanism controlling limb movements operates not only by insuring that the muscle groups of a particular joint are innervated, but also insuring that the appropriately timed sequence of muscles is activated by the appropriate order of motoneuron activities.

All of the work so far presented is consistent with the idea that specificity of function exists in different segments of the spinal cords in chickens and salamanders; that this specificity of function is determined very early during development, even prior to innervation of the musculature; that this specificity of function develops even without the presence of sensory input, both proprioceptive and exteroceptive.

Landmesser and Morris (1975) present evidence that the contribution that various peripheral spinal nerves make to the innervation of individual muscles of the chick embryo hindlimb is already present and stable (non-changing) from the earliest times that muscles can be caused to contract by nerve stimulation. In fact, they have shown that the correct pattern of innervation precedes the division of the primary dorsal and ventral muscle masses into the individual hindlimb muscles.

The chick hindlimb is innervated by the lumbosacral spinal nerves 1-8. Spinal nerves 1, 2 and part of 3 which form the more cranial crural plexus, innervate the thigh musculature exclusively. Part of spinal nerve 3, and spinal nerves 4-8 form the ischiatic plexus which innervates some muscles in the thigh before forming the large sciatic nerve which supplies all the innervation of the lower leg and foot. Stimulation of lumbosacral nerves 1-3 results in movement of the sartorius, femur tibialis, and adductor femoris muscles. Stimulation of lumbosacral nerves 3, 4 and 5 results in movement of the peroneus muscle. Stimulation of lumbosacral nerves 5, 6, 7 and 8 results in movement of the gastrocnemius muscle. Prior to stages 27-29 (Hamburger-Hamilton series) there has as yet been no individualization of these muscles, and the entire musculature of the limb exists as two simple muscle masses in the hindlimb, one dorsal and one ventral. By stage 33 (8 days) all of the above muscles are anatomically distinct and can be seen. Spinal nerve stimulation, whether performed at stage 25 or 38, led to identical patterns of muscle movements. Thus, throughout this entire developmental period, the pattern of functional nerve representation for a given muscle remained the same. No observations were made to suggent that spinal nerves initially innervate the limb differently or randomly, with later emergence of the adult pattern (Landmesser and Morris, 1975).

As a result of the work of such authors as Landmesser and Morris (1975) in which a fairly precise functional relationship exists between the spinal nerves and activation of limb musculature, can we assume a like relationship between strictly anatomic patterns of nerve-muscle connections and coordinated limb muscular performance? As the following discussion indicates, we must practice restraint in making such a generalization.

After regeneration of the facial nerve in man, the loss of
separate control of muscles (synkinesia) may be so bad as to throw
the whole face into a grimace on each attempt at movement. A blink
becomes a twitch of the mouth and a flaring of the nostril. People
with these disabilities can compensate only through conscious recognition of the defect and by learning to use disorganized contractions to the best advantage or, in the case of bad facial synkinesia, by not using facial expression at all (Mark, 1974). We
conclude from these results that the correct correspondence between
motoneurons and the musculature is lost during regeneration. In
contrast, amphibians, salamanders and newts do recover the coordinated movement of the whole leg following the cutting and regeneration of the motor nerves. Weiss (1955) reports that this coordinate
movement of the whole leg appeared even though the anatomical re-
innervation did not look normal. Grimm (1971) agreed with Weiss'
observations and extended the results. He exchanged (crossed) the
nerves supplying the forearm flexor muscles with those supplying
the forearm extensors in Axolotls. After recovery, the movements
of the forelimb were the same as those of normal limbs. Dissections
showed that the nerves remained crossed, and electrical stimulation
of the crossed nerves close to the muscles they supplied showed that
the nerves were functionally connected to the foreign muscles. However, further work showed that a few fibers from the crossed nerves
do find their way back to their original muscles, and this is indeed
enough to produce normal movement. We have here an obviously abnormal histological pattern of spinal nerve distribution within the
musculature and yet, normal limb movement.

In goldfish, rolling movements about the optic axes are produced by the two oblique extra-ocular muscles. Gravitational reflexes allow the action of these muscles to be observed in the
intact animal, and so progress, after denervation, of re-innervation
can be assayed from day to day (Traill and Mark, 1970). The muscles
involved are the inferior and superior oblique muscles. These
muscles are innervated by the third and fourth cranial nerves, respectively. Marotte and Mark (1970a, 1970b) cut the branch of the
third cranial nerve to the inferior oblique muscle near its insertion, removed the muscle, and laid the nerve trunk alongside the
antagonistic superior oblique muscle. The superior oblique muscle
was denervated by crushing the fourth cranial nerve. The inferior
oblique nerve now innervates the superior oblique muscle, which now
contracts when the inferior oblique (third nerve) motoneurones
discharge. The result is that the gravitational reflex becomes
reversed. Eventually the original superior oblique branches of the
fourth nerve grow back to form connections in the muscle already
innervated by the antagonistic nerve. At this time there is a
disappearance of the reversed reflex movements and the resumption
of the normal orthodox reflexes. The now functionless third nerve
terminals remain in the muscle and are indistinguishable by electron

microscopy from normal function terminals (Mark, Marotte and Mart, 1972). The works of Weiss (1955), Grimm (1971) and Mark et al. suggest that though there is a mechanism for the re-establishment of precise functional and anatomical nerve-muscle connections, there is also the ability of nerves both to form and to maintain connections with muscles normally foreign to them. One must therefore show great caution in attempting to correlate strictly anatomic patterns of nerve-muscle connections with that of coordinated behavior performances.

I return now to an interest, stated earlier, in those unique neural mechanisms within the brachial, thoracic, and lumbosacral segments of the spinal cord that underlie wing flapping, twitching, or stepping behaviors respectively. We now enter the spinal cord proper to look for neuroanatomical configurations that make possible the functional differences above described.

Romanes (1964) with mammals, and Hughes (1968) and Cruce (1974) with anurans, have claimed that motoneurons within the adult spinal cord are arranged in columns, with the more cranial columns innervating proximal limb muscles and the more caudal columns innervating distal musculature. Landmesser and Morris (1975) review the literature claiming that there is a cranio-caudal differentiation of motoneurons in the spinal cord (Romanes, 1941; Hamburger, 1948; Langman and Haden, 1970) and proximodistal sequence of limb innervation (Romanes, 1941, 1946; Roncali, 1970). Finally, Romanes (1941, 1946, 1951, 1964), Székely and Czéh (1967), Cruce (1974) present evidence that the hindlimb muscles in mammals and amphibia are innervated by specific groups of motoneurons with characteristic positions in the spinal cord.

In the chicken, though, in general the relationship of spinal cord cranial-caudal, limb musculature proximal-distal representations hold true, there are exceptions to the rule. The most proximal musculature will be the thigh musculature, followed distally by the shank musculature, with the most distal being the foot musculature. The lumbosacral spinal cord gives rise, as earlier stated, to 8 spinal nerves (1-8), number 1 being the most cranial, and number 8 the most caudal. Though, of the thigh musculature, the sartorius, femorotibialis, and adductor femoris are all innervated by the most cranial nerves (1-3), the caudilio-flexorius, still a thigh muscle, is innervated by spinal nerves 7 and 8. While the peroneus muscle (in the shank) is innervated by lumbosacral spinal nerves 4 and 5, another shank muscle, the gastrocnemius, is innervated by spinal nerves 5-8. As predicted, the intrinsic digit flexors of the foot are innervated by the most caudal lumbosacral spinal nerves 7 and 8, yet other foot musculature, the intrinsic digit extensors, are innervated by more medial nerves 4 and 5. Therefore, though a general cranio-caudal proximodistal relationship exists, it probably does not occur at a sufficiently fine level to account for a central mechanism for control of co-ordinated behavior (Fig. 5, Landmesser, 1976). For example, lumbosacral cord segments 4, 5, 7, and 8 all contribute to innervation of the thigh, shank, and intrinsic foot musculature. Although Landmesser (1976) and Landmesser and Morris (1975) report a slight cranio-caudal difference in the time of motoneuron proliferation and differentiation, both the crural and ischiatic plexuses form at approximately the same time. Most of the limb musculature is functionally innervated at the same time in no apparent proximodistal sequence.

Though a cranio-caudal, proximodistal representation is not apparent, it is still possible that particular groups of cells distributed within the segments of the lumbosacral cord of the chicken selectively send their axones to certain muscles within the hindlimb during development and therefore establish synapses with the appropriate muscles. Here, an assumption is made that both motoneurones and musculature show a specificity for one another. Supernumerary limbs were transplanted anterior to the normal limbs in chick embryos. This procedure allows motoneurones lying in a certain place in the spinal cord to grow into the supernumerary limbs from a position different from normal. For example, lumbosacral spinal nerve 1 which normally innervates the sartorius and adductor femoris, now finds itself entering the supernumerary limb from a new position. Electrical stimulation of the lumbosacral spinal nerve 1 showed that not only did it grow to muscles in accord with its new position (flexorius, gastrocnemius), but also that it actually formed functional synapses with them. Therefore, though in normal development different motor fibers may functionally synapse with predictable groups of muscles, they may also grow to and innervate "foreign" musculature (Morris, 1975).

Hollyday et al. (1977) used the same preparation as did Morris (1975). A supernumerary leg primordium was transplanted rostral to the host limb in chick embryos. After the transplants became fully functional, the origin of the nerves innervating the gastrocnemius (primarily an ankle extensor) were identified. Normally, the motor cell pool innervating the gastrocnemius is located in the caudal segments of the lumbosacral region. If, Hollyday argued, a prespecification exists between certain motoneurones and certain muscles, and this prespecification is unmodifiable, then one would expect the caudally located gastrocnemius motor pool to supply both the host and the transplant gastrocnemius muscles. This requires the assumption that some caudally originating axons would find their way across the plexus and enter the rostral nerves Hollyday identified the motor pool that gave rise to the innervatio of the transplant gastrocnemius, using the method of retrograde

axonal transport of horseradish peroxidase (HRP). She found the
motor pool for the transplant muscle located in rostral lumbosacral
segments 1-3 separated by a considerable gap from the host gastrocnemius motor pool in the more caudal segments 5-7, with no overlap.
Clearly, rostral motoneurones that normally supply thigh musculature
have changed their destination.

We certainly have not derived the principles of spinal cord
functional organization from considerations of either a fixed predetermined correspondence between motor cell pools and musculature,
or from rostral-caudal - proximodistal considerations. Perhaps the
results of the work with mapping of retinal representation upon
visual areas of the brain in different groups of animals can be of
help to us in our considerations of neuromotor control mechanisms.

Sperry (1965) emphasized the invariant nature of retinotectal
connections. Yoon, in a series of experiments involving the mapping
of retinal representation upon the optic tectum of goldfish, brings
into question Sperry's thesis.

Yoon (1972a) demonstrated that the separation of rostral and
caudal visual tectal areas in goldfish by either a piece of tantalum
foil or absorbable gelatin barriers led to the whole retinal field
being represented across the rostral tectum in front of the barrier.
This compression of the entire retinotectal input into only half a
tectum was reversible. Removal of the tantalum foil or resorption
of the gelatin barrier was followed by the expansion of the retinal
input to cover the entire tectum (normal situation). Yoon (1972b)
and Horder (1971) demonstrated that after removal of the temporal
half of the retina, the remaining nasal half of the retina spreads
its connections over the entire tectum. It appears that each
retinal element does not have a unique image in the tectum, but
rather that the mapping function is such that the most nasal
retinal cells available connect with the most caudal tectal elements available, the most temporal retinal cells present connect
with the most rostral tectal cells available, and the intermediate
retinal cells connect with the proportionately intermediate tectal
positions (Keating, 1976). The implication from Yoon's work is
that the organizing principle around which the retinal elements
are represented upon the optic tectum is topological in character.
That is, there is a significance of order of representation of the
elements one with another, rather than an exact specification of
location of each retinal element upon the optic tectum. The difficulties involved in finding support for a fixed positional
correspondence between motor cell pools and musculature, or a
fixed positional relationship between cranio-caudal spinal cord
structure and proximodistal innervation of musculature should make
us consider the possibility of topologically organized motor
neural control mechanisms that underlie behavior. Wyman (1973)

postulates a type of topological connectivity in the spinal cord,
and Landmesser (1976) further discusses the concept.

We have already spoken in some detail of spinal cord control
of both timing and the quality of single limb coordinated movement. The next step is to discuss factors involved in the coordination of behavior of pairs of limbs. Székely (1976) reports that
if two limbs are grafted onto the dorsal fin in a common tunnel with
a transplanted brachial section of spinal cord in urodeles, the two
limbs move in exactly the same rhythm, similar to oar-strokes. This
indicates that though the existing structure in the spinal cord at
the limb level can control stepping movements (as earlier described)
of individual limbs, it cannot control alternating movements of
limb pairs. Brändle and Székely (1973) transplanted various lengths
of the body of newts, including the prospective limb segments of the
medullary tube, into the sides of whole newt embryos. The transplanted limbs performed synchronous, oar-stroke movements if the
graft contained only brachial or only lumbosacral segments. If
either the medulla or a piece of the thoracic spinal cord was grafted
rostral to the transplanted brachial segments, alternating movements
by the grafted limbs were observed. Note that the medulla and
thoracic segments were interchangeable, but they had to lie rostral
to the limbs for the appearance of the alternating movement pattern.
It was determined that a critical length of the spinal cord (medulla
+ brachial segments, or more than 2 thoracic segments + brachial
segments) was required for the control of alternating leg movements.
This length is about one-third of the length of the medullo-spinal
neuraxis. Nikundiwe (1972) demonstrated that the alternating leg
movements in chick embryos (19 days) was lost after a lumbosacral
mid-saggital section (separating the lumbosacral spinal segments
into left and right halves). This indicates, if the newt and
chicken results prove to be comparable, that alternating leg movements not only require a minimal length of neuraxis for its performance, but also that the structural integrity of the right and
left half cord connectives be intact.

There are several models of neuronal networks involving the
motor cells, the interneurones, and commissural neurons proposed
to account for both the timing of and quality of motor performance.
They are all highly speculative (Székely, 1976). The firm ground
upon which neuronal network models must be built is sorely lacking.
This is, accurate descriptions of the neuroanatomic organizations
of those spinal segments that control the timing and quality of
motor performance should be vigorously pursued. Useful tools in
this endeavor will continue to be, (1) the "developmental" tool
in which segments of spinal cord and embryonic limbs are transplanted to either a dorsal fin or into different regions of the
neuraxis; and (2) continued use of electrophysiological measurements and the silver stain, horseradish peroxidase, and cobaltous

chloride (Pittman et al., 1972) techniques for the mapping of motor-interneuron - commissural neuron cell pools. It is on the basis of these results that neuronal functional models can be most directly tested.

REFERENCES

BEKOFF, A., P. STEIN, and V. HAMBURGER. Coordinated motor output in the hindlimb of the 7-day chick embryo. *Proc. Natl. Acad. Sci. U.S.* 72:1245-1248, 1975.

BRÄNDLE, K, and G. SZÉKELY. The control of alternating coordination of limb pairs in the newt (*Trituris vulgaris*). *Brain Behav. Evol.* 8:366-385, 1973.

COGHILL, G. E. *Anatomy and the Problem of Behaviour.* Cambridge: University Press, 1929.

CRUCE, W. The anatomical organization of hindlimb motoneurons in the lumbar spinal cord of the frog, *Rana custebiana. J. comp. Neurol.* 153:59-76, 1974.

DETWILER, S. R. Experiments on transplantation of limbs in Amblystoma. The formation of nerve plexuses, and the function of the limbs. *J. Exp. Zool.* 31:117-169, 1920.

DETWILER, S. R. Experiments on the transplantation of the spinal cord in Amblystoma, and their bearing upon the stimuli involved in the differentiation of nerve cells. *J. Exp. Zool.* 37:339-393, 1923.

DETWILER, S. R. *Neuroembryology.* New York: MacMillan, 1936.

DETWILER, S. R., and R. L. CARPENTER. An experimental study of the mechanism of coordinated movements in heterotopic limbs. *J. Comp. Neurol.* 47:427-447, 1929.

FAMBROUGH, D. M. Specificity of nerve-muscle interactions. In: *Neuronal Recognition*, edited by S. H. Barondes. New York and London: Plenum Press, 1976, p. 25-67.

FOELIX, R. F., and R. W. OPPENHEIM. Synaptogenesis in the avian embryo: Ultrastructural and possible behavioral correlates. In: *Behavioral Embryology*, edited by G. Gottlieb. New York: Academic Press, 1973, p. 103-139.

GRIMM, L. M. An evaluation of myotypic respecification in Axolotls. *J. Exp. Zool.* 178:479-496, 1971.

HAMBURGER, V. The mitotic patterns in the spinal cord of the chick embryo and their relation to histogenetic processes. *J. comp. Neurol.* 88:221-283, 1948.

HAMBURGER, V. Regression versus peripheral control of differentiation in motor hypoplasia. *Am. J. Anat.* 102:365-410, 1958.

HAMBURGER, V. Some aspects of the embryology of behavior. *Q. Rev. Biol.* 38:342-365, 1963.

HAMBURGER, V. The developmental history of the motor neuron. *Neurosci. Res. Prog. Bull. Suppl.* 15:1-37, 1976.

HAMBURGER, V., M. BALABAN, R. OPPENHEIM, and E. WENGER. Periodic motility of normal and spinal chick embryos between 8 and 17 days of incubation. *J. Exp. Zool.* 159:1-13, 1965.

HAMBURGER, V., E. WENGER, and R. OPPENHEIM. Motility in the chick embryo in the absence of sensory input. *J. Exp. Zool.* 162: 133-160, 1966.

HARRIS, A. E. Differentiation and degeneration in the motor horn of the foetal mouse. Ph.D. Thesis, University of Cambridge, 1965. (Cited in Székely, 1976.)

HOLLYDAY, M., V. HAMBURGER, and J.M.G. FARRIS. Localization of motor neuron pools supplying normal and supernumerary legs of chick embryos. *Proc. Natl. Acad. Sci. U.S.*, 1977. (Discussed in Hamburger, 1976.)

HORDER, T. J. Retention by fish optic nerve fibers regenerating to new terminal sites in the tectum, of "chemospecific" affinity for their original sites. *J. Physiol, London* 216:53P-55P, 1971.

HUGHES, A. F. *Aspects of Neural Ontogeny.* London: Logos Press, 1968.

KEATING, M. J. The formation of visual neuronal connections: An appraisal of the present status of the theory of "neuronal specificity". In: *Neural and Behavioral Specificity,* vol. 3, edited by G. Gottlieb. New York, San Francisco, London: Academic Press, 1976, p. 59-109.

LANDMESSER, L. The development of neural circuits in the limb moving segments of the spinal cord. In: *Neural Control of*

Locomotion, edited by R. M. Herman, S. Grillner, P.S.G. Stein, and D. G. Stuart. New York, London: Plenum Press, 1976, p. 707-733.

LANDMESSER, L., and D. G. MORRIS. The development of functional innervation in the hindlimb of the chick embryo. *J. Physiol.* 249:301-326, 1975.

LANGMAN, J., and C. C. HADEN. Formation and migration of neuroblasts in the spinal cord of the chick embryo. *J. comp. Neurol.* 138:419-432, 1970.

LEVI-MONTACINI, R. The origin and development of the visceral system in the spinal cord of the chick embryo. *J. Morphol.* 86:253-283, 1950.

MARK, R. F. Selective innervation of muscle. *Brit. Med. Bull.* 30:122-125, 1974.

MARK, R. F., L. R. MAROTTE, and P. E. MART. The mechanism of selective reinnervation of fish eye muscles. IV. Identification of repressed synapses. *Brain Res.* 46:149-157, 1972.

MAROTTE, L. R., and R. F. MARK. The mechanism of selective reinnervation of fish eye muscle. I. Evidence from muscle function during recovery. *Brain Res.* 19:41-51, 1970a.

MAROTTE, L. R., and R. F. MARK. The mechanism of selective reinnervation of fish eye muscle. II. Evidence from electron microscopy of nerve endings. *Brain Res.* 19:53-69, 1970b.

MEYER, R. L., and R. W. SPERRY. Retinotectal specificity: Chemoaffinity theory. In: *Neural and Behavioral Specificity,* vol. 3, edited by G. Gottlieb. New York, San Francisco, London: Academic Press, 1976, p. 111-149.

MORRIS, D. Development of motor innervation in supernumerary hindlimbs of chick embryos. *Neurosci. Abstr.* 1:753, 1975.

NARAYANAN, C. H., and V. HAMBURGER. Motility in chick embryos with substitution of lumbosacral by brachial and brachial by lumbosacral spinal cord segments. *J. Exp. Zool.* 178:415-432, 1971.

NIKUNDIWE, A. M. The ontogeny of coordinated limb movements in prehatched chicks: Effects of central nervous system manipulations on the frequency and patterns of movements. Ph.D. Thesis, Michigan State University, 1972.

OPPENHEIM, R., I. W. CHU-WANG, and R. E. FOELIX. Some aspects of synaptogenesis in the spinal cord of the chick embryo: A quantitative electron microscopic study. *J. comp. Neurol.* 161:383-418, 1975.

PITMAN, R. M., C. D. TWEEDLE, and M. J. COHEN. Branching of central neurons: Intracellular cobalt injection for light and electron microscopy. *Science N.Y.* 176:412-414, 1972.

PROVINE, R. R. Neurophysiological aspects of behavior development in the chick embryo. In: *Studies on the Development of Behavior and the Nervous System,* vol. 1, edited by G. Gottlieb. New York: Academic Press, 1973, p. 77-102.

ROMANES, G. J. The development and significance of the cell columns in the ventral horn of the cervical and upper thoracic spinal cord of the rabbit. *J. Anat.* 76:112-130, 1941.

ROMANES, G. J. Motor localization and the effects of nerve injury on the ventral horn cells of the spinal cord. *J. Anat.* 80: 117-131, 1946.

ROMANES, G. J. The motor cell columns of the lumbosacral spinal cord of the cat. *J. comp. Neurol.* 94:313-363, 1951.

ROMANES, G. J. The motor pools of the spinal cord. *Prog. in Brain Res.* 11:93-119, 1964.

RONCALI, L. The brachial plexus and the wing nerve pattern during early developmental phases in chicken embryos. *Monitore Zool. Ital. N.S.* 4:81-98, 1970.

SPERRY, R. W. Mechanisms of neural maturation. In: *Handbook of Experimental Psychology,* edited by S. S. Stevens. New York: Wiley, 1951, p. 236-280.

SPERRY, R. W. Embryogenesis of behavioral nerve nets. In: *Organogenesis,* edited by R. L. Dehaan and H. Ursprung. New York: Holt, 1965, p. 161-186.

SZÉKELY, G. Functional specificity of spinal cord segments in the control of limb movements. *J. Embryol. Exp. Morph.* 11:431-444, 1963.

SZÉKELY, G. Developmental aspects of locomotion. In: *Neural Control of Locomotion,* edited by R. M. Herman, S. Grillner, P.S.G. Stein, and D. G. Stuart. New York, London: Plenum Press, 1976, p. 735-757.

SZÉKELY, G., and G. CZÉH. Localization of motoneurons in the limb moving spinal cord segments of ambystoma. *Acta Physiol. Hung.* 32:3–18, 1967.

SZÉKELY, G., and G. CZÉH. Activity of spinal cord fragments and limbs deplanted in the dorsal fin of urodela larvae. *Acta Physiol. Hung.* 40:303–312, 1971.

SZÉKELY, G., and J. SZENTÁGOTHAI. Experiments with "model nervous systems". *Acta Biol. Hung.* 12:253–269, 1962.

STRAZNICKY, K. Function of heterotopic spinal cord segments investigated in the chick. *Acta Biol. Hung.* 14:145–155, 1963.

TRAILL, A. B., and R. F. MARK. Optic and static contributions to ocular counter-rotation in carp. *J. Exp. Biol.* 52:109–124, 1970.

WEISS, P. Further experimental investigations on the phenomenon of homologous response in transplanted amphibian limbs. II. Nerve regeneration and innervation of the transplanted limbs. *J. comp. Neurol.* 66:481–455, 1937.

WEISS, P. Nervous system (neurogenesis). In: *Analysis of Development*, edited by B. H. Willier, P. A. Weiss, and V. Hamburger. Philadelphia: W. B. Saunders Co., 1955, p. 346–401.

WINDLE, W. F., and D. W. ORR. The development of behavior in chick embryos: Spinal cord structure correlated with early somatic motility. *J. comp. Neurol.* 60:287–307, 1934.

WYMAN, R. J. Somatotopic connectivity or species recognition connectivity. In: *Control of Posture and Locomotion*, edited by R. B. Stein et al. New York: Plenum Press, 1973, p. 45–53.

YOON, M. G. Reversibility of the reorganization of retinotectal projections in goldfish. *Exptl. Neurol.* 35:565–577, 1972a.

YOON, M. G. Synaptic plasticities of the retina and of the optic tectum in goldfish. *Am. Zool.* 12:106, 1972b.

DISCUSSION OF THE TROPHIC FUNCTIONS OF NERVES AND THEIR

MECHANISMS IN RELATION TO MANIPULATIVE THERAPY

Marcus Singer, Initiator of Discussion

Instead of beginning with a presentation, I prefer, first, to initiate the discussion and then, in the remaining time, review some of my material on trophic phenomena in regeneration of body parts.

Classically, we look at the muscles and bones as mechanical and metabolic devices to express the wishes of the nervous system. Classically, we have also considered muscle and its attachments to be dependent upon the nerve for maintenance and growth. The development of functional control of muscle by the nervous system was well summarized in the embryological information which Dr. Balaban presented. He showed that the set, the "tape", of the spinal cord which is read out in musculoskeletal activity, is patterned early in development, before suprasegmental control and even before sensory input into the cord, and that there is relatively little modulation of that set. A major embryologic problem is what controls its development and the constant fiber patterns which form it.

In recent years, however, we also have learned that in addition to the functional importance of the relation between a nerve and muscle, there is another nervous control. This second activity of the nerve was well expressed by Dr. McComas in his presentation, an activity also emphasized by Dr. Nigro in his numerous clinical examples.

That something else we have classically called trophic. For many years, following the demonstration of electrical conduction in the nerve, this second function was either ignored or denied, but I think there is now a consensus that in addition to functional control of muscle, the nerve provides something directly to the muscle for its well-being, growth and maintenance. This trophic function seems logical as a supporting one for the function of conduction, for if the muscle is to respond adequately to nervous stimulation, its metabolic and structural machinery must be attuned and maintained intact.

The difficulty in separating the trophic nervous function from that of conduction in studies on nervous control of muscle is that trophic activity of the motor neuron coincides in direction with impulse conduction, namely, they are both centrifugal in the motor axon and simultaneously impressed on the muscle fiber. Sometimes the two can be separated clinically, as Dr. McComas and Dr. Nigro pointed out, and experimentally, as was done, for example, by Miledi and by Buller and Eccles.

There are two model systems which have yielded much more information on the trophic activity of neurons than has muscle. They continue to yield more information about the nature of the trophic phenomenon. One is the maintenance of taste buds, a phenomenon discovered about 1873. Taste buds degenerate after the innervating fibers are destroyed, and reappear upon reinnervation of the epithelium. In this instance, the trophic influence is in reverse direction to conduction, being centrifugal, whereas sensory conduction is centripetal. Therefore, the phenomena of conduction and trophic control are readily separated and studied.

The second phenomenon with which I have been long concerned is the most classical one. It was the first scientifically demonstrated one, and was reported by an English medical doctor, T. J. Todd, in 1823. Todd performed his studies while in Naples, and showed that the salamander, ordinarily capable of regenerating a limb, fails to do so when the amputation stump is denervated. Johannes Mueller, in his textbook of 1830, recognized the significance of this work even though he had learned about it by hearsay. At that time there was considerable debate whether trophic activity of nerves really existed. I might add that the term "trophic" was not used. Instead, terms like "spirits", "vital forces", and "humors" were employed. Mueller notes that the experiments on the salamander were the first, to his knowledge, to prove that nerves also control the growth and maintenance of peripheral structures. I will discuss this later, but I should open the floor to discussion.

First of all, I shall call on Dr. Zalewski to comment, since he has been working on the trophic phenomena as they apply to taste buds.

DR. ANDREW A. ZALEWSKI: Previous speakers have clearly shown that material is synthesized in the nerve cell body and transported

peripherally. I think the question that we would like to answer
is, what does this material do, and in fact, what is this material
biochemically. Of course, some of the material that is transported
peripherally is needed for the nerve to maintain itself. Some of
the material is used for synaptic transmission. That leaves the
third category which is the one that is the present topic of discussion, the trophic chemical. Is there really any evidence that
there is a chemical passing down the nerve fiber that can maintain
and endorgan?

    In this regard, I would like to present not my work but some
of the work of a colleague of mine, Dr. Oh, previously at the
National Institutes of Health, who is now at the University of
Maryland. Working with chick muscle cells in culture, Dr. Oh has
been able to make an extract of peripheral nerve taken from the
chicken. When he adds this extract to his chick muscle cells, he
can maintain them indefinitely. In other words, he has something
taken from a nerve extract that apparently can substitute for the
nerve. As the work of Dr. Stanley Crain shows, if muscle cells
are cultured just by themselves, they will develop to form mature
myofibers, but then, if the nerve is not present, will undergo
degeneration. But if at this point, the Oh peripheral-nerve extract is added to the culture, these cells can be maintained virtually indefinitely--six or seven months or more. The question is,
is there a single chemical factor or are there multiple chemical
factors? Dr. Oh and his colleagues have been trying to purify this
nerve extract, and have isolated a fraction that has only two, or
perhaps three, proteins that they can identify.

    This brings up another question. Of all the various ways we
measure trophic effects of, say, motor neurons on muscle, there
must be a half-dozen or more different parameters that are measured
--cholinesterase, morphology, electrical properties, binding of
various toxins, acetylcholine receptors--one wonders how many different trophic factors there are. Is it just one, or are we dealing with multiple factors? From the data that Oh has at present,
we would have to think that there are not a great many trophic
factors.

    Now, just to mention some research that I have been doing with
the taste buds, it is rather curious that you can take virtually
any sensory neuron and by transplanting grafts to the anterior
chamber of the eye--the model that Dr. Thoenen mentioned--you will
find that taste buds will in fact regenerate. One of the characteristics, at least of the muscle work, is that if you switch
various motor nerves to various muscles in situ you can convert one
muscle to another type. If you take a fast motor neuron and put it
into a slow muscle, the slow muscle looks now like the fast nerve.

There aren't as many parameters to measure in taste buds as in muscle. But, again, trying to find out how many chemical factors we might have to postulate for taste buds, Dr. Oh found that if one switches innervation, say, between the front and back of the tongue--which, as you know, differ in response to taste solutions-- the response does not change. In other words, the taste bud is still maintaining its own specificity. We decided to see whether taste buds would change histochemically after this type of cross-innervation. Fortunately, within the same animal, taste buds are histochemically alike. But there is an animal that one could use to combine tissues from different animals, and this is the immunologically-deficient nude mouse. This animal has no thymus gland, and therefore, you can transplant virtually any tissue from other species of animals, and these tissues will survive. So, we took tongue tissue that had taste buds of different histochemical characteristics, combined these with ganglia from other animal species, and found that, again, the nerve did not change the histochemical characteristics of the taste buds.

The impression that I get from this work is that probably the only visible effect--by no means an unimportant one--of the nerve on the taste buds is that it induces the taste bud. From there on, however, the taste cell expresses its own gene activity. Perhaps the explanation for this phenomenon is that there really is only one trophic chemical that the nerve cells pass on to the end-organ. During these isolation procedures that Dr. Oh is using, perhaps he really is beginning to isolate a trophic factor that will in fact perform all the phenomena that we can measure.

DR. P. W. NATHAN: There is a similar experience in plastic surgery. Skin and the hair growing thereon, transplanted from one part of the body to another, retains its regional characteristics, even though reinnervated by the local nerve supply, resembling your taste bud studies.

DR. ZALEWSKI: I think in those particular situations, connective tissue is the determining tissue. If you were to split epithelium from underlying connective tissue, and take just the epithelium from the palms, which have a thick keratinized layer, and place it over the body trunk, that epithelium would change. And I think evidence from transplantation work indicates that connective tissue is a regulator. Perhaps it is something we ought to consider, too.

DR. HANS THOENEN: Is it possible to transplant taste buds from one area to the other? You have transposed a nerve. But if you transpose taste buds, do they adopt the properties of the new location?

DR. ZALEWSKI: The taste bud will disappear when you initially transplant, because it is denervated, and now a new one will have to form. We tried to maintain taste buds in the culture using the various nerve extracts that Dr. Oh has, and so far, we haven't been able to do that.

DR. HARRY GRUNDFEST: What kind of taste specificity were you talking about? As I recall, each taste bud seems to have a mixed pattern of responses of practically all the four main modalities. Are you checking that with sensory properties, or in some other way?

DR. ZALEWSKI: There doesn't seem to be any specificity among sensory neurons in inducing taste buds. For example, by using the transplantation techniques and putting grafts into the anterior chamber of the eye, and adding a spinal ganglion which presumably never had anything to do with taste, you'll get taste buds to form. Whether Dr. Thoenen's results might indicate that there is something in the tissue which is being transported back to the nerve cell body causing it now to produce the trophic substance, or whether this material has been there all the time, is not known.

It's also possible to take muscle from different species of animals and transplant it to the nude mouse and get muscular re-innervation. In this case, using the motor nerve fibers of the nude mouse, you can take muscle from rats and get essentially as good a reinnervation as if you took the mouse's muscle. It also would be possible, I presume, to take human muscle and get it to be reinnervated, too. This may make it possible to study some neuromuscular diseases of which the origin is uncertain.

DR. OTTO APPENZELLER: Dr. Zalewski, I am sure you are famil-iar with the syndrome of dysgeusia, in which man can lose his taste in a very short period of time, in which taste buds degen-erate histologically and in which regeneration of taste buds can be induced by the administration of zinc. I wondered whether zinc has been tried in your preparation or what it might have to do with the trophic factor.

DR. ZALEWSKI: I know that there is some work on zinc proteins and taste buds, and at one time we tried to look for zinc in taste buds and didn't find it.

DR. C. M. GODFREY: My question is directed to Dr. Ochs and Dr. McComas, in regard to reversibility and return to normal of nerve function following compression, and its relation to neura-praxic lesions. We know that many radial nerves do not recover functional ability for many months after the actual incident, and may never recover it. How do we combine that clinical finding with your reversibility study?

DR. SIDNEY OCHS: I think the answer may be in the way in
which the compression was done. If you apply a tourniquet or a
compression by similar means to the soft tissue of a limb, you
have an edge effect, so that the pressure is not uniform, but is
focused at the edges. There, the force may be great over a unit
area, and then you can have compression effects on the nerve and
all the consequences of nerve compression. However, if you use a
broad tourniquet, which distributes the pressure, then you are
more likely to occlude blood vessels and produce a somewhat simpler
anoxic effect. I think that is true because you get an almost immediate return of function even after 3 to 4 h at 38°C. By an
"immediate" return I mean return of action potentials within an
hour or less. So it appears that with this particular set-up you
are not dealing with compressive effects such as intussusception--
one node going into another node--which take a long time for
recovery.

DR. FRED SAMSON: Dr. Zalewski, when you make an extract of
the nerve, you are extracting more than axons. How do you know
that the trophic materials have been axoplasmically transported?

DR. ZALEWSKI: Experiments are now in progress to look into
that question--whether these materials could be Schwann cells, for
example. No, we don't know yet.

DR. JOHAN SJÖSTRAND: I would like to mention a condition in
which you can have a prolonged conduction block and still get instantaneous recovery. In a patient with chronic pharyngeal tumor,
a cyst was formed which refilled rapidly after repeated drainage.
The patient was blind--he could just count fingers--when the cyst
was full. And the patient could sometimes be blind for a week.
But when that reservoir was emptied he had recovery of 20/20 vision
and the complete visual field, within ten minutes. So I think it
would be possible just to "hit" the conduction and still have maintenance of the axons, with very rapid reversal.

DR. NIGRO: Was the problem at the optic nerve or at the
colliculus?

DR. SJÖSTRAND: It was just underneath the chiasm.

DR. NIGRO: It's unusual to have such a rapid recovery with
so total a visual defect.

DR. SJÖSTRAND: It was unusual in that we had a patient who
was awake, but I think it has been shown in other cases of nerve-
compressing tumors that there has been an improvement as soon as
the patient wakes up after surgery.

DR. APPENZELLER: There is even better evidence of that in patients who have had tumors pressing on the optic nerve or the chiasm for many years, and who are operated on with some specific lights put on the cornea to elicit visual-evoked potentials, recorded posteriorly during surgery. The patient doesn't have to be awake. So even during surgery, as the tumor is removed, the activity in the occipital cortex responds to stimulation and can be seen within minutes. In fact, this system is used by the surgeon to monitor the blood supply to the optic nerve and chiasm to be sure that his dissection does not interfere with the blood supply to the structures.

DR. McCOMAS: Dr. Brimijoin is one of the few who have studied axoplasmic transport in man, and I wonder if he would tell us where his present studies are.

DR. STEPHEN BRIMIJOIN: I wasn't going to bring those up, as they relate to hereditary neuropathies, which perhaps are less relevant to the present questions than compression lesions. For some time we have been studying axoplasmic transport by looking at human biopsy samples. The technique, though imperfect, is the best we could devise. It amounts to measuring, in vitro, the redistribution of endogenous enzymes that we can detect in these biopsy samples. We began with the marker enzyme for the sympathetic nervous system, dopamine-β-hydroxylase. We have now added acetylcholinesterase to our paradigm to get some idea as to what may be happening in other fibers, especially cholinergic ones. We have now accumulated some 50 cases--though not yet in a very systematic manner--most of them hereditary neuropathies. The largest series is in the Charcot-Marie-Tooth disorders of which there are several types. There is a somewhat smaller series of Déjérine-Sottas neuropathies, of which we saw a brief example in Dr. Nigro's talk, and a variety of other conditions. It has been striking to us that in certain of these disorders, most especially Déjérine-Sottas neuropathy, but also the Charcot-Marie-Tooth, we see marked changes in the redistribution of the proteins. These changes could be inferred to reflect either an impairment of the axonal flow of protein in these nerves, or, possibly, a combination of impaired flow and reduced synthesis and delivery into the axons, or, conceivably, just a primary reduction in synthesis. It's hard to separate these things out, and that is what we are trying to accomplish at the moment.

The Déjérine-Sottas neuropathy is a very interesting case. I think most "transportologists" would agree that the transport system is important for the health and function of the nerve. The question is, whether its impairment always results from an axonal pathology or whether it can be a manifestation of Schwann cells pathology. The Déjérine-Sottas neuropathy is strikingly similar

to the trembler mouse pathology, which has now been proved by some
rather elegant experiments--I think, involving the nude mouse--to
reflect a purely Schwann cell effect. But a number of studies suggest that Schwann cell disease does not affect transport, and it is
likely that in the human condition the situation is somewhat more
complex.

DR. SINGER: At Dr. Korr's request I will now present some of
my work on the trophic control of body-part regeneration with
which I have dealt for many years. What seems to be coming out of
my work and that of some others is that we are beginning to recognize the trophic phenomenon as a general biological phenomenon involving chemical conversation between cells. The conversation is
not just one way; it is a two-way conversation. For example, in
the case of the neuron and its target cell, the neuron speaks by
way of a chemical agent to the synaptic and peripheral structure
and, as Dr. Thoenen pointed out, a retrograde conversation also
goes on in which muscle, as an example, talks to the neuron. Some
evidence was presented in the course of the workshop discussions
that muscle must tell the nerve about its state and its activity.
The only way we can conceive of this conversation in modern terms
is by chemical means. My own feeling is that one of the next big
drives in the biomedical field is to try to uncover the nature
and language of the "whisperings" between cells.

Heretofore, we've confined ourselves largely to contact inhibition as a mechanism of cellular interaction expressed in mechanical contact and surface molecular mechanisms. In addition,
we must examine in the future the chemical interactions between
the nerve and the end structure. The classical animal in regeneration studies is the newt or salamander, Triturus. It is also the
classical animal in studies on embryogenesis.

If one amputates the limb or tail, it regrows rather rapidly,
and repeatedly after successive amputations. In its sequence the
growth repeats embryonic development and forms all the missing
parts of the structure, finally developing a fully functional
limb or tail. During regeneration of the arm, there is a stage of
wound healing, and a bud appears after about 10 days. After rapid
growth and then differentiation, histogenesis and morphogenesis
set in. After a few weeks, the various parts of the limb, including the fingers and hand, are recognizable and functional.

From the start, during wound healing, nerve fibers regenerate
into the wound area in great numbers, even invading the regenerated
epithelium in fascicles. Scar tissue is formed, but after about
8 days following amputation the scar is dissolved and mesenchyma-
tous cells take its place. The epithelium then thickens, and
underlying muscle and connective tissue of the stump near the wound

are dissolved, contributing a flood of cells to form the early bud. There is rapid cellular multiplication enlarging the bud into a cone. At this stage the regenerate looks much like a benign tumor, but shortly tissue differentiation takes place and the bone is completed in cartilage and missing skeletal elements appear, as do muscle, tendon, joints and so on.

Now, if the nerves supplying the amputation stump are cut at the time of amputation (e.g., for the forelimb in the brachial plexus so that the whole stump is denervated), no regeneration occurs; there is only wound healing. The skin forms over the surface, and skin glands appear. If the denervation is done in the early bud state, the regenerate bud withers and wastes, and is converted into fibrocellular scar tissue.

In the case of the larva, as Butler and Schotté showed in the early 1940's, there is not only no regeneration after denervation, but the entire limb is resorbed in a distal-proximal direction. But if the nerve fibers reinvade the resorbing structure, then resorption stops and the limb regenerates anew. Although resorption does not occur in the adult, regeneration will resume once nerve fibers have regrown into the stump, provided the original wound is refreshed.

What is the nature of this nerve control of regeneration? Many things have been learned over the years. First of all, all neurons are trophic. In other words, all neurons can accomplish this growth in the absence of others. Regrowth occurs in the presence of a pure motor supply, sensory supply or central nerve fibers. This must mean that the trophic quality is unrelated to the conduction function since it is always centrifugal in direction, whereas in the sensory neuron the conduction is centripetal, and in the motor, centrifugal. Moreover, it doesn't depend on any reflex connections, because one can cut all the motor fibers, cut the dorsal root proximal to the ganglion, and still obtain growth with an isolated sensory system. Or one can ablate the sensory ganglia and implant them into the early regenerate after cutting all other innervation and still obtain a regenerate.

It has also been learned that the nerve apparently controls the mitotic rate of the regenerate cells and the appearance of these cells, as well as their accumulation to form a blastema. The nerve does not control differentiation of a structure, or determine whether it is going to be a limb or a tail. Apparently it is involved in growth only. Quantity of fibers in the wound area is very important in this action. There must be a critical threshold number of fibers in order to induce regrowth. A subthreshold number is an inadequate stimulus for regeneration.

This finding helped resolve the question of why animals above the urodele amphibians cannot regrow the amputated limb. These animals, from the frog up to the mammals, apparently cannot regrow their limbs because there are not enough nerve fibers in their limbs. The mass of the limb outgrows the numbers of fibers, and the newt happens to have a very rich innervation of its limbs-- much more than higher forms do. In the course of evolution the higher forms apparently put their chips on the central nervous development at the expense of the peripheral one. If one increases the innervation of the postmetamorphic frog's limb, the limb regenerates in almost all instances. Similar evocation of regeneration in nonregenerating forms was also caused in the lizard limb and in the newborn opossum, by Mizelle.

There are two major questions concerning the nervous action on regeneration: (1) what is the character of the response of the regenerate cells to the nerve action, and (2) what is the nature of the neurotrophic agent? Recent biochemical analyses have yielded considerable information concerning both of these questions. As for the first, the responding mechanism to the neural influence, denervation during the early phase of regeneration causes an immediate outburst in RNA, protein and DNA synthesis in that order, followed by a decline, just as rapid as the outburst, to a plateau of about 50 to 60% of the control innervated side by about 48 h after denervation. Further analysis of this phenomenon, via studies on protein synthesis, showed that it is apparently the absolute rate of synthesis which is affected by the nerve. These studies showed that the availability of the precursor pool for amino acid incorporation is not affected, nor is the rate of turnover of newly synthesized protein. We found also that the nerve has nothing to do with the rate of translation of a protein.

A major question is whether the nerve controls the kinds of proteins formed. That is, are there regenerate-specific proteins controlled by the nerve? No differences in the kinds of protein produced before and after denervation could be found. Autoradiographs of slab-gel electrophoresed regenerate proteins or of two-dimensional gel analyses revealed a similar pattern of newly synthesized proteins. Therefore, the nerve is not concerned with the kinds of molecules produced, only with the quantity. This is further evidence that the neurotrophic activity is concerned with the rate of events that go on in the cell, it doesn't cause something new to occur. In other words, the cell is doing these things all the time, but it cannot do them at a fast enough rate to construct the regenerate. This is the way it appears to us at the moment.

The nerve influences the metabolic activity inherent in the cell. So, applying it to muscle, we would say that the muscle has the mechanism to sustain its metabolism and structure; it is just

that the nerve raises it to a level high enough to give expression
to the innate ability. I do not have time to go further into the
nature of the response to the neurotrophic agent and its theoretical interpretation. Instead, I refer you to some recent papers
(references appended).

We also addressed ourselves to the second problem, the nature
of the neurotrophic agent. We found that we could infuse the denervated regenerate with various test substances to see if we could
reverse the effect of denervation. Since, as previously noted,
protein synthesis declines rapidly after denervation, extracts of
nerve tissue were infused into the denervated regenerate and protein synthesis was studied 4 h later.

We were able to recover 100% of the lost protein synthesis
with a brain extract obtained by homogenizing newt brains and
clarifying the homogenate by centrifugation overnight at
140,000 g. The results showed that the extract duplicated the
action of the nerve on protein synthesis. A similar result was
obtained on DNA synthesis. Similar homogenates of liver and spleen
did not yield such results. To my knowledge this was the first
demonstration that the neurotrophic effect is mediated by a chemical substance and the first assay method for the agent. Since
then, there have been other assay methods using tissue culture
which Dr. Zalewski mentioned, including those of Lentz and Oh.

In our studies we found, too, that a synaptosome preparation
from the frog brain also restores the lost protein synthesis. This
is of great interest because a synaptosome preparation is relatively clean neuronal tissue, more so than our gross homogenates of
brain which include myelin, glia and whatever else one finds in
nerve tissue. Therefore, the active agent is in the neuron. Moreover, the synaptosomal results show that the neurotrophic agent is
not specific, at least between the newt and the frog.

The ultimate test of the effectiveness of a molecular fraction
extracted from nerve tissue would be to obtain or maintain regeneration of the body part in the absence of nerve. This has not
been done, although there have been various claims and presumably
many unsuccessful attempts, including our own. It is difficult to
apply the substance in the way the nerve does, directly and continuously, to the cells of regeneration. Perhaps this is the
limiting factor in current efforts to evoke regrowth in the
absence of nerve.

Another aspect of this story is the historical side. I am
prompted to remark upon this because of the interesting conversations about it I have had here with Dr. Magoun. The thing that
impresses both of us in historical studies on the nervous system

is the unity of thought, in terms of trophic functions, that existed over the centuries, going back to the Greek philosophers. Ancient Greek philosophers and others since then, including Galen and Descartes, thought that the nerves are conduits carrying "humors", "vital spirits" or an otherwise-termed flow to the structures in which they ended. They said or implied that the flow had various qualities, and that one of its functions was to maintain the peripheral structure (e.g., muscle). They did not, of course, know the details of microscopic structure and they assumed that the nerve fused, for example, with muscle.

The diagrams of Descartes depict a mechanistic model of how the nerve works. The Cartesian view was that the objects of sense, for example, enter the nerve, are carried into the ventricles of the brain, where some are stored for memory purposes and others, after modification, return through the nerve and are impressed on muscle for movement and, according to the works of many early philosophers, to maintain the peripheral structure. The unity of thought with present concepts is obvious: We project into the axonal level what they ascribed to the whole nerve, namely, that there is flow of axonal substance, a component of which carries the trophic agent, and instead of particles of motion and sensation, we speak of motor and sensory impulse conduction.

REFERENCES

DRACHMAN, D. B., editor. Trophic functions of the neuron. *Ann. N. Y. Acad. Sci.* 228:1-423, 1974.

SINGER, M. Neurotrophic control of limb regeneration in the newt. *Ann. N. Y. Acad. Sci.* 228:308-322, 1974.

SINGER, M., and J. ILAN. Nerve-dependent regulation of absolute rates of protein synthesis in newt limb regenerates. *Devel. Biol.* 57:174-187, 1977.

DR. MICHAEL PATTERSON: If the main influence of the nerve on the endorgan is simply to regulate the turnover or production of protein, how would this square with the ability of the nerve to change the characteristics of red and white muscle when interchanged?

DR. SINGER: I do not have the answer to that question, but have given it some thought. Perhaps the nerve, as I think, controls only the rate of macromolecular synthesis, and when the rate is increased, the character of muscle biochemistry changes. For example, if there is more trophic substance in the fast fiber than

in the slow fiber, and more delivered per unit time, it may be that
something may appear that we don't see in the muscle in great
amount. Fast and slow muscle really do about the same thing but
one does more of it than the other. That's my very speculative
answer to your question.

DR. GRUNDFEST: I was intrigued by the fact that you have
synaptosomes doing the same thing as the nerve extract, because in
the case of sensory nerves and motor nerves, you have entirely
different kinds of chemicals at the terminals and different effects on structures in the innervated limbs. Hence, we're dealing
with different synaptosomes.

DR. SINGER: Now you are talking in terms of mediators. But
we are talking about something common to sensory and motor, in
terms of the trophic substance. That is, both of them have it.

DR. THOENEN: I have a comment on this cross-transformation
of fast and slow muscles. I think it is not necessary to transpose the nerve. If you impose on a motor fiber the rate-pattern
of the other type—fast or slow—you change the expression of specific genetic information. You actually change the kind of heavy
or light meromyosin which is being newly synthesized by releasing
genetic information for fast muscle which, in the slow muscle, for
instance, is dormant. And this is turned on only by changing the
rate of the activity in the nerve. It is a specific regulation.
While I am fascinated by the phenomenon of transsynaptic induction
in neurons, I think that, with respect to regulation, it is more
interesting to see that you regulate specific molecules and not
simply a general growth. By only changing the rate-pattern in the
same neuron, you can turn on one macromolecular mechanism and turn
off the other.

DR. SJÖSTRAND: How much is known about changes in the muscle
membrane? In denervated muscle, it seems that different membrane
molecules become diffusely located in the membrane and when you
get reinnervation you have a concentrated localization of receptors and precise organization, requiring less synthesis. Is there
any evidence that part of the trophic effect is a control of the
receptor organization of the muscle membrane?

DR. SINGER: Yes, it may be. On the basis of other studies I
didn't mention, we think this whole change in synthesis goes by
way of an adenylcyclase system, which means receptors in the membrane affecting the biosynthetic activity. But it acts, we insist
at the moment, by way of rate. It doesn't create anything new,
for example, in the muscle, different from its genetic characteristic. All the nerve says to it is "more", or "keep it at this or
that rate". What does this have to do with manipulative therapy?

Well, if we'll accept the view that there is a two-way conversation between muscle and nerve, we could understand the value of
some of the other thoughts here. That is, the muscle is telling
the nerve certain things. It is at least telling it what its
state is. And the nerve is supplying something which the muscle
has anyway. I might point out one additional thing, without going
into all the evidence. The trophic substance, from our point of
view, is not unique to the neuron. All cells are trophic. All
cells have this substance. It is only that the neuron, when it
grows, imposes itself on the other cells, quenching to a certain
degree their production of a substance which they need, so that
they become, as I said years ago, addicted to the nerve, or at
least dependent upon the nerve. That was shown beautifully in experiments of Yntema, and then by Thornton here at Michigan State--
on limbs that had developed without having ever known nerve. Such
a limb will develop in the amphibian, as Harrison showed 60 or 70
years ago, with all its muscles, but then secondarily degenerate.

If, however, you amputate the limb, it can regenerate without
the nerve. But, as Thornton showed, once you let the nerve come
in, regeneration immediately becomes dependent on the nerve. Thereafter, the tissues must have what the nerve gives them. Once they
become dependent, the nerve maintains complete control, including
metabolic control, on these structures.

DR. SIDNEY OCHS: There is a nice example of that, the work
of Miledi and Thesleff. Later on Albuquerque showed clearly that
in the early stages the receptor for acetylcholine is spread out
over the whole muscle. In the adult you find the receptor is
located densely, for the most part, in the endplate region. Now,
if you cut the nerve, you find, as a function of days and weeks,
that the receptors themselves begin to appear further and further
away from the endplate region until after a while the whole muscle
becomes sensitive to acetylcholine. This is part of the clinical
information that Denny-Brown and others picked up early on, that a
denervated muscle is sensitive to acetylcholine, that it has now
reverted to an earlier state.

If you reinnervate that muscle, then the extrajunctional receptors get lost and the receptors concentrate again in the junc-
tional area, as in the mature adult stage. Further, it has been
shown that actinomycin-D will block receptor-spread following
denervation, which indicates that whatever that trophic substance
is, it is acting as a repressor; then when you cut the nerve, you
lose that and allow this synthesis of receptor protein to go on.

DR. APPENZELLER: I was wondering what relationship there
might be between this neurotrophic factor and the angiogenesis
factor or angiogenesis-trophic factor that was demonstrated by

some surgeons in Boston and the fibroblast-stimulating factor,
more recently demonstrated. These are all substances that seem
to stimulate profuse growth of the specific tissues. The angiogenesis factor is one that stimulates the growth of blood vessels
into tumors, for example, and the fibroblast-stimulating factor is
another substance that stimulates tremendous growth of fibroblasts
in tissue culture. Is there any relationship between these?

DR. SINGER: The nerve-growth factor, NGF, is another one of
those remarkable molecules that one could speculate on. One thing
they seem to have in common is that they are low-molecular-weight
peptides.

DR. KORR: Haven't we prematurely dismissed the question of
specificity, raised especially by Hans? There is abundant evidence
for the neural control of genic expression, and I wonder if that
isn't worth exploring further. It occurred to me, after I heard
Dr. Nigro, that the nude mouse might be a useful model to use to
transplant tissues of other species, nervous and others, to see if
there is any degree of transformation of species-specific properties.

DR. SINGER: I would like to know what Dr. Nigro's views are
in terms of these myopathies. Do you think, Dr. Nigro, that the
genetic deficiency is predominantly a nervous one, or is it reflected in the muscle, too?

DR. NIGRO: Most of the diseases, in my opinion, were primarily
nerve diseases. Exceptions are biochemical disorders which are
rather diffuse and multisystemic, which would make it difficult to
say there is any primary source of defect. Dr. Appenzeller was
talking earlier about some nerve work he is doing with transplants.
Maybe he could relate the nude mouse idea to his nerve transplants.

DR. SAMSON: About the extract, Dr. Singer, how do you know it
is a protein?

DR. SINGER: Heating it or digesting it with proteolytic enzymes destroys the activity. So it's undoubtedly a protein, and I
think the others who are working with it, like Oh, have reached
the same conclusion.

DR. ZALEWSKI: Just to make a few comments about epidermal
growth factor and fibroblastic growth factor. I'm not sure whether
this angiogenesis factor is in fact fibroblastic growth factor, but,
judging from the ways the authors treat their protein, it's different from procedures you would use on epidermal or fibroblastic
growth factor. So it would seem it's distinct from those particular factors, though all of them are protein.

DR. SINGER: I should remark that the fibroblastic growth
factor is obtained from nerve tissue. Its effect was originally
found on fibroblasts in culture, but it's an extract of nerve
tissue.

DR. THOENEN: In isolating such a factor, we always ran
head on against the barrier of the quantity. Have you tried to
use extract of neural tumors to see whether they induce regeneration?

DR. SINGER: That is, the embryonic neural tumor? No, we
haven't. There is a quantitative aspect involved; it would be
worth doing that. We do know, for example, that ependyma alone
can cause regeneration in the tail of the lizard. But of course,
ependyma is nerve tissue, although one might call it the glial,
since it gives rise to the neuroblasts and so on. I suspect that
this factor can also be extracted from other nerve tissue. It
would be worth trying embryonic tissue; I suspect that embryonic
tissue is loaded with this factor.

DR. HORACE MAGOUN: I wanted to ask something in that same
direction, but with a different focus. Now that you have worked
out your protocol and technical manipulability and so on, could
you start a parallel program on the effect of neural tissue on
neuron differentiation or regeneration, which would explore at
what point the neural tube loses its capacity to generate a central nervous system? In phylogeny you see the beginnings of the
drop-off at some point between the newt and the frog. And by the
time you get up into the mammals, reptiles versus mammals, this
capacity is essentially eliminated, compared to what it is in the
fish and the salamander.

Similarly, because ontogeny recapitulates phylogeny, the
original neural tube in the young fetus has this potentiality;
it can regenerate a whole central nervous system. At some age
after the beginning of this development, this ability diminishes
and by adulthood it's gone. Is anybody attempting to explore
what that neural tube factor is? Can it be cultured or preserved
somehow and utilized, not from nerve to muscle, but from one part
of the central nervous system to another part of the central nervous system, for the regeneration, restoration and functional
restitution of injured parts of the central nervous system? Take
paraplegia, for example, and the need for regeneration of the
spinal cord. You can do that in some of these primitive animals
and in the earliest stages after embryogenesis. Where is it lost,
and can it be retrieved? Can it be injected into the severed
spinal cord, for example, and do what is done in newts, regenerate
the rest of the spinal cord?

DR. SINGER: Well, it is an important question. We have been
examining the regeneration of the cord in the newt, because we want
to see how it does it. And what we learned is that it does it because it retains a primitive ependyma into the adult animal. In
other words, if you cut the tail off the newt, it will regenerate
its tail. If it regenerates its tail, it regenerates the whole
contained spinal cord--new neurons, new ganglia, and so on. It's
truly remarkable. Now, when you look at the sequence of development you find the first thing formed is the ependyma which grows
out just as you see it in the embryo. You have a primitive ependymal tube with its radiating processes; these cells divide and
give rise to the glia and the neuroblasts. But the interesting
thing we discovered is that these ependymal processes form channels
in advance of the growth of fibers. In other words, the ependymal
processes channel the pattern for the descending fibers from the
old spinal cord. Not only that, we recently found the pattern determining where the motor roots are going to emerge. The processes
themselves grow out of the cord at these points, and the motor
fibers follow it along. So the important thing is, if we could
wake up the ependyma in the higher forms, and get it to go back to
the embryonic state, it could do all this. Now how to do that--
we don't know. Some day, we will know.

DR. MAGOUN: Who could better find out than yourself?

DR. SINGER: Well, you know how basic science works. You
study everything along the way, and then some day one makes a leap.
I don't think we are ready for a leap with the trophic substance at
the moment. It is worth trying, as you mentioned.

Now we don't know why the higher forms lost the ability to regenerate the cord; we can only speculate. I think, because it
wasn't of great survival value, and their energy went into something else that was of great survival value. For example, if the
cord is injured, in the mammalian form, that animal has practically
no chance for survival. It can't escape its predators. But if it
has a good central nervous system, and can make its muscles and
limbs move fast, there is greater survival value in that. So in
the course of evolution, what the mammal has done is decrease
the peripheral innervation tremendously compared to the newt and,
for the conservation of its own energy, lost the regeneration-
inducing ability of the ependymal cell, but developed this extraordinary apparatus that allows us to use our musculoskeletal system in many more ways than a newt can, with its stereotyped sort
of movement.

Well, these are fundamental biological questions. And I
wish I could live long enough to see them answered.

Concluding Discussion

Chairman: Irvin M. Korr

DR. IRVIN M. KORR: I have asked each session chairman to summarize, from his perspective, what happened in his session. I trust it will not be merely a repetition of what was said, but an assessment of the new insights and especially the new questions that have emerged. As Dr. Goldstein reminded me, the main purpose of this Conference--and particularly this session--is to sharpen the questions for further exploration. Murray, will you start with your own summary of the session on Clinical Observations and Emerging Questions?

CLINICAL OBSERVATIONS AND EMERGING QUESTIONS

DR. MURRAY GOLDSTEIN: I must congratulate our Planning Committee for putting together an interesting and provocative group of people to open our session. Namely, using the format of informed, inquiring clinicians who face the reality of everyday life to pose the problems which they see, and challenge the scientists, including themselves (some of whom are also scientists), with the forced explanations which they are required to use in order to rationalize the basis for their therapy. One of our participants put it all in proper perspective when he described the continuum from fact to fantasy to fiction. I have elaborated on that by trying to understand the differences between fantasy and fiction, and came to the opinion that fantasy is speculation, and essentially what, in scientific terms, is hypothesis formulation. Fiction, on the other hand, is quite often what the clinician is forced to resort to in his efforts at explanation or rationalization, given the few facts he has. He also has the responsibility of applying those facts to a real-life clinical situation which he does not have the prerogative to walk away from--namely, the patient who presents with a real, acute problem.

Dr. Lewit opened our discussion quite properly by trying to acquaint us, in the wealth of his own clinical experience, with what he considered some of the cardinal rules of manipulative

429

therapy, as these rules relate to the conceptualization and the
fantasy--the speculation -- namely, what reflex mechanisms are the
rule, the mechanical nerve lesions being, in his view, the exception. He further pointed out that in his experience nerve compression usually produces numbness rather than pain. I must say
that later on in the discussion there was some question about that,
in that some clinicians felt that in fact nerve compression did
produce pain, rather than numbness. I suspect that we are in a
terminology argument in terms of the differences between paresthe-
sias and pain, and how the patient describes this unusual feeling.
Whether the tingling fingers, the uncomfortable arm, or the uncomfortable back which the patient in his terminology describes as
pain, perhaps the neurologist would describe as paresthesia. But
I retreat from that, because there was a brief but heated debate
about that question.

     Dr. Lewit then posed the $64,000 question in his presentation,
as to what is the "cause", as he called it, of the reflex, because,
he said, "a reflex without a stimulus is an absurdity." He then
shared with us his own clinical experience in terms of case
studies, of actual problem areas, organic disorders, in which
he had felt manipulation had a major therapeutic role.

     Dr. Greenman then approached the same issue in terms of total
health care. He shared with us an abbreviated history of manipulative therapy, and pointed out a matter that I think all of us would
agree to, and that is the horrible confusion of terminology. As
this method of approach to health and treatment of disease evolved,
individuals and the schools of therapy that appeared developed
their own terminology.   Like the Tower of Babel mentioned earlier,
this essentially assured that there would be little communication
among groups and probably none at all from the clinical group to
scientific.

     Dr. Greenman offered one definition which is now used, at least
in osteopathic groups, and which has been introduced into international terminology as it relates to the coding of diseases and
disorders and to health insurance plans. I refer to the term
"somatic dysfunction" which is defined in his paper and utilized
there. But the key point that Dr. Greenman made, at least to me,
was that the manipulative therapist does not treat pain. Although
the patient often presents with a complaint of pain, at least the
skilled therapist, the experienced clinician, is directing his attention not to the treatment of the pain, but rather to the treatment of the disorder, with the expectation, as Dr. Lewit would put
it, that if the "stimulus" is removed, the pain will disappear.

     It was at that time, I think, that we got into a bit of a dis-
cussion of what the stimulus is. Dr. Greenman and others offered

the point that the primary stimulus--the disorder, if you will--
was one of restricted motion, at a joint. He discussed a number
of the joints and the vertebral column as potential sites for that
restriction of motion.

We then moved on to Dr. Haldeman. Or, rather, Dr. Haldeman
moved on to us, and gave us all, I thought, a very lucid presentation of constructive criticism of the literature. He offered us a
parallel to the Koch postulates, the Haldeman postulates, that a
clinical investigator, particularly, would have to satisfy before
the data, and certainly the conclusions, could be accepted in the
literature and by the rest of us.

Then he summarized by giving us, I believe, two illustrations
each of some of the hypotheses that have been put forward in the
literature for the etiological factors and the results related to
manipulative therapy and the restricted joint motion.

The main point for me in Dr. Haldeman's presentation was the
real danger of what is euphemistically called "library research",
where some investigators go to the library, pick out findings and
pieces of information from various papers and weave them together
into a lovely story which, it is proposed, explains the entire
matter. The real danger of being so self-satisfied that we can
now explain everything--since the "facts" are in the literature
and it is just a question of their integration (Dr. Haldeman correctly pointed out this is probably more homogenization than
integration)--is that library research too often becomes an end
rather than a beginning.

I then used my prerogative as chairman and set up Dr. Buerger
as a straw man, asking him to describe the controlled clinical
trial, the first phase of which was being completed at University
of California-Irvine. I had done this with the idea that we would
get into a discussion of some of the pros and cons of the controlled clinical trial. Instead, the participants, as one might
have foreseen, started actively to redesign Dr. Buerger's trial,
to answer the questions which they were interested in solving.

The controlled clinical trial, of course, is a monstrous experimental instrument, now available to the clinician, and like
the laboratory research plan, has its strengths and weaknesses,
does it not? As a methodology, it is obviously good, the results
being valid and reasonably reproducible. The problem, of course,
is to find the question to which the controlled clinical trial is
applicable. One of the dangers I think we face, particularly at
this stage in development of the conceptualization of manipulative
therapy as it relates to health and disease, is to frame the meaningful question, and frame it carefully. Were it not precise

enough, the trial would give us results that don't fall on a bell-
shaped curve. And so our first session was spent, I think, in defining some of the overall problems and some of the concepts, and
focusing on some of the terminology, as viewed from the real-world
viewpoint of the practicing clinician.

I now invite your corrections, comments and additions to my
summary. Scott, did I either overdo or underdo the message con-
veyed in your presentation?

DR. SCOTT HALDEMAN: I don't think you did either. I think
you presented it very well. My concern has been, as I have said,
that throughout the field of manipulation certain clinical results
have been consistently observed even by conflicting professional
groups. In its battle for recognition, and in competition with
the others for the right to practice this art, each group has
formulated theories to try to justify what they are doing. Because much of the effort of the leaders and the educators of these
groups has been towards political recognition, with a neglect of
science and of research to the point where the theories, or the
fantasies, started being accepted as fact. This form of dogma
brought some discredit to the field as a whole.

I hope we have reached a stage where we can start distinguishing dogma from facts, and listening to the scientists, as we
have here, tell us where we are right and where we are wrong;
where we just don't know, and where the gaps are. One hopes that
the clinicians will go back and do the necessary research to fill
their part of the picture, and that the scientists will then get a
different approach or see how their methodologies and results have
been used. We will then, perhaps with minor changes or adaptations in some of the techniques, be able to help in determining
the validity of some of these theories.

DR. GOLDSTEIN: I would take only one exception to something
you said. I think it is unfair to charge scientists--and I assume
you mean basic scientists--with the responsibility of telling the
clinician whether he's right or wrong. That may be a judge-and-
jury situation. I would hope that the scientist tells the clinician whether he's right or wrong not by addressing that question
in itself, but in fact by substantiating what the real facts are
in terms of basic mechanisms, and that the clinical investigator
tells us whether our methodology is right or wrong.

Dr. Grundfest, do you feel that, in our opening session, the
explanation of the problems that the clinician faces offers enough
of a base to be of interest or stimulus to the preclinical or
basic science community?

DR. HARRY GRUNDFEST: In applying the "scientific method" you often have to squeeze your data until they scream. And the person who can squeeze the data in this particular way is the clinician. I agree with you on what you've just said about the judge and jury. The clinician has to take the data and really squeeze them, and come up with the validations, the hypotheses. I didn't get enough of that aspect, in either the opening session o r the following one. We really did not face enough of a data bank for us to make any judgments about how this relates to basic science. Perhaps I can comment further about this in our discussion of the next session.

DR. GOLDSTEIN: As Editor of the *Journal of the American Osteopathic Association*, Dr. Northup has had a great deal of experience with data bases, in terms of authors submitting manuscripts with a great deal of data in them. I wonder if he would like to elaborate further on the availability of data and making the data "scream".

DR. GEORGE W. NORTHUP: In the first place, before I get down to specifics, I think that what has impressed me most about this conference is that it is one of the few interdisciplinary conferences that I have attended through the years where manipulative therapy was discussed, not on the basis of trying to prove or disprove it, but to talk about some of the possible mechanisms through which it is manifest.

I agree with Dr. Grundfest that the data base is lacking, and one of the reasons that we come to you is to learn how to construct a data base perhaps in an area in which data bases have been somewhat differently constructed. We have the unusual situation of trying to analyze a subjective physician and his performance with a subjective patient, when the physician himself is part of the treatment. And this poses problems. So one of the features of the Conference that especially pleased me was that not only did we not come to disprove or prove anything, we came to discuss something that clinicians have observed through the years on an empirical basis. They have not always been clear and have come up with fanciful theories that did not hold up, as Scott has reminded us. We may not have discovered answers to some of the questions we are asking, but we learned something else: that perhaps we weren't asking the most appropriate questions. It seems to me that in our discussion, several areas came into scrutiny that had not been mentioned before, and which, it is hoped, people are now stimulated to discuss.

To most clinicians this whole area of axonal transport is a brand-new world. It is like suddenly seeing the other half of the world that you didn't know was there. It brings into sharp focus a much more close and sophisticated interrelationship between the nervous system and the musculoskeletal system. I am persuaded that there is much going on in the muscular system that has clinical implications that we are only just now beginning to discern.

Going to the other extreme, we have clinical observers who are looking at what Janet Travell refers to as trigger points. We have a man in Canada who says that trigger points are actually motor points. Another one says--authoritatively--that the so-called acupuncture points are nothing more than the accidental finding of putting a needle somewhere near a motor endplate. All in all, one gets the impression that there is some phenomenon here that different people are looking at and being awed by, then hastily creating a theory, without examining and comparing the observations of others.

Hence it seems to me that this conference has done many things. One of them--perhaps I emphasize it because of my bias-- is to focus on what is going on in a joint, and not just what is going on outside it. There is so much we clinicians don't know about the things that have to do with the internal milieu of a synovial joint and its relation to other matters discussed here, that I think we do need help.

As Murray said, several hundred papers cross my desk each year, and sometimes I have to look the other way with tongue in cheek, because clinicians are only human and, feeling like outsiders in the scientific community, sometimes when they come into print, they show a tendency to want to be "scientific". So they rush in with statistics, but without professional statisticians available, they try to become instant statisticians themselves. They want to show that they have read everything, so they append a bibliography of 300 references. In fact, I sent a paper back recently with the suggestion, "How about writing an article according to you?"

It seems to me that clinicians need help in two particular areas. As has come out here time and time again, first with the discussion of Dr. Buerger's and Dr. Godfrey's projects--and I want to compliment them for having the courage to enter the lion's den--I think it is an admirable thing. What happened is an example of what I have in mind. May I tell a short anecdote that is another example? I was once asked to do an organizational job, but I didn't have any idea how to start, so I consulted the man responsible for assigning me the job. He said, "I haven't the faintest idea, George, but I'll tell you one thing, I'll tear the hell out of your report!" And he did! It's easy to be critical of honest efforts at clinical research, when what clinicians need is help, not criticism. In a job such as mine you can see many examples of good, sincere people struggling to report their clinical research. I believe we need to elevate the standing of the straightforward report of clinical observation. Certainly, clinical observation has often led the way to fundamental knowledge, and in unanticipated directions. What the physician, with his trained, skilled eye, sees in his patients, but can't always explain, and is encouraged to report in an accurate outline fashion, is in our opinion a contribution to the literature. I certainly have appreciated the opportunity of being here to listen to men I have read about and greatly respect. And I think if you've done nothing more than give us an insight into what is going on in this interesting and amazing field of neurobiology, then you certainly have done us clinicians a great service. Knowing what goes on perhaps helps us at least to organize our confusion, and to get a clearer view of some of the more appropriate questions we should be asking.

DR. C. M. GODFREY: I thought the Conference got off to a good, if confused, start, because we sat down with eminent basic scientists and asked them to explain what we do, when we failed to agree on a definition of what it is that we do with manipulation. As we heard in the opening clinical papers, the term "manipulation" was, by one speaker, restricted to specific manipulation for the reduction of a joint dysfunction; others included various forms of soft-tissue treatment and even the nonspecific manipulation which had to do with a variety of diseases or internal disorders. And I felt a bit of guile in inveigling people like Dr. Magoun to sit down with me and explain something I hadn't clearly identified in the first place. So I was a little disappointed that we started running in all directions at once. The questions before us are all very important, but we must address one question at a time. I say let's solve the joint problem first.

DR. GOLDSTEIN: Dr. Godfrey, I think what the opening session did was accurately describe the state of the art. Namely, the confusion: the fact that people are using different terms for the same thing, and the same terms for different things. In that respect, I thought the Conference was particularly accurate that morning. It identified the issue that we may need to be more specific, though I'm not sure we have to select one issue as more important than another. I would hope much of this research can go on in parallel. I would also hope that we could be specific enough so that when others read our research or try to duplicate it, they know precisely what procedure we are talking about, rather than the broad generality of manipulative therapy.

I apologized last night to Dr. Koizumi for using my Chairman's prerogative to short-circuit the discussion of her very important question. She wanted to know what manipulative therapy was. That is, in some respects, what the whole conference is about. Yet we use the term for countless specific activities and for many generalities. This problem, I must emphasize, is by no means peculiar

to manipulative therapy. There is no field of science, whether it
be clinical or basic, in which preciseness is inherent in the system. Precision is the result, I think, of a lot of hard work.

So we should not be discouraged because clinicians cannot yet
define and because clinical data seem, therefore, in some respects,
to be random.

DR. PHILIP E. GREENMAN: I agree. But my interchanges with
colleagues in the chiropractic profession as well as with colleagues in the medical profession who do manipulative therapy and
colleagues in the osteopathic profession, convince me that we all
are dealing with the same basic phenomena going on in the musculoskeletal system, however we may describe it, with whatever terminology. So once more I take the opportunity to plead for the
development of good terminology for these phenomena. I agree that
it will not be easy. Certainly, commonality of procedures, descriptions and terminology has not yet been achieved within the
osteopathic profession. Commonality is being sought by a small
group of osteopathic physicians here at Michigan State, who work
together in the classroom, in research and in the clinic, even
sharing patients, all under the scrutiny of each other and that of
a group of bioscientists. They still have not achieved commonality
of description of what they actually do, apart from improving mobility. I merely wish to emphasize to our basic science colleagues
here that we are dealing with a monstrous language problem that
must be solved before we can address the issues of statistical
analysis of the changes that occur when manipulative therapy is
used.

DR. MARTIN E. JENNESS: Really, the basic thing, as I see it,
that Dr. Greenman is referring to is two concepts in measurement:
one of course is referred to as reliability or precision of measurement, and the second is referred to as objectivity, or the
ability of two different investigators to arrive at the same conclusion in their observations or measurements. I have been doing
work on this issue with respect to the clinical procedures that are
in common use by all of the health professions. The literature
doesn't give me much help in this area. Such common things as taking blood pressure, as I'm sure many of you know, are subject to
varying interpretations. So, my objective is to try to state in
some type of operational definition the methods that should be
used, or ideally could be used, in some of the work that we do as
clinicians. I think that this is imperative before we can consider meaningful clinically controlled trials. I see the purpose
of this workshop, in part, is to enable us to better design our
clinical trials for manipulation.

Now, we heard from Dr. Buerger and Dr. Godfrey about the clinical trials they were doing, and I felt a great empathy for the situation that they find themselves in. If this conference can provide us a stronger basis for properly designing clinical trials, I feel it will have accomplished a great deal. We also heard from Dr. Coote, Dr. Koizumi and Dr. Korr relative to autonomic influences. In particular, Dr. Koizumi showed us the effects of even skin stimulation on certain internal activities, the intestinal motility. So, in trying to design controlled clinical trials, it is desirable to develop a clear-cut control group, or placebo group, as was attempted by Dr. Buerger.

But the work of Drs. Coote, Koizumi and Korr demonstrates just how difficult this is. For example, if stimulation of the skin can affect internal activity, then certainly we would expect massage, which was used as the control in Dr. Buerger's experiment, perhaps to be a second--though unwanted--experimental group, not a placebo. So I would like to ask the question of this body, how can we properly design a placebo or control group such that we can be sure it is in fact the control and not an additional experimental group?

DR. GOLDSTEIN: Dr. Jenness, I think that is a good question, but I suspect that in a summary session it might take more time than we have available. As a matter of fact, it might be in some respects a conference subject in its own right. With your permission, I would like to shelve that question as too big and too important for this brief summary session.

DR. KAREL LEWIT: I would like to comment in a slightly more optimistic way. I was surprised that there was one aspect in which there was less confusion than I expected. However different the terminology used, all the clinicians got to the same problem-- however differently they explained it--that we are dealing with impaired joint function, that manipulative therapy is really therapy to restore joint function. Therefore, I would point out that the concept of somatic dysfunction is a concept which expresses something important. (In Europe we call it the segmental lesion, and some call it the pseudoradicular lesion, because it is a reflex phenomenon.) But it has too many facets: it has a muscular side which can be dealt with by massage; it has skin changes which may be dealt with by needling or other techniques which act on the skin receptors directly. But I think we could define the lesion which we treat by manipulative techniques with some word which really defines the restrictive movement. In Europe, the word "blockage" has come into wide usage, and you will now find it in most of the literature. Some prefer the word "binding", some, "fixation". I don't think this matters, but I think one crystal-clear conclusion could be that manipulation acts on--pick your term--movement restriction, fixation, binding or blockage.

DR. GOLDSTEIN: I agree with you, that we are all dealing
with a single phenomenon of reduced mobility, however we describe
it.   But my concern, and I think perhaps the concern of the basic
scientists, particularly those in biomechanics and biophysics, is
whether the phenomenon exists.   It may satisfactorily designate
what is _perceived_ to be going on, but the real hard evidence of a
quantitative sort is still very thin.   That doesn't mean that the
phenomenon doesn't exist, but I am concerned that if we prematurely
lock into a single term that we all agree on, it may come to represent a concept that has not yet matured in demonstrated biophys-
ical and biomechanical terms.

SIR SYDNEY SUNDERLAND: Just a few comments on that delightful
presentation of Marcus Singer's yesterday afternoon.   He mentioned
the meaningful dialogue that is going on continually between nerve
and muscle and muscle and nerve, using a code which still eludes
us.   We have now passed to another phase, where we have the clinician on the one side, and the "fundamentalist" on the other, with
a dialogue passing between them which is not always meaningful.   In
other words, there is a great deal of static about, and I don't
think we have yet managed to break the code.   This, I think, is
partly a question of terminology; the Book of Corinthians says,
"Unless you utter by the tongue words easy to be understood, how
shall it be understood what is spoken?"

Let's look at this problem in another way.   The fundamentalist
is obliged to satisfy only his curiosity.   The clinician is not
only inclined to satisfy his curiosity, but he is also obliged to
satisfy a clinical need.   So he has a dual task.   To me, one of
the problems, particularly those relating to the first morning's
discussion, was that maybe we did not allow sufficient time for
the clinicians to put their point of view.   But, as that great
Frenchman, Maurice Chevalier, said, "At our age, we must be
reasonable."   There is a dilemma here, you see.   If you think back
to medicine, say in the United Kingdom in the 18th Century, treatment was based essentially on history-taking, and analysis of
symptoms.   And I think we owe to the French the recognition of the
importance of physical signs in clinical diagnosis.   But it was
only finally when you could combine symptoms and signs, by studying the problem in the postmortem room, that you could bring some
sound basis to therapeutic procedures.   And it seems to me that in
this area--and I don't want to be misunderstood when I say this,
because I recognize all of the difficulties--but in some respects,
in this field at the clinical level we are still back in the 17th
or 18th Century.

In other words, we do not know the basic pathology; we speculate on what the pathology might be.   We are meticulous in taking
a history, in listening to the patient, in eliciting physical signs,

signs, but from that point onward, we are manipulating in the dark.
This is the dilemma of the clinician, and I think what the clinician
must do is to specify more clearly to the basic scientist what the
core of the clinical problem really is.   It's not initially a problem directed to the basic scientists, it's one that comes up in the
course of clinical practice.   And now, we go to the scientist to
see what he can do to assist in reaching a solution to the little
experiments that nature, from day to day, is carrying on, where we
are regrettably unable to code the message that nature is trying to
transmit.

DR. GOLDSTEIN: Thank you, Sir Sydney.   That was well put in
terms of the first session.   Final comment, Dr. Gitelman.

DR. RONALD GITELMAN: I believe we as clinicians have misled
you somewhat.   You define our problem quite well, but in terms of
clinical signs.   You tell how we all methodically come to our conclusions through a detailed examination.   The interesting thing is,
that although that is true, we all do different detailed examinations.   And the real issue is that this subject of palpation has
never really been established as a valid method.   We have never
taken a half-dozen palpators to palpate the same patients to see
how well they correlate.   So that one of the things that we do not
have is a basic standardization of the examination procedure.
Hence, if we are making decisions on questionable information,
our conclusions obviously are questionable.   And our ability to
communicate with each other is limited.   In short, we must
standardize.

DR. GOLDSTEIN: The time has come that we must bring this
discussion to a close.   Obviously, one of the major problems is
communication, both between and among disciplines and, as
Dr. Gitelman is pointing out, even between and among clinicians.

DR. KORR: I think the important parts of the Conference--the
most valuable ones, perhaps--are the conversations that take place
during the recesses.   Conversations with a couple of my fellow
senior citizens a few minutes ago really made it clear that objective number two in the design of the workshop was quite unrealistic.   The first one was identifying new questions emerging
from clinical experience; the second one to seek answers in the
research findings that are already available.   We should not be
expecting answers.   I think the best we can say we have achieved
is that we have identified mechanisms that may be implicated in
what the manipulating clinician does.   And that brings us to objective number three, which is, as Murray said, to "sharpen the
questions", to identify and project needed lines of research that
one hopes may provide some answers and, one also hopes, will raise

a new series of sharper questions. As James Thurber said, it is
better to know some of the questions than all of the answers.

I now call on Dr. Magoun to summarize and moderate discussion
of impulse-based mechanisms.

IMPULSE-BASED MECHANISMS

DR. HORACE W. MAGOUN: For me, the opportunity to summarize is
an opportunity rather to generalize. First, however, I want to
call attention to what I thought was the beginning step in the
impulse-based part of the program, and that was, in the classic
British tradition, Sydney Sunderland's definitive exposition of
the anatomical organization of the vertebral column and its relation to the spinal cord and the roots, forming the peripheral
nervous system for the body. It was a beautiful presentation of
fundamental material relevant to the whole substance of what is
going on in and is envisioned for the future in spinal manipulative
therapy.

The balance of the presentations in that part of the program
elaborated features of the irritation or injury of two functional
components of these spinal nerves, as a step toward understanding
the relief which spinal manipulative therapy can provide when
these nerve components are irritated or injured. The first of
these functional components to be discussed were the sensory ones
consisting of the small myelinated and unmyelinated fibers of the
dorsal spinal roots, excitation of which is experienced as pain.
In particular, emphasis was placed on the posterior ramus of the
exiting spinal nerves, which innervate the deep and cutaneous
structures surrounding the vertebral column, irritation of which
is thought by some to be responsible for some of the tortures of
back pain.

The second of these functional components, on the motor side,
consisted of the preganglionic autonomic fibers of the ventral
roots of the thoracolumbar region which, relayed by the peripheral
ganglia of the sympathetic nervous system, innervate the smooth
muscles and glands of the viscera throughout the body. It was
proposed that irritation of these fibers contributes to such
chronic disorders of visceral function as hypertension, gastric
and duodenal ulcers, colitis, diseases of gallbladder, kidney,
and other viscera.

With these two simple but fundamental summary generalizations
of the middle part of the program, I would like next to respond to
Murray Goldstein's question as related by Dr. Korr, "You've had
your workshop--what should you do next?" The usual response of

people who organize workshops--and I can say this because I have in
an earlier period had some responsibilities like this--is to hold
more such workshops. Indeed, some foundations or organizations in
this country have put their entire resources and facilities into
conference series, and I'm sure they have contributed something to
the development and advances of the health sciences. But in the
present case, I would like to propose an alternative route that
would have the advantage of bringing the concepts and issues discussed here, together with the physicians and scientists concerned
with them, out of the relatively circumscribed and isolated environment of a shut-in workshop, into broader associations with the main-
streams of advance in the health sciences. These are to be found
in the annual meetings, conferences and symposia of already-
established societies that have grown up around the various interdisciplinary areas of contemporary scientific research.

In the case of the problem of pain, there is a rapidly growing
international association for the study of pain, with national
chapters, one of them an American chapter. The meetings of this
society have drawn together anesthesiologists, dentists, physiologists, neurologists, surgeons, a range of people from a variety of
backgrounds and views, all concerned with the attempt to develop
means for pain control. The spinal manipulative therapist could
provide a valuable input into the programs and activities of this
society, and doubtless benefit from interchange with its ranging
membership. My first suggestion would be, then, that the way to
go next might be to get in touch with the program committee of the
American chapter or other national chapter of the Association for
the Study of Pain, and see if they can't join with you in providing
more and wider ranging opportunities for the exploration of control
of back pain and of spinal manipulative therapy in its amelioration.

In the case of the problem of disordered visceral functions,
there are still more varied associations and opportunities for
joining with them in existing societies, where specialty groups
have been assembled in this area over at least the past half-
century. A number of these have had the special feature of interrelating the scientists and therapists with visceral physiologists
and physicians. An important early development in this direction
was that which took off from the appointment of Alan Gregg as the
Vice President of the Rockefeller Foundation in the beginning of
the 1930's. Gregg seized this opportunity to utilize the Rockefeller Foundation's funds to advance the field of neuropsychiatry
in this country and in Canada. Among the programs which were supported was that of Stanley Cobb and his associates at the Massachu-
setts General Hospital at Harvard, that of Franz Alexander at
Chicago Psychoanalytic Institute, that of Flanders Dunbar at Columbia, Howard G. Wolfe at Cornell Medical School in New York--and a
number of others in areas identified at the time as psychosomatic

medicine. A society was established, a journal was initiated, and
the people involved in this program presumably were concerned with
effective therapy by manipulation of the patient's psyche.

In relation to this same area, there was established a field
identified as psychophysiology, of which Chester Darrow at the
Juvenile Research Center in Chicago was a key promoter. The current president is David Shapiro, a colleague at UCLA. The particular focus of interest of this group lies in applying the techniques
of electrophysiology to the study of the EEG, the psychogalvanic
reflex, electromyography, studies of vasomotor activity, heart rate
and other visceral behavior. Again, a growing society has been
established, and it publishes a journal.

In a somewhat analogous direction is the specialty called
psychobiology, fostered by Adolf Meyers in the Phipps Psychiatric
Institute of the Johns Hopkins Medical School. Two early associates
were Curt Richter, who I think has exemplified what the field of
psychobiology can lead to, and Horsley Gantt, who was an early
leader in the development of the Pavlovian Society of America. The
goal of this society was to introduce and utilize conditioned reflex
techniques for the investigation of both visceral and psychovisceral
functions, and also to advance their therapy.

In this direction, two psychiatrists specialized in introducing
conditioned reflex studies, first in monkeys and then in the relief
of visceral disorders in patients. I believe one of these was a
South African psychiatrist named Volpe, now in this country. The
other, doing all of his work in this country, was Jules Masserman
in the Department of Psychiatry at the University of Chicago, and
I think more recently at Northwestern.

I should name one more organization. The early-established
society in this broad field, the American Psychiatric Association,
has, like the American Medical Association and other such major
organizations, had its general focus on a variety of therapies.
Most of them were so clinically oriented that the basic science-
oriented people attending these meetings early established a
Society of Biological Psychiatry which used to meet the day before
the APA meetings to provide an opportunity to get together.

Out of the specialties that I have mentioned was developed the
concept of behavior modification, with roots in the areas of learning function, drive reduction, and emphasis on either positive or
negative reinforcement. The Yale psychologist, Clark Hall, was
prominent in this movement. It has roots also in the work of Neal
Miller and others, in the conditioning of visceral function, both
as an investigative methodology and also as a therapy. One of the
most impressive developments in this direction is presently given

the specialty term of biofeedback, which claims to enable the patient to utilize, for therapeutic purposes, the principles of
physiological information that have been developed in this area.

Well, the generalization I would make as to future meetings
to succeed this workshop, or perhaps concurrent with subsequent
workshops, would be the effort to interest such broader and more
widely disciplined organizations in the issues and problems of
spinal manipulative therapy, and to attempt to interrelate them
in the more general goal of improving therapy for disease and injury in this direction, as contrasted with the holding of a succession of self-contained workshops.

I can't resist the opportunity to comment on the concluding
part of yesterday's program and that marvelous presentation of
Marcus Singer on regeneration in the newt. This seems to me to
be the take-off and breakthrough in this general field of neuro-
plasticity and the restorations of structure and function after
injury to the nervous system. In groping for a way to comment on
this, I found an article by R. P. Bunge, of Washington University,
on the changing uses of tissue culture from 1950 to 1975. It appears in Volume I in the Basic Neurosciences of the 25th anniver-
sary publication of NINCDS, a three-volume collection of papers on
The Nervous System, of which Donald Tower is Editor-in-Chief.
Bunge states, "To this writer, the most attractive hypothesis is
that, in general, neurons, during some stage in their development,
acquire a critical defect in some vital function (e.g., their
ability to transport certain nutrients). This deficiency must be
corrected by an outside agent--a trophic factor--if the neuron is
to survive and function. This trophic factor may be provided to
the neuron from its synaptic input and/or by supporting glia and/or
by contact with target tissues. If we provide adequate glial support or target tissue the neuron may survive in culture, even
though the specific agent or agents being provided by these cells
to correct its deficiencies are not known. If the trophic factor
is known (and NGF is certainly such a factor), then the neuron can
be maintained indefinitely in complete isolation. . . ."

Bunge ultimately focuses on the culture of a specific supporting cell, free of other cell types, which has also been accomplished.
A recent report indicates that essentially pure Schwann cell popula-
tions may be obtained from rat sensory ganglia in explants. Using
special methods of explant preparation and so forth, the possibility exists for turning out normal Schwann cells in large numbers.
I think Dr. Singer commented on the importance of attending to
these along with the preservation of the regenerative capacity of
neural tissue proper, because the combination of the two seems to
be essential in the restoration and regeneration of structure and
function.

It seems to me that of all of the marvelous presentations we
have heard at this workshop, this one of Singer's introduces a
field and a prospect for the future that has significance not
simply for spinal manipulative therapy, but for the entire spectrum of diseases, disorders and injuries to the nervous system,
from which such large portions of the American population suffer.

DR. MICHAEL M. PATTERSON: In the discussion about manipulative therapy our emphasis seems to have been on shorter-term sorts
of problems, such as the "blocked joint"--a mechanical thing which
may occur very rapidly, and be rapidly corrected. But we have the
interesting obverse question. We go through our lives doing all
sorts of things to our spines and musculoskeletal system in general.
The question is, "Why don't these problems occur more often than
they do?" I would like to offer a possibility that has not been
emphasized much here yet, namely that the spinal cord itself may
play a central role in protection against the problems we have been
talking about that are amenable to manipulative therapy.

I have in mind the ability of the cord and its reflex circuits
to respond in a plastic fashion, with habituation, for instance, as
a protective mechanism against input that is aberrant. That is, if
some mechanical problem occurs, or receptors are overactive, the
spinal cord itself tones down their impact through habituation
mechanisms, and therefore protects against the vicious cycle that
would produce pain and dysfunction. The possibility then occurs
that we get the problems we have been talking about only when certain prepotent or terrifically overactive inputs occur, that cause
the opposite process of sensitization. And then, some of these
longer-term conditions, axonal flow problems, and problems of entrapment and so on, can begin to occur. I think, therefore, that
we should not neglect this possible role of reflex plasticity
itself in the phenomena that we are looking at--especially when we
think of the short-term situations where manipulation can be used.

DR. MAGOUN: Do you have a suggestion as to how this could be
cultivated by clinical maneuver? I mean, how would you try to
suppress the sensitization?

DR. PATTERSON: I think that the rapidity with which some of
the problems seen by manipulators can be altered would indicate
that the manipulative procedure may simply allow the spinal cord
to begin the process of reflex habituation.

DR. MAGOUN: Is there anything in addition to the routine
manipulation that you can think of to advance this habituation,
some suppressive activity?

DR. PATTERSON: Sleep, for example, or other forms of psychic relaxation, might be thought of as reducing the overall level of activity in the system. Certain drugs also exert similar non-specific effects. But it is one of the beautiful features of manipulative therapy that it can be so specifically directed to the problem area or segment.

DR. GOLDSTEIN: In listening to the papers the last day and a half, I was impressed by one omission, except for Dr. Singer's impressive presentation, and that was that there was no mention of the use of an animal model in which variables could be studied under more controlled conditions. I couldn't help but wonder whether it was just the preselection of our participating group or whether, in fact, there was a shortage of this technology in our science, as it relates to this problem. Since Dr. Korr invited us to discuss deficiencies, I just wondered whether this model did not exist at all, and if it didn't, is there potential value in developing models for use in a laboratory situation and of teasing apart and identifying specific problems with that model. It would give us the opportunity to examine some of the biologic phenomena related to manipulative therapy. I think we would all agree that if the clinical aspect is a phenomenon unique to the human, we would all feel quite uncomfortable about the validity of the phe-nomenon. One hopes we are dealing with a more generalized bio-logical issue. And so, I did want to introduce into the discussion the question, "Is there a lack of an animal model; if so, why; and what are the consequences of such a lack?"

DR. MAGOUN: Dr. Weaver, do you have a suggestion to make here?

DR. LYNNE C. WEAVER: Certainly there is one animal model for low back pain that I can think of immediately. If that is one of the pathological situations that manipulative therapy is used to approach, there is a superb animal model--the dachshund. The dogs which are relatively long have the same sort of difficulties as humans do with upright posture, in supporting their spinal struc-tures. The dachshund, the beagle, other breeds of dogs and many species of animals have, with advancing age or even at maturity, tremendous difficulty regarding their bony structure. I would think that, particularly on this campus, we have an ideal environ-ment to use this particular animal model to try to ascertain some possible mechanisms of manipulative therapy.

DR. MAGOUN: This response is a beautiful illustration of in-terrelating fields around this problem, because I happen to know that Dr. Weaver's background has been in veterinary medicine, where, I believe, I heard her mention she had earlier treated back pain difficulties in dachshunds, brought to her by their owners.

DR. WEAVER: But never with manipulation.

DR. MAGOUN: Well, you certainly have an opportunity here at Michigan State to develop a program of this sort. It may help in many directions.

DR. JOHN H. COOTE: There aren't models that relate particularly to the clinical problem. But there is work that experimental "fundamentalists" do with regard to the afferent fibers coming from muscles and joints, and what their effects might be on the somatomotor system as well as the autonomic system. I did mention some of my own work on this, in which we showed it is the small myelinated and nonmyelinated fibers involved in the autonomic nervous systems. These are fibers which cause excitation when the joint moves. It's possible that these endings can be sensitized under some circumstances. I think I did try to point out that we don't know as yet-- and it is an experiment that still needs to be done with regard to these joint fibers--what, under normal circumstances, is stimulating those fibers to send their information to the central nervous system. What sort of movements are required in order to activate them? We can experimentally do something with them, as I described in the cat, but it is an extreme situation in which we put the legs on a bicycle and twirl them around and measure their angles and movements. But nobody, as yet, has recorded from those small fibers and shown the adequate stimulus to them. That is an area that needs to be studied.

DR. MAGOUN: Dr. Coote, may I ask if it would be any more difficult for you to undertake these experiments in dachshunds than cats? You are a lot closer to Germany, the source of the dachshund.

DR. COOTE: They would also be much cheaper, actually. Cats are very expensive.

DR. MAGOUN: I take this opportunity to say that, in this field of the spinal organization for visceral motor function, it appeared to me that Dr. Coote's presentation at this workshop was an epoch-making beginning in the study of this field, and in the pattern established more than a century ago by Sherrington in the somatic motor organization of the cord. It seems to me that, not only for spinal manipulative therapy, but for the whole field of visceral physiology and medicine, the work that he is doing is laying the kind of foundation that one would like to see in every facet of what we have talked about at this meeting.

DR. GRUNDFEST: Models are important, I think, where one is subjecting the model to some kind of destructive processes. If one uses nondestructive methods, the human being is just as good a model as anything else. The problem then comes up, what kind of data can be gathered, given the limitation of nondestructive approaches? This is a problem of ingenuity and of concentration of resources, such as engineers, physiologists, mathematicians, electronics people and others. This would yield the methods for examining things nondestructively. There are common and successful non-invasive procedures in many fields now. Models like the dachshund are valuable and should certainly be pursued, especially where, as Dr. Weaver points out, you can have collaboration between a leading school of veterinary medicine and one of osteopathic medicine. But one needn't simply throw up one's hands if one doesn't have an animal model.

Now, I would like to come back to a subject Dr. Goldstein raised earlier this morning, and asked for my comments. I wanted to elaborate a little, and Dr. Korr has already made some good points with which I agree. I would like to point out that what the basic scientist can do is express what can and cannot be done with his knowledge. But where a specific hypothesis must be developed to explain the data, say, of manipulative therapy, it must come from the therapist himself. I mean that, as a neurophysiologist, I can't tell the clinician what will happen if we have a nerve lesion of such-and-such kind, in a particular situation. All I can say is, given the lesion, such-and-such things might happen; given another set of conditions, something else might happen.

Dr. Coote's analysis of the autonomic organization gives information about what kinds of pathways there may be. He doesn't know yet what other kinds of pathways there may be. There may be many more. The question now is, can you formulate a hypothesis on the basis of current knowledge? And then, can you make those data on which the hypothesis is formed scream loud enough?

DR. KORR: May I respond to the question about models? It certainly is an important one which has plagued us for a good many years. This is not to question the validity of what you had to say, Harry. There have been, throughout the history of research in the osteopathic profession, a number of attempts at models which, at least from my viewpoint, have been unsatisfactory and not worth my own pursuing. Many years ago, Louisa Burns, a distinguished osteopathic physician, created what she thought was a model of the "osteopathic lesion". Working with rabbits, she would apply, at least as I saw the technique applied, shearing force between two consecutive spinous processes and hold the pressure until palpation of the paraspinal muscles and the responses of the animal told her that spasm and other self-sustaining changes had been induced. She studied those animals for weeks and months on end after inducing these "intervertebral strains", as she called them. Her approach was to study histological changes in the paraspinal tissues, changes in the vascularity of the muscles and changes in viscera that were "segmentally related" in comparison to those that were not segmentally related. This was pursued for many years by

Dr. Burns and a number of her collaborators at a research institu-
tion in California. It was associated with the former College of
Osteopathic Physicians and Surgeons in Los Angeles. This was the
college that was converted in the 1960's to the California College
of Medicine at Irvine.

More recently, J. S. Denslow, my colleague at Kirksville, has
for some years been studying motor reflexes associated with what he
regards as a naturally occurring osteopathic lesion in dogs. In
the lower thoracic spine of the dog there is a reversal of the direction of the spinous processes. He discovered, having worked
with dogs for years, that that is a very tender spot. He uses
that as a sort of trigger or pushbutton for eliciting EMG-measured
responses of various trunk muscles. It's a kind of model. But
how closely it corresponds to "the lesion"--the somatic dysfunction
--that arises in the human lifetime, in the course of battling and
adapting to gravitational forces is, in my opinion, most uncertain.
I do not think it is a good model of what the clinician is concerned with, useful as it may be for the study of certain reflexes.

Now, more recently, I am told, Dr. Denslow has been joined by
Elliott Hix in an approach to the visceral responses to vertebral
stimulation. During a recent visit, I was told that the EMG
changes, in trained dogs, were accompanied by an abrupt decrease
in renal blood flow and glomerular filtration. If the pressure is
applied at other segments, unrelated to renal innervation, it does
not happen. Hix has also shown by other techniques--by the application of cold, for example, to selected dermatomes--that there are
potential reflex pathways between the kidney and corresponding
dermatomes. This seems related to the counterirritation hot-pack/
cold-pack methods well known to ancient medicine.

But a more direct approach such as used by Dr. Coote is much
less feasible because access to appropriate roots, rami, nerves,
etc., for recording requires that you destroy or disorganize the
very thing you are trying to study. This is certainly out of the
question for humans--even heroic humans. You've got to remove or
sever the muscles, ligaments and their attachments, remove laminae
and disrupt joints in order to place the electrodes. That's the
reason that, as a long-time investigator in this area, I was at-
tracted to the work of Coote and others, because it has already
yielded much relevant information about sensory inputs, pathways
and reflexes. I couldn't help being amused yesterday when he tried
to answer a question as to how his work on the effect of stimulating this or that sensory nerve might relate to manipulation, he
had to be reminded that he himself had done very relevant studies
indeed on the joint receptors and muscle receptors, also.

I don't know what the answer is, but my own feeling, as reflected in my work of many years, is that we have to study these
phenomena in their natural habitat, as they develop in the course
of individual human history; take it as we find it and study that.
Of course, it is immensely difficult, and it hasn't yet yielded a
great deal of information, but it has given us a few clues with
which we can begin to use such contributions as those that have
been made during these three days.

DR. HALDEMAN: Dr. Magoun, I would also like to refer to
Dr. Weaver's suggestion of the dachshund as a good model. Many
people who practice manipulation have done so on dogs, specifically on the dachshund, and have claimed good results. Some
veterinary surgeons bring all their dachshunds with back pain to
a chiropractor for manipulative care.

DR. MAGOUN: But it has never previously been utilized by the
physiologists and neuroscientists to attempt to analyze these
things in more experimental detail.

DR. P. W. NATHAN: May I comment about dachshunds and
beagles? They really represent a form of achondroplasia, and of
course there have been studies about humans with achondroplasia.
They are known to have narrow intervertebral foramina, particularly
in the lumbar and lower thoracic spine, and also prolapsed discs.
There are many papers on the back disorders in achondroplasia.

I would like to say also that that outlook is quite different
from Dr. Korr's about doing electromyography in humans, and the
thing disappearing under your eyes. I have done a series of
studies with Dr. Dimitriovitch on spasticity in man. We would
place the spastic patients, undressed in a warm, quiet room, and
by the time we got, say, 15 pairs of surface electrodes in place,
the patient was no longer spastic. So, we were faced with the
problem of how to bring the spasticity back. We found that it can
be done by rubbing the skin vigorously. Then you can get a whole
study of which stimuli in skin induce which muscle reflexes.
Muscle spasm seems to be an important issue in manipulative therapy
and trigger-point therapy, but it is vaguely defined. So what is
muscle spasm? I mean, we all hold our heads upright, so our
muscles are working. But what is the difference between that
and muscle spasm?

DR. MAGOUN: I think you are pointing to the need for further
study and knowledge of these abnormalities of somatic neuron and
skeletal muscle that were emphasized analogously by Dr. Korr,
needed in the field of visceroneural activity. You are pointing
to the need for much additional study in the somatic part of these
syndromes, as well as in the visceral part.

DR. KORR: May I comment on Dr. Nathan's comment? A group at
Kirksville also made electromyographic studies. We plastered the
whole back with surface electrodes, and studied EMG activity of
paraspinal musculature in various postures, mainly quiet standing.
As the subject stands, gradually relaxing, there is a progressive
subsidence of muscular activity. But we never found complete electrical silence in any individual. Always there was some residual
muscular activity somewhere, in one or more areas of the back--
some high, some low, some in the neck, lumbosacral area, and sometimes quite diffuse, or all down one side. This pattern of persistent muscular activity was quite characteristic to each individual.
We could recognize the patient from his EMG pattern. If you asked
the subject to try to "get that silent", by changes in posture, he
often would end up in grotesque positions. He'd often achieve
silence, but at a terrible price.

I want to make one point, though, that illustrates the importance of the conceptual viewpoint from which you start, the bias,
if you will. At the time we were doing these experiments, several
other groups were also doing the same thing, studying posture electromyographically. They reported complete electrical silence in
the back, although with alternating activity of flexors and extensors in the legs. When we questioned them, they said, "Oh, we
make the same observations you do. But since these active areas
are exceptional, we ignore them." What was the focus of interest
for us was noise and nuisance for them.

DR. MAGOUN: Dr. Nathan, I think you need equal time.

DR. NATHAN: Just very briefly, I didn't mean complete silence.
I agree, it is very difficult in normals, or anybody, to get complete EMG silence. I meant just a very slight activity. I was
reminded of another interesting observation when you talked about
recognizing the record. We were working mainly on complete transverse lesions of the cord--paraplegics--and we found individual
differences. So that if you produced a flexor reflex, say, in one
patient, the gastrocnemius would always be the first muscle to
start off. And in another, the tibialis anterior. And this difference was so clear, that individual patterns could be discerned.
So, although there are universal patterns of flexor and extensor
reflexes, there are, even in the total spinal lesion, individual
differences. That is quite an interesting thing to study.

DR. ROBERT E. KAPPLER: I would like to relate one clinical
observation I made on a student of ours who had a thoracic sympathectomy for hyperhidrosis of the hands. (I think human subjects
can be used when traumas or surgical procedures have occurred.
they make good models to compare with normal.) This student had
sympathetic ablation above T4; above T4 there was no sympathetic

activity. With the kind of palpation that I do, there was no activity that I associate with spinal somatic dysfunction in the
sympathectomized area. At the junction, there was excessive activity and extreme sweating; almost always there was a line on the
patient's shirt where the skin above that point was warm and dry,
and then a tremendous hyperresponse, pain, hyperalgesia, restriction
of motion; the area below that was what I would find in any patient.

This observation had a lot of impact on me in my assessment
that there has to be a distinct relationship between function of
the sympathetic nervous system and what I feel in tissue texture
change. I just can't dismiss that.

DR. GRUNDFEST: In continuation of human models, I think there
is a good model for muscle spasm, and that is muscle cramps. I
wonder if Dr. McComas can tell us something about the mechanism of
it, and some of the details.

DR. ALAN J. McCOMAS: I think the most elegant work on muscle
cramps, of the variety we have all experienced, has been done by
Lambert's group at the Mayo Clinic. They were able to show, in
people who were predisposed to these, that they could induce them
quite easily by stimulating the appropriate nerve distal to a local
anesthetic block. It looks as if you may have generator sites in
the nerve fibers quite close to the muscle, and certainly, when you
put a recording needle into a muscle which is undergoing cramp, the
activity you see is characteristic of motor units rather than of
individual muscle fibers. Now, as is so often true in biology,
that may be a simplification.

There may well be other cramps which may have their generator
in the motor neuron, and I am rather struck by the fact that many
of us also have fasciculations from time to time. These are isolated twitches of muscles, which can be easily removed in most
cases by stimulating an area of skin, usually immediately over the
muscle. That sort of spontaneous activity isn't a cramp, but it
obviously is coming through the motor neuron, rather than the motor
nerve lower down.

DR. GITELMAN: A related clinical observation is that individuals who have had a history of sciatica on one side are predisposed
to more cramping on that side than on the opposite side.

DR. LEWIT: That would be in accordance with a clinical observation I have been making recently. After sciatica, people
frequently incur cramps. The true sciatica has a slight nerve
block which may persist; the ankle jerk is lost and never returns.
With a certain type of examination, we usually find joint blockages,
in the foot or on the fibula, that would be the source of stimulation.

Treating these small lesions of the foot is the best way to improve this cramp. It would be a corollary of what you have said.

DR. SUNDERLAND: One has a feeling that the final answers in this regard will come from the physiologists and chemists. Concerning the morphological background, there is just one point I would like to stress. I wouldn't like to leave you with the impression from my morphological presentation that I thought we had the answers to the problem. I don't believe that we do. I was merely pointing out the morphological parameters within which you must consider the problem. But it seems to me, following the discussions of the last few days, that we are using physical methods to cure an inferred physical lesion. I wonder if perhaps there are not other, nonphysical, factors operating here, which could be responsible for the condition for which the patient seeks treatment.

I am thinking here in terms of chemical agents and their liberation into tissues—I am thinking also of infection. I wonder if, for instance, in myalgia paresthetica and suboccipital neuralgia, it is not common to have an associated intercurrent infection, just prior to the incident. In many cases, there is such an incidence. Wharton drew attention to this many years ago in an elaborate study. One wonders if there is not some chronic latent virus operating in collagen, so to speak, which is activated by even minor trauma not in itself responsible for all the disability.

As a simple illustration, if I go out and do rock work, as I often do, I can come in in the evening and wash my hands, and for the first time feel pain, and notice the skin off my knuckles and the scratches on the back of my hand, which during the day's activities I haven't noticed or felt at all. If, however, in the course of my activities I disturb an ant's nest—the big jumping ants that we have—there is an agonizing sensation of pain at the instant of being stung by one of these ants, a very compelling pain. This is strictly chemical; there's very little in the way of physical trauma. The sting apparatus of this ant is quite sharp, very fine. Yet, this relatively minute quantity of presumably formic acid or whatever it is, produces the agonizing pain. The immediate response, of course, is to rub it violently; presumably, gate-control people would say, that is done to flood the cord with afferent impulse. On the other hand, it could be to dissipate the noxious agent through the tissues, to cause it to be carried away in the blood. Perhaps the physical effects of the manipulations are to improve the circulation to a region, and in this way to bring about some effective response.

DR. GREENMAN: I would like to support what Dr. Sunderland said about one of the things that I attempted to focus on earlier, namely, the role of manipulation in total health care. In my opinion it influences much more than the nervous system. I am personally persuaded that change in circulation is a large component of what happens under manipulative care. Therefore, I would support what you are saying, that there are more mechanisms operative than those which we have covered in this workshop.

I would like to direct a comment to Dr. Coote and Dr. Koizumi and others who are doing work on the somatosympathetic reflex. From the clinical perspective, much of what we appear to deal with in patients with chronic rather than acute disease states are the influences of chronic stimulation through the sympathetic nervous system. Any work that can be done to help give some explanation for the influence of chronic stimulation in this area would certainly be of value.

I am reminded of a comment that Dr. Weaver made to me yesterday: This is such a complex mechanism, and we know so little about it normally, that we have a problem dealing with what the abnormal aspects of it are. And yet, we talk about the things we do to change the abnormal toward a normal we don't understand. The more work that fundamental scientists can do to find out what the normal is, both acutely and chronically, the more understanding we could bring to future discussions of this same nature.

DR. JOHAN SJÖSTRAND: Discussing physical factors and possible influences on the circulation or manipulation, I have been struck that we haven't talked much about tissue pressures. Have any studies been carried out to measure tissue pressure? For example, Dr. Sunderland spoke about the importance of the intrafascicular pressure. It would be possible to measure the pressures experimentally and to estimate the effect on the pressure of different compressions or lesions. That is important since we know that pressure will affect perfusion in that area. It is a measurement that could be done in humans, too.

DR. MAGOUN: I am glad that you asked this, but I am not able to ask anyone to answer it now because we have just come to the end of our time. Perhaps, in some conversation later. I simply wanted to respond to Murray. He asked the question, what is a good animal model? He got not one answer, but two. Man and his dachshunds.

DR. KORR: Before calling for the last summary, I would like to comment on your questions, Dr. Sunderland and Dr. Sjöstrand. As Murray will confirm, our grant application to NINCDS proposed three workshops at two-year intervals, on the general theme, Biologic Mechanisms in Manipulative Therapy. The first one in the proposal was the neurobiologic. The second one would deal with hydrodynamic or body-fluid mechanisms--blood, plasma, lymph, cerebrospinal and

endoneurial fluid, interstitial fluid and edema. Presumably, intraneural circulation would be included, Dr. Sjöstrand. The third
workshop would be on the biomechanics of the musculoskeletal system. In its wisdom, NINCDS decided that we had enough to do with
neurobiologic mechanisms.

It is now my pleasure to present Dr. Samson to summarize the
session on nonimpulse-based mechanisms and to moderate further
discussion.

NONIMPULSE-BASED MECHANISMS

DR. FRED E. SAMSON: There are two aspects, as I see it, in a
summary. One, you've already heard in yesterday's session. The
second is before us now: What does what we have heard mean for
manipulative therapy? Now I am not going to try to recapture the
excitement or the power of what you have heard. As a matter of
fact, I am in an anticlimactic situation. What does stand out in
my mind is that we saw documented the ongoing chemical biological
interactions, so-called "talk", from neuron to neuron, neuron to
effector cell, effector cell back to neuron. And yet, we got only
a glimpse of the iceberg tip of potential in such matters as
Dr. Thoenen's nerve growth factor, Dr. Singer's turn-on factors,
and many others. I think we all would agree at this point that
nonimpulse mechanisms deserve a little more attention than they
have received in the past.

It is easy to recognize why that has happened. The tools for
impulse-type mechanisms have been with us for a long time, and
continually improving. Those for nonimpulse mechanisms are more
recent and we are now beginning to have such wonderful methodologies as radioimmune assay and others. We certainly have added to
the list of potential mechanisms that could be examined, not only
in a third conference, but in many conferences. It could outlast
our need for employment.

Now I am reminded of the importance of structure in osteopathy,
and of the saying that structure determines function. That structure, of course, extends down to the molecular level. We have to
bring into consideration now the necessity for coherent structure
at the molecular level--every molecule having to be in its right
place at the right time. A nerve cell is not a bag of enzymes and
other components. It has a highly ordered structure, involving
such components as the microtubules and the neurofilaments. Certainly Sid Ochs' transport microfilament is a structure that had
better be in its place at the right times.

Axoplasmic transport has been a major theme in the Workshop. As a person who likes physical models, I want to use one to illustrate some things related to axonal transport. [*Editor's note: Dr. Samson used as his model a fishing reel, the line of which was pulled out by another participant walking the length of the conference room while Dr. Samson held the reel. In the model, the reel represented the perikaryon; the line, the axon; and the participant, the effector in which the axon terminated.*] This obviously is a simplistic model, but it will serve to illustrate relative sizes. If the line, representing a relatively thick axon in a long nerve, were correctly proportioned to this, the perikaryon, then the line, with its countless terminal branches, would have to be carried not to the other side of the room, but practically to the airport. Now, the synthetic machinery needed to support this enormous surface and volume in the axon and terminals is incredibly immense. That machinery has to be turning out essential materials for the maintenance of the entire cell at a great pace, and they have then to be delivered. In addition, that machinery has to receive information back from the terminals, telling it what to do. So that axoplasmic transport is a critical and possibly vulnerable process. I merely wanted to illustrate it visually.

Well, what does this interaction mean? Two things: On the one hand, it means a tremendous capability for adaptation, response, homeostasis; but on the other hand, it means the probability of domino effects. So we really have two sides to look at in these interactions.

Now Dr. Ochs pointed out how small changes in the microenvironment of neurons can modify—in his instance—axoplasmic transport. So I would like to return a little later to the importance of this microenvironment in which all the neuronal processes are carried on. This means, in chemical terms, an uninterrupted flow of free energy, despite the operation of the second law of thermodynamics—the tendency toward a state of randomness. Hence a biological system has to be an open system, and there has to be a continuous flow of substrate, fuels, oxygen, and so on. The role of circulation in carrying substances to and from the tissue has been pointed out a number of times here. Maintaining this highly ordered dynamic state puts a tremendous burden on the directed flow of free energy. The second law is with us all the time. What emerges is that there are many Achilles heels, many vulnerable points, and you have heard about a few of them.

I would like to comment briefly about other areas of our discussion—first the need for better definition. I had the feeling during the discussions about manipulative therapy that it was a moving target. Among the things that people in the laboratory have to have are reproducible kinds of phenomena. Unless we have something reproducible, it's terribly hard to put it into what we are

seeking, a scientific framework. But there are some problems with
experimental, fundamental science itself. One of them is that it
tends, by and large, to be reductionist in approach. And in reduc-
tionism you have some serious problems. One is that you can purify
the important thing away. We have an important classical example
in recent biological science--the fantastic DNA story. In their
quest for the fundamental element, the early investigators had
purified that beyond the point where the information was contained
--in the organization of those elements. I think the only answer
is to run up and down the levels of organization and try to
examine the subject in that fashion.

Another problem: science deals with generalizations, while
the clinician deals with a specific. That is a wide divergence.
It may please the scientist to know that a given reaction or effect
goes in a predictable direction 80% of the time, but that merely
puts the clinician in the ballpark. Unfortunately, he has to hit
the ball. But that is all that basic science is going to give the
clinician, some kind of a fundamental basis from which to draw inferences and try to do what he can in the context of the total
situation--the patient, for instance. I know in our own work with
neuropathies and the involvement of axoplasmic transport in neuropathies, I came to the conclusion that we can never prove it,
but only provide enough evidence by strong inference, if we're
right, of what has to be taken into account, or that there is a
line of thinking to follow.

Well, what about the future? I am impressed by what functional neurochemistry can offer. I think the problem here is that
manipulation is viewed as a physical kind of treatment, and therefore the disorder must be a mechanical type of thing. It is my
feeling that the chemistry of it may be much more important than
the gross physics of it. Neurochemistry has been moving more and
more away from extractive, analytical neurochemistry toward the
functional, as illustrated repeatedly at the recent neurochemistry
meetings in Copenhagen. Improvement in technology obviously makes
it possible to do experiments we couldn't do in the past. But the
conceptual basis from which we can think has also improved. Nucleotides and their derivatives have emerged as one exciting area.
Adenosine, in particular, has been shown to be released in large
quantities from stimulated brain; it is axoplasmically transported,
and is one of the strongest stimulants to cyclic-AMP, and so on.
The concept is emerging that adenosine is probably a synaptic modu-
lator. I think modulation of synapses is possibly a topic most
relevant to the area of this conference. Another potentially relevant molecular category is the neuropeptides which are relatively
simple molecules, and powerful in minute quantities. Their bio-
dynamic qualities are such that there is a possibility they could
be involved in phenomena considered here.

We have heard a lot about pain. Let me identify some other advancing areas in neurochemistry that may have a bearing. The current great search for the naturally occurring endogenous ligands for receptors is one example. Further, there is indeed a system which is concerned with how one deals with pain, and which may be involved in such pain phenomena as we heard described--doing garden work and not discovering that you've chewed up your hands until you get in, or suppression of the intense pain that a football player must be exposed to. Now in the search for the ligands for the morphine receptor, such systems are being identified, as you know, as endogenous opioids, endorphins, encephalins, substance-P, and others, which are fitting into a clearer pattern. It has been shown recently that there are opioid active substances in human blood and urine. Keeping in mind the need for a human model, as emphasized by Harry Grundfest, I wondered whether it is possible that manipulation changes the level of opioids in blood or urine. These are aspects that can be examined now.

DR. GREENMAN: Yesterday afternoon, our topic was the trophic function of nerves in relation to manipulative therapy, and we didn't fully address that. I would like to make some to-whom-it-may-concern comments based on "anecdotal" experience. Members of our osteopathic and chiropractic professions have found that appropriate, well-diagnosed and well-dosed manipulative care seems to have a powerful influence on the maintenance of health in individuals, as distinguished from treatment of disease. When I was in active practice I had the experience of having a certain patient population that would come to me on a regular basis, not because they were sick, but because they wanted to stay well. I had inherited some of those patients from previous generations of osteopathic physicians. It was interesting to me that a number of them did stay remarkably well, and functioned very well. When I first began to hear about the trophic influence of nerves, I said to myself that in all probability the kind of thing that was going on in those patients over that period of time was that the therapy was affecting a whole variety of systems, not just the nervous system; it seemed to improve the "trophicity" of those individuals to live out the positive aspects of whatever their genetic heritage was. It would appear to me that this is one area, although it is global in its scope, that we ought to look at, and particularly in view of the statistics from various studies indicating that 20% of the population have 80% of the disease states that we treat. Maybe we ought to be looking at what has gone wrong in that 20% segment of the population, and see if we can do anything that will improve their trophicity. Experience indicates that one way is through appropriately designed manipulative care of the patients, to maintain their health, rather than just treat disease.

DR. SAMSON: Can you teach people to treat themselves for the benefits that you feel people accrue from this?

DR. GREENMAN: Certainly individualized instructional programs for the health maintenance of patients are appropriate. Of course, one of the most difficult things that a clinician has to do with patients is to get them to comply with any kind of structured maintenance program, including exercise, but that is an important component of this type of approach. I know that Dr. Lewit has some strong feelings about mobilization and self-treatment, and perhaps he would like to comment on the instruction of patients in self-treatment.

DR. LEWIT: I think we have to treat the motor system as a whole, and the joints are the passive part. One cannot reduce oneself to that passive part, if one wants to achieve results which hold for a longer time. This question of general health care may have to do with one of the things Dr. McComas was saying, that we really don't use our motor system, and in teaching patients the proper use of their motor system actively, we promote their health. We try to help the patient to have some motor program which is appropriate to the individual.

DR. KAPPLER: I would like to second Dr. Greenman's observations, that there may be a neurotrophic effect in the maintenance of health, in the maintenance of vitality of target organs--and, perhaps, vice versa. Some of the results which I have observed from manipulative treatment are hard to explain on the basis of impulse-based mechanisms, or on the basis of circulation. I have long felt that there is something that happens to improve the vitality of the nonvital endorgan. A lot of answers may come from trophic, nonimpulse-based mechanisms. I think this area has great clinical potential.

DR. SAMSON: One reaction I have is that I need to be convinced that these patients were healthier because they did this in a routine way. Would you like to comment on that, Scott?

DR. HALDEMAN: That is a hard assignment. I would like to answer a question which has come up in basic science discussions both here and outside, and that is, why am I here? Why is the basic scientist who has no concept of manipulation being invited to a manipulation conference? And has he anything to offer?

To use the metaphor of switching on the light in manipulation, there has been very little research, and participants may never know the consequences of their contributions here. As one who spends much of his time promoting, trying to motivate people to do research, especially in the chiropractic field, I know that the

NINCDS manipulative conference of 1975 was such a powerful stimulus
to the sciences in the manipulative field that there are now science departments in every chiropractic college. The more established science and research departments in osteopathic colleges are
becoming reactivated. At least four foundations in the chiropractic
profession, collecting funds for research, have been set up in the
last two years. What these conferences serve to do is, not switch
on the light, necessarily, but point to the fact that there is a
light switch and show us which way we have to move to find the
light switch. This, I think, is going to be the greatest outcome
of this type of meeting, and the reason why I believe further meetings of this type are essential.

It's a meeting like this that puts the pressure on the clinician to ask new questions which will cause him to have another look
at answers which he has been accepting as fact. So, I'd like to
emphasize to everyone that each new input is essential to development of this field, and the comments of each one here will carry a
great deal more weight than they realize.

DR. SAMSON: This was summarized in a comment that someone
made last night, "We've got a lot of answers, can you think of
some questions?"

[Editor's note: At this point there ensued an extraneous
discussion of the publication of research on spinal manipulation
and about the "contraindications" and hazards of manipulative
therapy.]

DR. WEAVER: I wanted to get back to science, because I have
one other comment that I thought might be relevant, in view of the
interest in finding a scientific basis for this form of therapy.
One thing we might be tempted to do is review basic science literature retrospectively. I would like to suggest a warning about
that sort of thing. In the literature, I am sure it is possible
to find articles, experiments which have been done, which would
support any hypothesis that one might want to propose related to
possible theories of manipulation. I'd like to suggest that each
experiment done in each individual laboratory is subject to the
experimental conditions set up by that experimenter; the truth obtained by that experiment is dependent upon the experimental situation. Hence, the truth in one place might be very different from
the truth in another. Though it is critical to learn from past
literature, one must also generate and test hypotheses directly
related to manipulative therapy, not depending too much on what
has been done for another purpose in the past.

CHAIRMAN'S CONCLUDING STATEMENT

DR. KORR: This has been a most gratifying experience for me.
In one of my recent letters to all participants, I said that the
Planning Committee was looking forward to an exciting experience,
which it has been. I predicted also that it would be a *gemütlich*
experience, and it certainly has been that, beyond our expecta-
tions. We have, indeed, been a most congenial group.

Among the good things that have happened was the coming together of professional groups who ordinarily do not meet together.
I mean the clinicians--a very special and mixed group of clinicians
--and the scientists, also of very special kinds. I mean also two
groups of neuroscientists who go to separate sessions at scientific
meetings and who ordinarily have little to say to each other about
their work. One group records impulses and other high-speed phenomena, measured in seconds and milliseconds. The other times its
phenomena by calendar as well as by clock. One is predominantly
physiological in its orientation; the other, no less functional, is
predominantly chemical. Vocationally, one might be more closely
related to the electricians, the other to the plumbers; one to the
radio-TV industry, the other to the postal system.

Despite the diversity of their interests and methodologies,
all these groups did talk together here for two and one-half days.
The dialogue has not only been pleasant, it has been productive.
We have shown that the field of manipulative therapy, even when
vaguely defined, is an area needing and meriting fundamental investigation. It has been shown that clinical experience in that
field raises unique kinds of questions in basic neuroscience; that
recent and current lines of investigation offer some valuable clues,
but that new lines of investigation need to be opened. At least
some of these seem to be in the DMZ, the demilitarized zone between
impulse-based and nonimpulse-based phenomena--a zone for which
there is no basis in the nervous system itself, as we have seen.

What next? I have been asked this question by several of you.
Should another conference be planned to continue on this topic or
on some aspect especially ripe for exploration? Or, having staked
out an area, would we better achieve our objectives by assimilation
and interchange, as Dr. Magoun eloquently urges, in established research and clinical organizations in contiguous areas? Or both?

It is too early to say. One thing is certain.   Much has
happened to each of us in the course of these intensive,
interdisciplinary conversations--new attitudes, new knowledge, new
insights and, perhaps most important, new and sharper questions.

We shall take these with us as we return to our offices, laboratories, clinics and classrooms. Over a period of time, perhaps
long after we have forgotten their origin, these will inevitably
have <u>some</u> impact on our thinking, our research, our practice, our
teaching. Perhaps some time in the future there will appear a
sudden hunch, a new way of looking at an old problem, asking an
old question--the seed of which was planted here by something
somebody said--that will launch a new kind of inquiry.

Through our teaching, our contacts with our colleagues, and
through the published volume of proceedings, these impacts will be
diffused to other fertile and receptive minds, with inevitable
effect on thought and action. Without resolving, at this time,
the question, "What next?", this seems achievement enough for one
workshop. The Planning Committee feels highly rewarded, and we
thank you, individually and collectively, for your valuable contributions to the Workshop.

Subject Index